A Textbook of Nursery Nursing

THE ESSENTIALS

A Textbook of Nursery Nursing

THE ESSENTIALS

Patricia Gilbert

Stanley Thornes (Publishers) Ltd

© 1997 Stanley Thornes (Publishers) Ltd

The right of Particia Gilbert to be identified as author of this work has been asserted by her in accordance with the Copyright, Designs and Patents Act 1988.

First published in 1997 by:
Stanley Thornes (Publishers) Ltd
Ellenborough House
Wellington Street
CHELTENHAM
GL50 1YW
United Kingdom

97 98 99 00 01 / 10 9 8 7 6 5 4 3 2 1

A catalogue record for this book is available from the British Library

ISBN 0-7487-3176-8

Photo Credits
Bubbles/Loisjoy Thurston (p. 91); Eureka! The Museum for Children (p. 1); Format/Jacky Chapman (p. 175); Lupe Cunha Photos (p. 221); Zefa (cover photo; p. 275)

Typeset by Best-set Typesetter Ltd., Hong Kong
Printed and bound in Great Britain by G. Canale & C.S.p.A.—Borgaro T. se—TURIN

CONTENTS

PREFACE

This book is primarily intended as a basic text for nursery nurses undertaking the BTEC qualification in nursery nursing. The aim is to provide a text giving the essentials of the course in one volume. For example, there are relevant chapters on legal, psychological and data investigative aspects in addition to more everyday child-care matters.

The 'core' modules of the BTEC syllabus are covered as well as some of the optional modules. Advice on further reading, for greater detail than can be contained in one volume, is given at the end of each chapter.

It is also hoped that much of the subject matter will be of value to students on other caring courses concerned with child welfare.

ACKNOWLEDGEMENTS

Thanks are due to many people who willingly have given their time, advice and encouragement. Rosemary Morris must be first on the list as the instigator of this book. Without her far-sighted encouragement, nothing would have been written.

Especial thanks are due to John Colvin, senior lecturer in IT; Eryl Copp, nursery nurse lecturer; Jenny Dill-Russell, special needs teacher; Judy Greaves, paediatric nurse; Natalie Turner, barrister; Joy Wellan, educational psychologist.

Finally, extra special thanks to my husband for the ever-cheerfully-given assistance with 'data' – in all its forms!

INTRODUCTION

The human infant and child, unlike most other animals, needs constant care and protection in the early years of life. Physical needs are paramount in the early days – shelter, food, warmth, all given with lashings of love. As the months go by, the need for mental and emotional care and guidance develops with the infant's unfolding abilities and personality.

Historically these needs were met almost exclusively within the family setting, with a few children being cared for almost entirely by a mother-substitute – the 'Mary Poppins' type nanny. The wider family (uncles, aunts, grandparents, cousins) also had a hand in caring for the new member of the family and moulding the personality. Today's altered social structure means that families are more mobile and widely separated. The extended family still exists in very few places, and has been replaced by the nuclear family of parents and one, two or three children. The past decade has also seen a rapid increase in the numbers of single parents facing the difficult, and unenviable, task of bringing up a child, or children, on their own.

In view of these changes – and at present there is no evidence of a swing back to the wider family unit – the need for child carers outside the family is increasing rapidly. Nannies and child-minders are in ever-increasing demand, and there would seem to be no likelihood of this demand diminishing.

In order to ensure that children, the citizens of tomorrow, are adequately, consistently and properly cared for, appropriate training needs to be given to these valuable and dedicated people offering themselves for this vitally important work. Knowledge of child development is a necessary part of ongoing care. No longer are children thought of as 'mini-adults' as was the case at the beginning of the twentieth century (even the clothes in which children were dressed reflected this view!). It is now fully recognised that children are indeed a 'race apart' needing special care and guidance if they are to grow into useful and well-adjusted adults. Each stage of development requires appropriate skills, activities and equipment.

Much has also been learnt in recent decades regarding the psychology of child behaviour and emotional growth. Broad aspects of this bank of knowledge needs to be understood by people having the day-to-day care of developing children. Play is also an important part of the learning activity of the growing child. By play a child's understanding of the wider world is gained. Child-care workers need to have a fund of enjoyable play activities, suitable to the child's specific developmental level, available as part of their knowledge base.

Physical safety and health are further aspects requiring knowledge and skills. Childhood accidents still take an horrendous toll of young lives and many of these occur in the home. Thoughts and actions of all child carers must always be on safety aspects in home, nursery and out in the wider world. Knowledge of first aid, for the inevitable times when preventative measures have failed, is also a must for all child-care workers. The actions taken during the first few minutes following an accident are often vital to the final outcome of a serious accident.

Childhood infections, too, need sympathetic and constant watch for signs of unwanted complications. For the best possible care, basic information on the natural course of such infections needs to be known.

Legal aspects of child care is a further necessity needing to be understood fully. The 1989 Children Act together with the 1988 Education Reform Act and the 1993 Education Act are recent important pieces of legislation. Equal opportunities, sex discrimination and stereotyping aspects which underpin all good quality child care are further examples with which all child careers should have at least a nodding acquaintance.

To be able to understand the wider implications of child care in, for example, hospital, day nurseries and infant school, a basic knowledge of data collection and interpretation is necessary. By the use of such knowledge different strategies of child care can be better understood.

The above outline may seem daunting at first sight, but when taught and practised in a logical sequence, aspiring child-care workers will soon adapt to a child-centred way of thinking. This book aims to present the essential material necessary to be studied in a practical and understandable way. The content closely follows the outline of the BTEC National qualifications in Caring Services. Thus the essential material for a range of careers in the caring service is covered. In the space available much detail has had to be omitted. Further reading on specific subjects is suggested at the end of each chapter. Along with the presentation of facts are suggestions for exercises, role-play and discussions. The exercises can be used as a basis for course work in conjunction with practices in the workplace. The scenarios suggested for the role-play will give the student practice in facing the many unusual – and sometimes difficult – situations they will find themselves in during the course of their careers. Discussion points can be tutor-led or used by students to underpin recently acquired knowledge. These activities will link theory to practice, and provide students with a sound base of understanding of the practice of their art, that of caring for children.

At the end of the book there is an appendix giving useful addresses and other information in connection with child care.

It is suggested that students, at the commencement of their course, start keeping a log/diary (in a ring binder for example) based upon the student exercises, role-play and discussions found throughout the book. Wherever possible all material should be finally presented by using a word processor, spreadsheet and/or any other suitable software. As a final student exercise, all the material should be indexed. This log will then prove of value for revision, reference and assessment purposes.

The use of gender throughout the book is random, except where there is a certain gender difference as in, for example, certain diseases. Haemophilia and Duchenne muscular dystrophy, for example, are diseases which affect only males.

THE BASICS

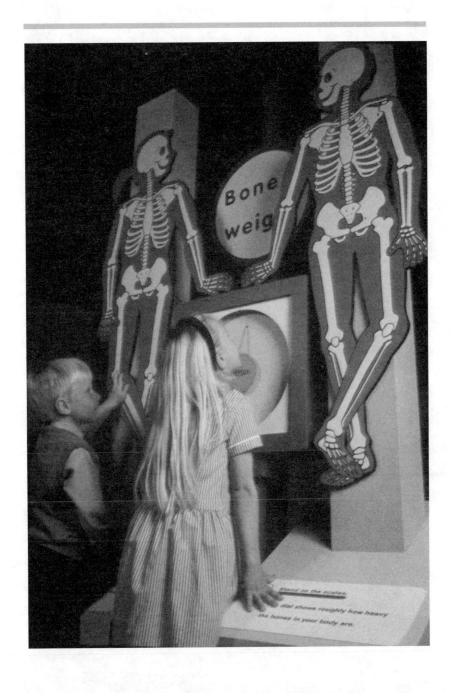

1. OVERVIEW OF GROWTH AND DEVELOPMENT

OBJECTIVES

1. Understand basic principles behind human growth and development.
2. Appreciate prenatal factors influencing development.
3. Appreciate multicultural issues in interpreting growth and development.
4. Understand basic tenets of observational skills.

Growth and **development** are quite different concepts. Whilst they are closely interrelated and, to some extent, dependant on each other, the two words should never be used to denote the same aspect of child care. Growth, as defined in the *Shorter Oxford English Dictionary*, is 'A stage in the process of growing' or 'Size or stature attained by growing'. Development, again as defined in the *Shorter Oxford English Dictionary*, is 'A gradual unfolding' or 'A further working out of detail'. To put it more succinctly, growth is an increase in size whilst development is an increase in complexity.

Growth would seem, therefore, to be a more objective and potentially measurable concept than development. It will continue in a preordained manner, almost regardless of external forces. Exceptions to this do, of course, occur as in the case of some genetically determined conditions where growth is retarded. But, by and large, growth proceeds – and ceases! – in a predictable form.

Development can be described as a variable process which occurs together with, and alongside, growth. It is dependant upon many internal and external factors – heredity, environment and opportunity – for its full flowering. Good, sensible and sensitively delivered child care can do much to ensure that developmental processes occur fully and at the proper time, helping the child to acquire full genetic potential.

Growth
Increase in size.
Development
Increase in complexity.

GROWTH

The most well-known aspect of growth is **linear growth**, i.e. the length of the baby and the height of the child. Seen over time growth seems to occur as a steady continuous process. But for much of the time, growth proceeds in a series of short, sharp bursts. Various life events, such as illness, bereavement, or even moving house, can affect a child's linear growth pattern. After the unsettling event has passed a 'catch-up' spurt of growth occurs. Final adult height is largely ordained by the child's genetic make-up, although, as will be seen later, environmental factors can also influence final height. Usually tall parents will have tall children, and short parents short children. The mechanism of linear growth is controlled by complex hormones, mainly from the pituitary gland situated deep in the brain tissue. Linear growth is wonderfully (it almost seems magically) terminated at around the age of 18 years in women and 21 years in men.

Gain in **weight** is a further aspect of growth This measurement is of special importance in infants and early childhood as a measure of satisfactory thriving. Again, over the long term weight gain appears to be continuous, but, as every mother or child carer can tell you, there can be periods of time when little or no weight is gained at all, only to be followed by an encouraging large weight gain.

Normal birth weight falls within the range 2.2 kg to 4 kg. A very rough 'rule-of-thumb' guide to satisfactory weight gain over the months is 'birth weight doubled by six months and trebled by one year'. (Small babies, for whatever reason, will have a greater 'catch-up' growth than their more average sized peers. So this rough prediction will not apply to their rate of growth.) Newborn babies can lose up to 15% of their birth weight in the first few days of life. Return to birth weight is usually achieved 10 days after birth. Genetic inheritance, as well as external factors, will have a bearing on rate of weight gain.

One further important measurement in the first two years of life is **head circumference**. This particular measurement is indicative of the steady growth of the brain inside the skull. The average head circumference at birth is 35 cm. At one year of age this will have increased to 46.5 cm and by two years of age to 49 cm. Minor variations to these, fairly consistent, measurements will occur, depending on the size of the baby and also on genetic predisposition.

Serial head circumference measurements are important clues in the diagnosis of certain problems; for example, hydrocephalus (in which there is excess fluid round the brain) and craniostenosis (a condition where the bones of the skull fuse together prematurely).

It is of interest when considering growth to note the variation in body proportions of children as growth proceeds (Figure 1.1). At birth half the baby's body is above the level of the umbilicus. By seven years of age these proportions have altered so that the half way mark is nearer the region of the hips. In the adult this difference is further marked.

Note also that, in a diagrammatic representation where the body is marked into quarters, the newborn baby's head takes up one quarter of the body. In the adult the ratio is reduced to around one seventh.

Centile charts

Measurement of these three important aspects of growth in early childhood are routinely recorded on special growth charts, called percentile charts, but more usually known as **centile charts**. On these

Figure 1.1 Body proportions at different ages.

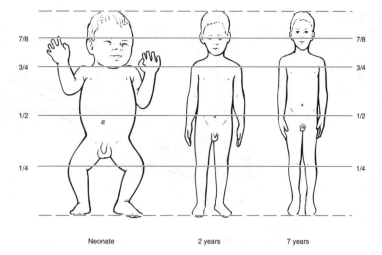

7/8

3/4

1/2

1/4

Neonate   2 years   7 years

charts the measurements are plotted over the weeks and months as the child grows.

They give vital information as to the **rate of growth**. Individual measurements at any one point in time are of less value than serial ones and will only relate the size of the child to the average and not give insight into individual progress.

The rate of growth of children has been measured for centuries. The oldest record in existence is a chart by a French Count. He measured his son's height every six months from 1759 to 1777. This record showed a continuous relatively steady increase in height as do the centile charts of today.

Rapid increase in height (or 'length' in babies up to the age of one year) is most marked during the first two years of life. (But even this spectacular rate of growth is surpassed in the rapid growth seen in the unborn baby. During the nine months of pregnancy, the baby grows from two fused cells, infinitesimally small, to a length of 50 cm at birth.)

Centile charts are graphs plotting height (or weight or head circumference) on the vertical axis against age on the horizontal axis (Figure 1.2). They have been derived by measuring a cross-sectional group of babies/children at varying ages. The midline of growth – or 50th centile – represents the 'average' rate of growth. The 3rd centile line of growth refers to those children whose rate of growth is slower. Only two normally growing children out of 100 will grow at a slower rate than this 3rd centile line. Similarly the 97th centile line refers to those children who have a relatively fast rate of growth. Only two normally growing children out of 100 will grow at a faster rate than those growing along the 97th centile line.

Weight and head circumference charts are derived along the same principles. Most of the growth charts used today are based on those originally proposed and designed by Tanner.

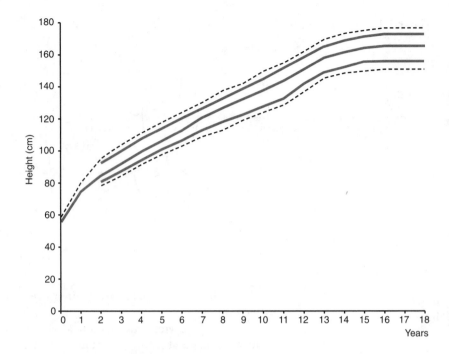

Figure 1.2 Normal height chart for girls.

Once set along a line of growth – be it on the 50th, 3rd or 97th centile – the vast majority of children will remain growing on this centile line. It is because of this fact that adult height can be fairly reliably predicted from reference to the charts. Most children reach a height roughly midway between those of their parents. Another way of predicting adult height is by adding both parent's height together, adding 13 cm for boys and subtracting 13 cm for girls, and then dividing by 2. The answer to this sum will give the expected adult height.

Student exercise

Try this prediction on your own, and your parent's height, or check on a friend's family. Make, and record, the predictions of final height of children in your place of work experience.

There are two important measurement changes which should alert carers to possible growth or thriving problems.
• When a child who has been growing along a specific centile line (for example, the 50th centile) drops to a lower line (for example the 10th centile) over a period of weeks or months. This applies particularly to height and weight measurements. An example of this is seen by the weight chart of a young boy over an 18-month period (Figure 1.3). The normal weight 50th centile growth line suddenly dips and remains

Figure 1.3 *Specific weight chart for a boy from birth to two years.*

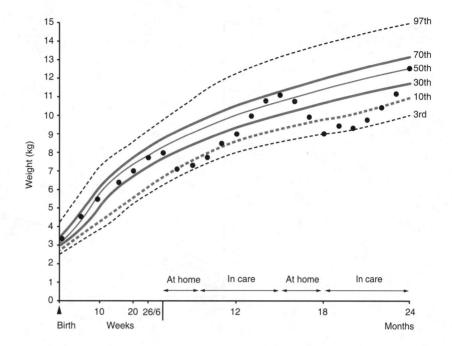

along this lower line for about three months. After this time there is a steady increase until the original growth line is reached. It remains at this level for about six months after which the whole pattern is again repeated. Along with other events and factors, it is found that the boy is being abused at home during the times when his weight falls off. During his six months' stay in a foster home – repeated again at a later date – his weight gain rises, each time, to the normal growth line. It was the evidence of this weight chart that helped the juvenile court to decide that the boy should no longer live with his natural parents. It was the dramatic change in growth levels that were so significant.

• When the lines of growth relating to height and weight diverge markedly over time. A simple example of this is seen by the height chart of a young girl (Figure 1.4). The height is proceeding steadily along the 50th centile growth line, but the weight gain shoots up, over a period of months, to the 90th centile. Under these circumstances it is found that the child's grandmother is feeding her grand-daughter vast quantities of ice-cream and sweets after school each day in an attempt to gain extra affection in order to assuage her own loneliness and sadness following the death of her husband. Again, the evidence of the weight chart gives objective evidence of continuing weight gain from a definite period in time.

The above are just two examples proving the value of plotting serial measurement of the various parameters of children's growth.

Figure 1.4 *Specific height chart for a girl from two to nine years.*

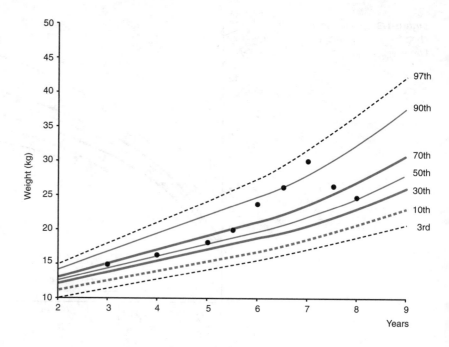

Student exercise

Copy, with permission, some typical centile charts in your place of work experience. Write some notes explaining why some of the differences you have observed could have happened.

Influences on growth

Genetic or environmental?

Both these factors will play a part in the rate of growth and the final size and shape of each individual child. Improvement of the environment in which children grow and live will certainly maximize their rate of growth. Final weight and height will, however, only be marginally altered by environmental factors. The genetic make-up, laid down at conception, is the most important factor in final size. But there are a number of other influences at work in aspects of growth.

Secular trends

In the last hundred years, children in America and Europe have become progressively taller and heavier. This is apparent early in life, the average birth weight of babies being higher than that of babies born a century ago. Even allowing for improved socioeconomic conditions, the trend is still upwards. It is the rate of growth, more than the final adult height and

Influences on growth
- Genetic
- Secular trends
- Racial characteristics
- Nutrition
- Disease
- Seasons
- Stress

weight, that has shown this marked increase. It is thought that the increased mobility of populations has some bearing on these facts – starting with the invention of the bicycle! A greater mix of genes has occurred with the decrease of inbreeding amongst fairly static populations.

Racial characteristics

Different races of the world have certain differing characteristics. Two of the most obvious differences are skin colour and eye shape. Race can also exert an influence on the pattern of growth, although climatic and nutritional factors are closely interwoven.

Babies with dark skins are ahead of their lighter coloured skinned peers in bone development at birth. As a result of this, these babies are often more advanced in the early years in their motor abilities of walking, running and climbing. This effect persists until around two years of age when this difference between the races is less obvious, although the success of dark-skinned athletes in later life is clear for all to see.

Given equal socioeconomic circumstances, dark-skinned children often reach a taller height, and physical maturity is gained earlier, than in Caucasian children. These differing rates of growth will have an impact on the way nursery personnel need to handle physical needs. Chairs and tables need to be suitable for bigger children. Objects out of reach of smaller children will need to be kept at a higher level if taller children make up part of the group. Activities will also need to be scaled to the needs of both groups.

Discussion

Note during your work experience any differences in the rate of growth in children from different races. Discuss with your group how differences in rate of growth could modify your handling of the children showing these differences. Summarize and write up your conclusions.

The eruption of teeth also follows the same pattern. As the basis for this aspect of growth is determined before birth, racial genetic factors would seem to be playing an important part.

Nutrition

This plays an important part in growth. Different effects are seen, however, when the lack of suitable food occurs for only short periods of time as opposed to long-term chronic starvation. Under the former conditions where, for example, there is an acute shortage of food for a limited period of time due to war or short-lived famine, children's growth slows or ceases. When food becomes readily available again regulatory mechanisms come into play, and 'catch-up' growth occurs. (To a lesser extent, this 'catch-up' growth is seen in children in an affluent society following a severe illness in which growth has temporarily ceased.) In chronic undernourishment, however, final adult size, in both weight and height, is less than would be expected.

Disease and nutrition

Disease is closely linked to nutrition in its effect on growth. When children are ill, from whatever cause, lack of appetite is commonly a prominent feature. So growth will be halted temporarily, but catch-up features will occur once the disease process has been controlled or burnt itself out. Disease on top of chronic malnutrition will have a greater, more serious and long-term effect on growth.

Certain congenital conditions can also alter the rate of growth. Children with Soto's syndrome (also known as cerebral gigantism) grow very rapidly in the early years and often reach a tall final height. Conversely, children with achondroplasia have short limbs from birth which do not grow in proportion to the rest of their bodies.

Seasons of the year

These can exert an effect on growth. Growth in height is greatest in the spring months, whilst the autumn months show the greatest increase in weight. Collected data have shown this to be the case in both America and Europe.

Psychological stress

This can undermine growth if continued in a severe enough form or any length of time. This has been shown to occur even in the event of the affected children eating an adequate and suitable food intake.

Many and varied are the influences affecting children's growth. In any one individual child's life it is probable that more than one of these influences will have some effect, even if only for a short time. This only goes to emphasize the importance for child carers to be aware of the child's whole environment, as well as the child as a whole.

DEVELOPMENT

In many ways development resembles growth. There is a well-defined sequence of events, each event preceded by a recognizable developmental stage. To take an extreme example, walking cannot occur until the child is able to stand. Similarly understandable speech will not occur until hearing mechanisms are fully developed.

Unlike physical growth development is not so easily plotted. A number of developmental profiles have been developed over the years, and many are the well-known names connected with research into this aspect of child care. All developmental profiles are based on four main areas of child development:

1. Posture and large movements. This involves the big, wide ranging movements such as walking, running, jumping, etc.

2. Vision and fine motor. This group tests finer skills involving smaller muscles and eye/hand co-ordination.
3. Hearing and speech. Speech and language development and testing of hearing.
4. Social and behavioural skills. General social behaviour, ability to play, understanding concepts such as time, sharing, affection and moral precepts.

Detailed assessment skills are vital adjuncts in the underpinning of knowledge of development in young children for all child-care workers.

It is important to understand clearly that there is no one special day, or even week, when a child acquires a definite skill. Developmental skills are reached at a time individual to each child, but within given parameters specific to the skill being tested. Developmental profiles will show different ages at which children can be expected to be able to fulfil certain activities and skills. For example, walking can occur as early as 10 months of age, whilst other children do not acquire this skill until 18 months of age, or even later in some unusual cases. Similarly, the development of speech varies, within given parameters, in each individual child. It is when these parameters are exceeded that there is concern about developmental progress. It is usual to test baby's and children's abilities at certain set ages, and all developmental profiles reflect this aspect.

It is important to remember, however, that these screening tests are useful as an aid to memory and also for recording purposes. Remember that there are relatively few checks at each age group compared to the skills children are learning all the time. Little allowance can be made when checking on development for either the speed or quality of performance used by the child when performing the given tasks. All tests should be used, therefore, as a guide to the progress a child is making and not as a 'pass' or 'fail'. If a task is not performed satisfactorily, further detailed investigations will be needed to see if there are any further added difficulties needing extra care and attention. (Detailed testing of developmental profiles are to be found in Chapters 3 and 4.)

Role play

A mother has brought her 2-year-old daughter for developmental assessment. The child has been unable to fulfil successfully some of the items of the assessment, probably due to the fact that she is just getting over a cold. The mother is very upset about this. With a colleague playing the mother, act as a nursery nurse to reassure her, both by giving possible reasons, e.g. infection, shyness, and by stating what needs to be done, e.g. checking at a later date. Write a report on the interview for the child's notes.

Influences on development

These are again both genetic and environmental, but it must again be remembered that every child must be looked on as a complete person. We

---

Areas of development

- Posture and large development
- Vision and fine motor
- Hearing and speech
- Social and behaviour

are all products of our genes and our environment. At varying times and in differing circumstances will these two aspects play a greater or a lesser part.

Genetic influences

At conception half of the genetic material to build a new individual will come from the mother and half from the father. This genetic material is contained in the genes. These genes are carried on the chromosomes and there are thought to be around 100 000 pairs of functional genes in human beings.

There are 46 chromosomes in every cell in the human body with the exception of the sex cells, the ovum and the spermatozoon. These specialized cells have only 23 chromosomes. So, at conception, when a sperm and an ovum fuse, the full complement for the new individual is made up.

So what effects do these genetic influences have on the newborn baby?

- **Physical effects** are the most obvious. Examples of this are basic shape of the baby's body, and hair and eye colour. Many mothers will recognize the comment: 'She's just like Auntie Jane!' and react with agreement – or irritation! Further environmental influences can do nothing to alter these genetic effects.

  The physical effects of inherited disease are also carried by the genes. A well-known example of this in Caucasian populations is cystic fibrosis, where a fault in a specific gene on chromosome 7 gives rise to malfunction of certain glands in both respiratory and digestive systems. This genetic physical effect will have life-long implications.

  Similarly a baby who inherits short sight or a hearing loss, due to genetic causes, will have difficulties in learning about spatial relationships and sound effects respectively. This in turn will affect later developmental issues.

- **Personality** has undoubtedly a genetic basis. Some babies are born placid and undemanding, whilst others shout loudly from day one. Probably more than physical characteristics, however, personality can be modified to a greater extent by environmental factors. The demanding baby can be soothed and quietened by appropriate and consistent handling. Alternatively, the quiet introspective child can be stimulated and encouraged to be more outgoing. Even so, basic personality traits will persist throughout life.

- **Intelligence**. The debate on whether intelligence is inherited or moulded by environmental factors has continued long, and, at times, acrimoniously. It is probable that genetic influences play a large part in intelligence, with environmental factors playing a part, some studies on twins suggesting that up to 80% of variation in intelligence can be attributed to genetic inheritance.

Environmental influences

These influences will, of course, work on the basic genetic material with which the baby is born. For example, a baby born with a physical disability in the hands will, sadly, never be able to be taught to be as manually dextrous as the baby without this problem. Similarly a baby born with a musical talent will benefit more from musical training than one born without this gift. But there are a number of broad environmental factors which will exert an influence.

Social

In the widest sense the impact of the culture into which a baby is born will influence development. Expectation regarding various skills will differ from culture to culture. Effects of these expectations will be seen in pregnancy and birth practices. In some societies first babies are always expected to be born in the grandparent's home. After the birth the care of the newborn baby and mother are largely in the hands of the older women in the extended family. In this way cultural practices and influences have an early effect on the new member of the family.

Later on in childhood, the influence of various cultural practices persist. For example, Caucasian children learn automatically to keep a certain spatial distance from each other whilst communicating or at play. Arab children expect be in close contact whilst speaking or playing. Similarly, simple everyday eye contact varies in different cultures. In an Anglo-Saxon culture inability to look, for example, a parent in the eye is automatically thought of as a sign of guilt about some misdemeanour. In Asian cultures eye contact with adults is considered to be an impertinence.

It is important that all people having the care of children from differing cultures should be aware of these, and many other, differences. Not that every cultural innuendo can be fully appreciated, but at least sympathetic understanding to other people's ideas, values and views are vital for every child-care worker.

In the microculture of every home, too, environmental influences exert their effects on development. The 'bonding' of mother and baby in the early days will have an effect on the interest and help mothers will give to their child later in childhood in the development of skills and relationships.

Bonding
Ability to retain a relationship over time, even in the absence of the other individual.

Premature babies, who need to be nursed in an intensive care unit for some weeks after birth can lose out on this initial bonding process with their parents by the lack of close physical proximity. So every effort must be made to fully involve parents with the care of their baby under these circumstances. This also applies to children who are hospitalized for long periods of time.

A child born into a home where alcohol or drug abuse occurs will suffer developmentally. Handling of the child will not be consistent under these circumstances as well as there being possible poor feeding and sleeping habits.

Ongoing continuity of care throughout the early years has a bearing on steady developmental progress. This care need not necessarily be parental, but regular daily care from one familiar adult gives stability to the child's developing world.

Economic factors

The child brought up in abject poverty will have few material objects on which to hone developing skills. Good, understanding parenting can help. A child can develop skills playing with a cardboard box, a spoon and a saucepan lid, for example, as readily as can a child with a far more sophisticated range of toys. (In fact imaginative processes can be better developed in the former!)

Overcrowding is frequently a common adjunct to poverty. This can restrict some aspects of a child's development. Later experience in playgroups and nursery schools goes some way to redressing these effects.

Nutrition

Diet, both in quantity and quality, will exert an influence on mental and physical development. To take an extreme example, deficiency of vitamin D can result in the disease rickets where bones are malformed. This will have an undoubted effect on the ease at which the child will be able to carry out various physical tasks. In extreme poverty, lack of sufficient calories in the diet will give rise to developmental delay as well as causing physical effects. Good parenting in an affluent society will ensure that children have adequate suitable food. Regular meals with time to eat in friendly surroundings can be good learning experiences for the developing child.

Illness

A further environmental, albeit physical, factor which can temporarily inhibit development is illness. The child who has an serious infectious illness during a particularly critical developmental period will be behind his peers in certain skills. These skills are, fortunately, rapidly picked up again once the infection has cleared, provided, of course, that no permanent damage has been done by the infection. This factor can be closely linked with social, nutritional and economic environmental factors.

The perception of illness also varies in different cultures. It is important that child carers are aware of, and sympathetic to, the expectations of mothers of sick children from other countries. Similarly child-care practices in general can differ from culture to culture and can possibly at times lead to ill-health. Examples of this include the application of surma (which contains lead – a known poison) to children's or mother's eyes to make them look big and bright.

Again, in some, cultures, the giving of the colostrum (the protein-rich secretion from the mother's breast immediately after birth) is frowned upon. Whilst this in itself has no harmful effects, this practice denies the baby important antibodies and protein from the mother.

Media

Many aspects of the media can influence children's development. Television exerts a particularly potent influence on today's children in developed countries of the world. It has been estimated that an average 1990's child will have watched around 15 000 hours worth of television and videos before school-leaving age has been reached! This, in anyone's book, is an enormous amount of potential 'learning' – for good or ill – experience. Child carers should be aware of the impact of some programmes on children. Research has shown that children as young as 14 months of age can imitate actions seen on television. This effect can be seen even after a lapse of time, showing that long-term imprinting has occurred. The horrendous shooting of a grandfather by his 6-year-old granddaughter shows how powerful this imitating procedure can be. If programmes cannot be viewed together, parents and carers should be sure that they keep a close eye on what their children are watching.

Other forms of media, such as early learning books, or comics in an older age group, also have an influence on development. Few children have to be persuaded to read comics and these do indeed have some value in providing reading material. They are basically short stories with powerful visual images stimulating children's imaginations.

It has been said that media activities of all types – and this includes computer games – can lead to wastage of time which could be spent in wider interactive activities with friends. On the other hand, being unable to discuss television programmes, comics or the latest in computer games can lead to isolation in a peer group.

Care also needs to be taken that marketing influences do not carry too much weight in children's minds. Similarly, unreal stereotyping of individuals and places can lead to prejudices when real-life situations are met.

The media in all its forms gives opportunity for positive health education, both directly and by role models of, for example, sports stars and 'Top of the Pops' personalities. So it is good to discuss various programmes seen with children. Many situations can be turned to advantage, on an individual basis, to instil healthy living habits.

Discussion

Ask several children of different ages about their television-viewing habits. List the replies you receive. Discuss with colleagues these replies and how much you think television has modified their behaviour and thinking. Summarize and write up the conclusions of the group plus any comments of your own.

Education

In its widest sense, education will also have a bearing on the acquisition of skills at the appropriate time. Education begins in the very early days of life at home when the child learns the basic skills of eating, crawling, walking, using a spoon, talking, to mention just some of the vast array of skills to be learned. Never again, in a whole lifetime, will a person learn as much as is learnt during the first two years of life. (Further discussion can be found on this topic in later chapters.)

Influences on development
- Genetic
- Social
- Economic factors
- Nutrition
- Disease
- Media
- Education

Environmental influences play an enormous part in children's development. How they handle these varying influences can be modified by their genetic inheritance. Nevertheless it is every child's right to grow up in the best possible environment – not necessarily the richest in economic terms, but richest in the sense of belonging, loving care with well-defined guidelines to show the way ahead.

OBSERVING CHILDREN

Over and over again the following message is repeatable: 'Observational skills and accurate recording in the assessment of children underpins all good educational practice'. Good observational skills do not often come naturally. Even those people who, from an early age, note details of people and their surroundings, need to sharpen up these inbuilt qualities. Effective record-keeping is certainly very much an acquired skill.

Historically, the first people to keep records of observations on their children were parents. In 1774 Pestalozzi wrote a diary of the activities of his $3\frac{1}{2}$-year-old son: *A Father's Diary*. In 1877 Charles Darwin, who wrote *The Origins and Development of Species*, published observations that he had made many years before of his son's activities and development. Much can be learned from looking back at these recorded observations, not least the knowledge of the vital part played by parents.

Permission and confidentiality

Before observation, and subsequent recording, are begun, the child-care professional must be sure that the child's parents or guardians know that they are being carried out as part of an assessment procedure for example. This will need to be clearly explained at an early stage. They must also understand that these observations must be shared by all the professionals working with, and for the benefit of, the child.

Issues of confidentiality must also be carefully explored at the outset. It may be that facts regarding the parent's health, for example genetic disease, which could have a bearing on the future health and development of the child, or practices, for example drug abuse, are relevant to a child's possible difficulties. These facts will need to be made public in the context of the case conference at the end of an assessment period. Parents must fully understand the need for this, and give their permissions for these aspects to be explored.

Practices vary in different parts of the country regarding the organization of the case conference, at which observations of a number of professionals are discussed. Parents can be a valuable part of this meeting, but may find it difficult to accept the objectivity of some of the observations that have been made. This whole issue needs sensitive handling. Child-care workers need to be aware of these facts as they make and record their observations on a child.

Discussion

Discuss with your colleagues and tutor possible issues that could cause distress to the parents of a child who is being observed as part of an assessment process. Write notes identifying the issues and how they might be handled.

Why good accurate observation is necessary

Assessment over time

Much of good assessment practice is performed over time. Observing a child playing at frequent intervals during a morning will give concrete ideas on the level of specific developing skills. Ask a child to perform a certain task, for example to build a tower with a certain number of bricks, and chances are that she will not do so! The reasons can be many:

- shyness;
- tiredness;
- hunger;
- onset of illness;
- just plain awkwardness.

Leave her alone with the bricks for a while, but still observing closely, and the task will often be completed quickly and readily.

Disabling conditions

Warning signs of some specific disabling condition can be noted by ongoing observation. For example, a child with Duchenne muscular dystrophy (in which, amongst other problems, is a weakness of the muscles of the pelvis and legs) will be noticed to be having difficulty in getting to his feet from a sitting or kneeling position. The very specific way in which he overcomes this difficulty – by 'crawling' with his hands up the front of his legs – is an important early clue in the diagnosis of the disease. (This way of standing up is known as the 'Gower manoeuvre'.) Accurate observation of such a child in a normal play situation can be the first positive fact noted. Reporting this, at first seemingly isolated, fact can be of enormous value to other professionals concerned with the child's development.

Developmental delay

Similarly, small early signs of developmental delay can be noted by a critical observer. If several signs, by themselves of little significance, are put together, the sum can point to an area of development where a child needs extra help. The child who does not play as readily or as competently as his peers with certain toys may just be shy. It is when another observation is made that the same child is unable to verbalize his needs easily that queries about possible overall (or 'global') developmental delay arise. Further investigation into other developmental areas can then be made by the assessment team. Without the initial observations being collated there could be a time lapse before specific help was given to the child.

Onset of illness

The onset of illness in a child often results in minimal differences in behaviour in the early stages. Maybe these changes are merely due to just one more of the upper respiratory tact infections to which young children are so prone, or maybe it is the beginning of some more serious infection. Other diseases too, for example juvenile arthritis, can show themselves in unusual behaviour or play patterns. Observations in detail, when shared with other care workers, can help with early diagnosis and hence help for the child.

Child abuse

The possibility of child abuse must, regretfully, always be at the back of a child carer's mind. Often early signs of this can be detected in a situation away from the abusing one, where the abused child feels safe. Many and varied are the signs, ranging from aggressive, noisy behaviour to the 'frozen awareness' of the repeatedly abused child. Many stages occur between these two extremes. A withdrawn, sad-looking child, sitting in a corner on his own, may indeed have reason to be looking sad.

Sexual abuse can also manifest itself by masturbation, an excessive interest in other children's genitalia or by acts of indecent exposure. Great care, of course, must be taken in the interpretation of such events. Many happy, well cared-for children exhibit unusual behaviour patterns at times. Sharing of observations will help to determine whether or not the situation is one needing further investigation.

Individual programmes

Individual care programmes, under certain circumstances, need to be set up and adhered to by everyone who has contact with, and care of, the individual child. Observations of both initial and changing needs, as well as the day-to-day working-out of a programme, are all vital.

Accurate observation necessary for:
- Assessment
- Diagnosis of disability
- Diagnosis of developmental delay
- Onset of illness
- Child abuse
- Case preparation
- Case conferences
- Court hearings
- Curriculum planning

Case conferences

Case conferences or court hearings all rely heavily on the observational skills of the people in daily contact with the child. By the weaving together of many small pieces of 'evidence', a full picture of an individual child can be gained. As an adjunct to these skills, accurate recordings will need to be available.

Curriculum planning

In a wider scene, observation of children's needs in a specific group are required to help with curriculum planning and the setting up of an appropriate environment to maximize available resources.

Types of observation

There are several main methods of observation that can usefully be made in differing situations. The nursery nurse needs to be aware of all these methods, and to be able to employ them appropriately at different times for differing reasons. As we have seen, there are a variety of reasons why accurate observations are needed, and each of the methods will be useful in specific situations.

'Snapshot' observations

As the name implies these are 'one-off' observations of what a child is doing at one particular time. This type of observation must be used in conjunction with other recorded events in the child's day, or wrong interpretations can easily be made, For example, a snapshot observation of a child with his hand raised could have a number of interpretations:

- response to an action game;
- asking for help;
- pointing at a distant object;
- in the process of hitting another child – or adult!

So it is important that this type of observation is used in context with other happenings.

Naturalistic observations

These are the observations made of children playing in a normal, usual situation. The children will be making their own rules and doing exactly as they please within the confines of their immediate physical situation. There must be no attempt on the part of the observer to structure the situation in any way. (Obviously if a situation is seen to be getting out of hand in a way that is unsafe for the group or an individual child, the situation must be controlled and the observation stopped.)

Structured observations

As the name implies this type of observation is one which the observer has arranged in order to gain specific information. A simple example of a structured observation is the jumping off of a low box onto a mat by a number of children of approximately the same age. Observation of the way in which this task is performed by each of the children is made. This gives information on the stability, the muscle control and the way in which the exercise is approached, i.e. fearfully, or with aplomb.

Longitudinal observation

This type of observation is one which is taken over a specified length of time. Either a specific child, a group of children or a sub-group of a class over, for example, a day or a week could be studied by this method.

Student exercise

You are to attend a case conference about a child with whom you have been working for the past month. The child has a language difficulty and the conference has been called to determine the child's overall developmental profile. Prepare a report, for presentation at the meeting, on what you think are the relevant observations about the language difficulty. Knowing, also, that the scheduled 'chair' of the conference is particularly fussy in questioning staff about the different types of observations used, defend your case, within the report, for your use of different types of observations.

Types of observation
- Snapshot
- Naturalistic
- Structured
- Longitudinal
- Comparative

Comparative observations

This is a definitive observational exercise set up to illustrate the range of variables in a given developmental situation. Examples would be:
- the dressing skills of children of approximately the same age;
- the drawing skills of the same group of children.

Practice in this type of observation can be carried out at any time and in any situation. A group of children at the swimming pool, in the park or out shopping can be observed during a weekend. Use these observations to discuss later with your colleagues.

Student exercise

In the park you have observed a group of 3-year-olds playing on the available equipment. Describe, in writing, how each child reacts to:
- being pushed on a swing;
- sliding down a chute;
- crawling through a tunnel.

List the factors that might be at work in the different attitudes you may have noticed.

RECORDING OF OBSERVATIONS

There are a number of methods of recording observations. It is advisable that students should practise all available methods to find out with which method they themselves feel most comfortable, although it may not always be possible to use this chosen method. Also, other partners in the team may request a specific method to be used in a certain situation.

It is important to remember issues of permission and confidentiality before recording observations. Permission must be obtained from the child's parents or guardians if the observations are to be made in the child's home. If a workplace is the venue for the observation, permission from the person in charge – teacher or nurse – needs to be obtained.

To ensure confidentiality it is usual not to write down the child's real name, but to use a letter, abbreviation or some other method of concealment. Written notes can easily be mislaid or even – as was the case a few

Remember confidentiality issues and use abbreviations or symbols for specific children – you could leave your notebook on the train!

years ago – turn up on a waste tip! Much heart-searching and upset was causes by this event as the child's real name and address had been used in a highly confidential report.

Always start a record of observations with basic information (sex, age, place in the family) and the time and place where the observations are to be made. Much of this information can be found and jotted down before the actual observation is started. Any equipment used will also need to be mentioned, as well as other children and adults who may be present in the room or playground.

The purpose of the recording needs also to be documented. For example, a specific purpose such as: 'Observation of a 2-year-old child playing alone with building blocks' could be a title.

Recorded observations must always be factual and objective.

Remember, too, that a record of observations should not contain the observer's opinion on either the methods or the result of the observation. Opinions can, of course, be given in later discussion between professionals or in a tutorial discussion group.

Always have a pencil and paper handy if possible when in the company of children. Small children never behave in a preordained pattern, and many unexpected and enlightening events occur at most unexpected times.

Finally, remember that the good observer will:
- know exactly why and what is being observed;
- know the method that is being employed;
- have ready at hand any equipment needed – getting up to sharpen a pencil will alter the observed situation;
- merge into the background (obvious activity will have an effect on the situation);
- avoid eye contact with the observed child as this can alter behaviour;
- not attempt to interpret results at the time – this must be done later;
- remember not to embarrass the child, or parent, by a too obvious observation.

Types of recording

Time sampling

This type of observation requires the observer to record what a child, or group of children, is doing for a specified length of time. This slot of time can be repeated at regular intervals throughout the day.

The observer will need to decide:
- the length of time the observation will take, e.g. 10 minutes/30 minutes;
- the frequency of the observations, e.g. three times during the course of a morning;
- when, or if, a similar exercise should be done, e.g. observing the same child two or three months later.

The chosen time must be strictly adhered to. It can be all too tempting to extend this if a child is beginning to do something really interesting just as the set time limit expires! If recordings are continued after the time limit, the whole point of time sampling lost.

Event sampling

This type of observation and recording requires the observer to record a predetermined event in the day of an individual child. Recording how many times a child had a temper tantrum or threw a toy at another child in anger is one example of this. The event chosen will of course be one about which there is concern in an individual child.

This method can also be valuable in assessing the success, or otherwise, of an intervention in an attempt to control challenging behaviour. Markers, e.g. red dots, can be placed on a time plan showing how many times a child jumps onto a table. Following the use of behaviour control techniques to stop this unwanted activity, a similar exercise in event sampling could be done again after various time intervals. Any decrease in the number of red dots will then give a quick visual clue as to the success of the technique used.

One problem that needs to be overcome in this type of recording is the necessity for the observer to be available to record the chosen event. Often other tasks and duties will be being done when the child has a temper tantrum, for example. Other workers will need to cooperate and take over quickly the observer's tasks whilst a recording is made.

Student exercise

List several aspects of children's behaviour which could be used as examples of:
- time sampling;
- event sampling.

Describe the difficulties that could arise in the examples chosen.

Using structured records

There are a number of published charts which all have the same basic format – that of marking expected behaviour at definite ages or stages of child development. Skills which the majority of children of a specific age should be able to do are listed. The observer records whether or not an individual child is able to perform the given tasks. The results will show the strengths and weaknesses of a child. It must never be used as a 'pass' or 'fail' test. These charts should be used as a guide to show where a child/parent/ nursery nurse needs to act in partnership in order to overcome any difficulties, or to build on specific strengths.

There are a number of charts available commercially having different formats each of which has its own merits. The Sheridan charts, Denver charts and Cash–Bellman charts are examples of these.

Student exercise

Prepare a table showing the benefits and limitations of the different types of chart with examples if possible.

Target child observation

This type of observation and recording focuses on one particular child within a group. The child can be one who has been noticed to be unusual in some particular way from her peers. The child picked for a target observation could be:
- showing challenging behaviour;
- having learning difficulties;
- noticed to be withdrawn;
- showing some signs of a special talent.

(A child with no special difficulties can, of course, be chosen. But in the early stages of learning about observational skills it is easier to have more obvious facts to look for.)

The target child is observed by both time and event sampling methods, the observations being specifically related to the difficulties suspected. Structured records can also be use to fill out the profile of the child.

Additional aids to recording

- **Video or audio tapes** can be used as a method of bringing extra life to reports. The equipment must be available and the observer skilled in using the technology to most advantage. It is a waste of time and resources playing a video or audio tape with no particular purpose in mind, but, if it is used with forethought, useful events and facts can be brought out.
- The keeping of a **diary** throughout a course in child care can give valuable retrospective information. Specific events and/or impressions of different children, recorded with no immediate purpose in mind, can yield useful information at a later date. This type of recording will need to be kept consistently to be of most value.
- **Anecdotal records**. Children's drawings and paintings can be added to give extra information. Photographs of the child can also be included.

Good observation of children together with adequate record-keeping are basic requirements in the assessment of children's abilities and need; as a result it is good educational practice.

Student exercise

Start a diary of events as they happen in your place of work experience. Look for, and note, the unusual events.

Types of recording
- Time sampling
- Event sampling
- Structured records
- Target child

Additional aids
- Video/audio tapes
- Diaries/log books
- Photographs
- Drawings and paintings

FURTHER READING

Bruce, T. (1993), *Getting to Know You*, London: Hodder & Stoughton (A guide to record keeping in early childhood education and care).

Illingworth, R.S. (1983), *The Development of the Infant and Young Child*, Edinburgh: Churchill Livingstone.

Lindsay, B. (1994), *The Child and Family*, London: Ballière Tindall.

2. THE HUMAN BODY

Anyone having the care of children will need to have at least an elementary knowledge of the structure and function of the human body. All organs are in place and potentially functional at birth. Throughout childhood changes in size takes place but basic function does not change. (There are one or two exceptions to this: for example, the thymus gland, situated in the chest, is relatively large and fulfils a function in childhood, but almost completely disappears at puberty. A further example is the reproductive organs in both sexes. Although present in basic form at birth, only at puberty do they attain full maturity and function.)

The basic units of the body are **cells**. These tiny structures consist of cytoplasm surrounding a nucleus, again with one or two exceptions: for example, some blood cells have no nucleus. A membrane surrounds each cell, giving it its distinctive character.

Similar types of cells combine together to make **tissues**, for example muscular tissue, bone tissue.

Organs are specialized groups of tissues which act as a unit with very specific functions, for example liver, kidneys. These organs further combine together as functional units, or **systems**, for example the digestive system, the cardiovascular system.

Anatomy is the study of the structure of the body and **physiology** is concerned with the function of the various parts. In this chapter these two facets will be looked at together as the various systems are described.

Before beginning a discussion on each system it is necessary to have an idea as to where the various organs are placed in the body (Figure 2.1).

The main trunk of the body is divided by the thick, strong sheet of muscle, known as the diaphragm, into two separate cavities: the **thoracic cavity** and the **abdominal cavity**. This latter cavity is further subdivided into the main abdominal cavity and the **pelvic cavity**. The brain is enclosed in a cavity inside the skull known as the **cranial cavity**.

SKELETOMUSCULAR SYSTEM

The skeletomuscular system consists of the bony skeleton providing a framework and the muscles attached to these bones enabling movement to take place. As well as these functions the bony skeleton supports and protects the soft underlying organs. The bone marrow in the centre of bone is concerned with the manufacture of blood cells. In young babies all the bones are involved in this process. Later in life, only the bone marrow in the sternum, ribs, vertebrae and the upper ends of the humerus and femur are involved.

Functions of bone
- Support and movement
- Protection of underlying organs
- Concerned with blood production

Bone

Bone itself is tough and strong, in spite of being made up of 50% water! The remainder consists of calcium salts and organic substances such as

Figure 2.1 Organs of the body.

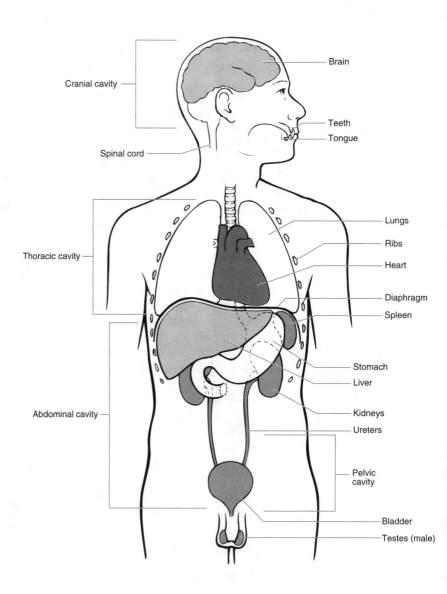

collagen and gelatin. All bones are covered by a tough membrane known as the **periosteum**. Bones come in many shapes and sizes:

- **Long bones** of the arms and legs. The main shafts of these bones are made of hard, strong compact bone with a hollow centre containing the bone marrow. The ends of these bones are made of a somewhat similar substance, cartilage. Cartilage is softer and more pliable than bone so allowing movement to take place at joints. In children there is a further specialized area in the long bones known as the epiphyseal plates. It is at this area that growth takes place, up to the age of 18 years in females and 21 years in males. At these ages growth ceases and the epiphyseal plates become fused.

Wrists and ankles, at the ends of the long bones, are made up of highly specialized and shaped bones to allow for fine movements. Fingers and toes are again made of specially shaped bones for their specific uses.

- **Vertebral column** or **spine**. This keeps the whole body upright as well as providing vital protection for the spinal cord. These bones all have a basically similar irregular shape which varies slightly up and down the length of the vertebral column (Figure 2.2).

Figure 2.2 Basic structure of vertebrae.

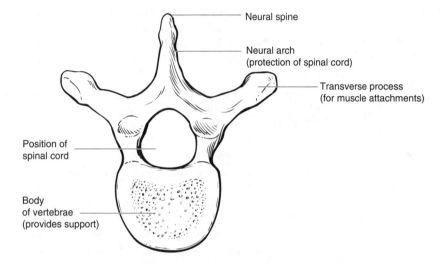

Neural spine

Neural arch
(protection of spinal cord)

Transverse process
(for muscle attachments)

Position of
spinal cord

Body
of vertebrae
(provides support)

There are 33 vertebrae in all: seven in the neck (cervical) region; 12 in the chest (thoracic) region; five in the back (lumbar) region and nine in the lower back (sacral) region. These latter bones are fused together to form the **sacrum** and the **coccyx**.

Between the vertebral bodies (or centra) are the **intervertebral discs**, soft pliable discs which cushion and allow flexibility of the spine. Ligaments join these bones, and others in the body, together.

- **Skull** or **cranium**. Situated at the top end of the vertebral column, the cranium consists of a number of small bones fused together to form a strong 'box' to protect the brain. These bones are fused together by flat joints known as 'sutures'. In babies and young children these sutures are flexible. This allows the 'moulding' of the baby's head in the journey down the birth canal. Until around the age of 18 months there are two main areas between the skull bones which are not fused and form the **anterior** and **posterior fontanelles**. In these areas the brain is covered by thick fibrous tissue. Between 1 year and 18 months these fontanelles close and the skull becomes continuous.

Also as part of the skull are the bones of the face, specialized to perform various functions such as: the protection of the eyes by the orbital bones; the bony upper part of the nose to protect the nasal passages; the specialized upper and lower jaws which contain the teeth and provide anchors for the muscles associated with speaking and chewing.

- **Ribs**. These are flat, curved bones attached at the back to the vertebral column and in the front to the flat breastbone, or sternum. This 'cage' provides important protection for the heart and lungs in the thoracic cavity.
- **Shoulder blades** or **scapulae**. These are placed on the back of the rib cage. Muscles attached to these structures and the collar-bones, or clavicles, allow movement of the arms. Together these bones are known as the **shoulder girdle**.
- **Pelvic bones**. These are attached to the lower part of the vertebral column at the back and joined together in the front in the pubic region. These bones are of an irregular shape, the most prominent part being the hip-bones. This group of bones together is known as the **pelvic girdle**.

All the bones, and groups of bones, are made into one whole by **joints**. Without these joints movement would not be possible. There are a number of different types of joint:

- **Fixed**, or **fibrous, joints** such as those between the bones of the skull – the sutures.
- Joints with a minimum of movement, or **cartilaginous joints**. Examples of these are the joints between the vertebrae and those which join the ribs to the sternum. (Cartilage is made of collagen and other organic substances similar to bone but has a lower calcium content.)
- Joints that are freely mobile. These are also known as **synovial joints**, and have a capsule in which there is fluid, the synovial fluid, which lubricates the joint.

  These synovial joints are further subdivided according to their function:
  - ball-and-socket joints (the hip and the shoulder), allowing wide ranging movements;
  - hinge joints (the knee and elbow);
  - saddle joints (the joints of the thumb), allowing the important 'pincer' movement of the thumb, so important in the handling of tools;
  - gliding joints (those between the articulating parts of the vertebrae).

Types of joint
- Fibrous joints
- Cartilaginous joints
- Synovial joints

Muscles

The muscles attached to the bony skeleton vary enormously in both size and shape depending on position and function. It is these muscles that give the body its basic shape as well as allowing movement to take place. All the skeletal muscles are made up of specialized tissue, **striated** or **voluntary muscle**, which is able to contract and relax under the voluntary control of the nervous system. Each muscle has its own nerve supply controlling its action. The muscles of a young child are of basically the same shape as in an adult, but the nervous control has to mature before full control is possible.

Student exercise

Watch the uncoordinated hand movements of a young baby. Compare these with the relatively skilled handling of objects – with a 'pincer' grip between thumb and fore-finger – of an 18-month-old child. Draw the different types of movements observed.

(There are other types of muscle apart from those attached to the bony skeleton. These are:
- **cardiac muscle** found only in the heart;
- **smooth, unstriated** or **involuntary muscle** found in blood vessels, intestines, and bladder. This type of muscle is under the control of the autonomic nervous system, i.e. not under conscious or voluntary control.

Types of muscle
- Voluntary, or striated, muscle
- Involuntary, smooth or unstriated muscle
- Cardiac muscle

These muscle types will be mentioned again under the various systems in which they are present.)

Muscles in many parts of the body are attached to the same bone and exert their action in a paired fashion. For example, relaxation of the triceps and contraction of the biceps (both muscles in the upper arm) creates the movement of bending the elbow. When the arm is straightened the opposite action occurs: the triceps contracts and the biceps relax (Figure 2.3).

Muscular action uses glucose and various enzymes for energy. This glucose is obtained from stores in the body, in the form of glycogen. Oxygen is necessary to convert this glycogen to a usable form. If there is inadequate oxygen available for vigorous muscular action, lactic acid builds up in the muscles. This lactic acid is the cause of aching muscles following vigorous or unaccustomed exercise. With rest the lactic acid disperses and the muscles become pain-free again.

CARDIOVASCULAR OR CIRCULATORY SYSTEM

This system includes the **blood**, the **lymph** and the **system of vessels** transporting these fluids throughout the body and the heart. The **heart** is the pump which, by its contractions, pushes blood through the arteries to the networks of capillaries (the very smallest blood vessels) enmeshed deep in the tissues. Blood is then returned to the heart via the veins, so making the blood system enclosed and complete.

Blood

Blood is the vital transport system of the body for the provision of oxygen and nutrients to the tissues and the removal of waste products arising from the work of these tissues. Oxygen is obtained by respiration taking place in the lungs. Nutrients are obtained from the digestive system. Waste products are passed in the blood to the kidneys for elimination in the urine.

Blood also has the important function of fighting disease by the means of cells specialized for this purpose.

Figure 2.3 Antagonistic action of muscles on arm movement.

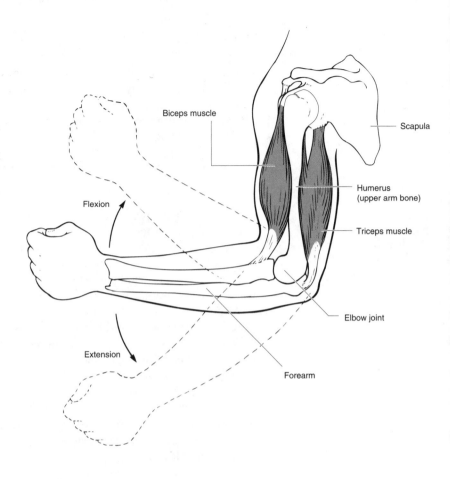

Hormones from the ductless glands of the body (see under endocrine system) are also carried in the blood.

Blood consists off different types of cells floating in a fluid known as plasma.

Cells
- **Red blood cells** have no nucleus and contain a substance called haemoglobin which is the oxygen-carrying part of the blood. This haemoglobin gives blood its red colour. Red blood cells are very numerous, about 5 000 000 in a cubic mm of blood.
- **White blood cells** have a nucleus and are involved with fighting invading bacteria and viruses. Different types of white blood cells have differing sizes and shapes. There are between 6000 and 8000 white blood cells in a cubic mm of blood.

The **plasma** is a straw-coloured fluid and consists of 90% water, the remaining 10% being dissolved substances such as minerals, glucose, hormones and various waste products.

- Tiny **platelets** are an important group of cells; they are intimately involved with the clotting of the blood following injury.

Blood groups

All humans have a specific blood group. These blood groups were discovered by Landsteiner in the early 1900s. Each individual is born with a specific blood group, genetically inherited, which remains constant throughout life. These groups are O, A, B and AB. (There are a number of subgroups in this major classification.) If a person is given blood from a group which is incompatible with their own blood group, serious (and often fatal) clotting will occur due to the interaction of the differing blood groups.

One further group which is of immense importance in baby care is the **rhesus factor**: 85% of people, both male and female, have a particular substance on their blood cells, known as the rhesus factor. They are termed to be rhesus-positive (+ve). The remaining 15% of the population do not have this particular antigen (a substance which produces antibodies in the human body) and are termed rhesus-negative (–ve). As with the other blood groups, the rhesus factor is inherited from the baby's parents. If both parents are rhesus +ve the baby will also have the rhesus factor in his blood. Similarly, if both parents are rhesus –ve their offspring will also be rhesus –ve.

Problems arise when a baby is conceived by a rhesus –ve mother from a rhesus +ve father. The baby from this union will be rhesus +ve – since the rhesus factor is inherited in a dominant way. As a result the mother will become sensitized to the rhesus +ve factor in her baby's blood and will produce antibodies. In the first pregnancy no problems will be encountered. But in a future pregnancy, without treatment, these antibodies will affect the baby's blood and cause a specific type of anaemia. Stillbirth can be the result or the baby can be born with a severe degree of anaemia and/or jaundice. Fortunately this tragic situation can be avoided by giving the mother an injection of anti-D globulin within 72 hours of the birth of her first baby to destroy these antibodies. (A rhesus –ve mother will also need the protection of anti-D if she miscarries a rhesus +ve baby.)

Lymphatic system

Lymph is a colourless fluid derived from blood. It is found in most of the spaces between the tissues and drains into tiny vessels which become larger and eventually drain back into the venous system via the thoracic duct. An important constituent of lymph are the **lymphocytes**. These cells play a vital part in the fight against disease. They are produced in the lymph nodes, or glands, which are found in a number of different parts of the body:

- in the neck: the **cervical lymph glands** which so quickly become swollen in children as throat infections are fought off;

- in the armpits and groins: these, too, become enlarged if damage or infection occurs in arms or legs;
- smaller secondary nodes found behind knees and elbows: these only become obviously enlarged with severe trauma or infection.

As well as these superficial lymph nodes, other masses of lymphoid tissue are to be found:

- as the **tonsils**: two large masses found either side of the throat; again these become rapidly red and swollen as throat and upper respiratory infections are fought;
- as the **adenoids**, which are masses of lymphoid tissue at the back of the throat and nose and which again are actively involved in the fight against infection, especially in children. (Tonsillectomy and adenoidectomy – removal of the tonsils and adenoids – needs to be done when these masses of lymphoid tissue become frequently infected. Today's thinking, however, considers that too early removal destroys an important aspect of the control of infection, and this operation is not performed as frequently as it used to be. As a general rule, children's tonsils are only removed if there has been more than four confirmed attacks of tonsillitis in any one year, or if the airway is almost obstructed by the grossly enlarged and chronically infected tonsils. Adenoids are usually removed at the same time as the tonsils.)
- in various parts of the **small intestine**: here, this lymphoid tissue is known as Peyer's patches; it can become swollen, giving rise to abdominal pain, particularly in children, during a bout of infection;
- in the spleen, tucked up under the ribs on the left side of the body.

As well as fulfilling an important part in the fight against infection the lymphatic system is involved in the passage of nutrients, hormones and waste products of metabolism between blood and tissues.

Heart

The heart is the pump which sends the blood round the entire body. This tireless organ beats at an average rate of 60–80 beats per minute, 24 hours a day, 7 days a week, 52 weeks a year up to 100 – or more – years of life!

The tissue making up the heart is a specialized form of muscle, known as **cardiac muscle**, and branches and interweaves in order to fulfil its unique function. The walls of the heart, made of this cardiac muscle, are thick and strong to perform this minute-by-minute pumping action.

The heart has a special blood supply of its own – the coronary arteries and veins. These blood vessels are tiny, no larger than a piece of string. It is blockage of these that gives rise to coronary heart attacks in later life.

The simplest way to think of the heart's action is as a double pump, with two distinct sets of chambers on either side (Figure 2.4).

The right side of the heart receives blood lacking in oxygen (deoxygenated) back from all parts of the body into its upper, collecting, chamber, the right atrium. From here the blood is passed, through the tricuspid valve, into the lower chamber, the right ventricle. The pulmonary artery then takes this blood out to the lungs where oxygenation takes place in the

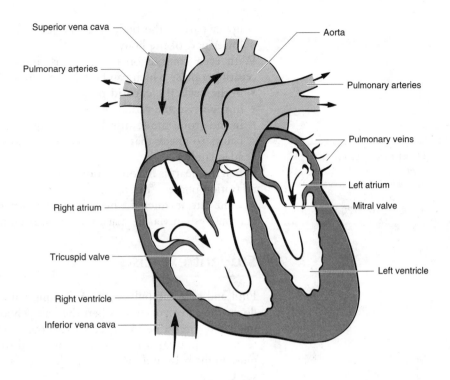

Figure 2.4 Heart anatomy showing direction of blood flow.

lung tissue through respiration. This freshly oxygenated blood is then passed back into the left side of the heart via the pulmonary vein. The blood enters into the left collecting chamber, the left atrium, and is passed through the mitral valve into the left ventricle. From here, oxygenated blood is pumped, via the largest blood vessel of all, the aorta, to all the tissues and organs of the body.

From Figure 2.4 note:

- right and left sides of the heart are completely separate;
- the thick, muscular walls of the ventricles: the wall of the left ventricle is thicker than that of the right ventricle, as it has to pump blood around the whole body; the right ventricle only has to pump blood to the lungs;
- the thinner muscular walls of the atria, collecting chambers only, with no pumping action;
- pulmonary arteries containing **deoxygenated blood**, the only ones in the body to do so (other arteries always contain oxygenated blood);
- pulmonary veins containing **oxygenated blood** (other veins always contain deoxygenated blood);
- tricuspid and mitral valves pointing into ventricles to prevent blood regurgitating back into the atria;
- superior vena cava taking deoxygenated blood to the heart from the

upper part of the body; the inferior vena cava taking blood from the lower part of the body.

With each contraction of the heart, blood is forced round the body, creating a pulse which can be felt in various places, most commonly:

- in the neck: the **carotid pulse**;
- in the wrist: the **radial pulse**;
- in the groin: the **femoral pulse**. (This is an important pulse to feel in babies to check that the blood flow to the lower limbs is functioning adequately.)

When the heart is in contraction, this is known as 'systole' and when in the relaxation phase – 'diastole'.

The rate at which the heart beats is under the control of the autonomic nervous system via the 'pace-maker' situated in the right atrium.

Heart rate average
- Adults: 60–80 beats/min
- Children (5–12 years): 80–100 beats/min
- Babies: 100–120 beats/min

Student exercise

Find and take the pulse rate of a young baby and an older child. Write down the rates you note when the baby/child is quietly resting and immediately after a period of activity. Note and record the time it takes to restore to normal when activity ceases and the easiest places to take the pulse in the baby and the older child. (For details on how to take the pulse, see Chapter 9.)

The direction of the blood flow in the heart is quite different in prenatal life from that after birth. Before birth, oxygen is passed to the baby via the placenta and umbilical cord – the baby's lungs not being used for this purpose at this stage. At birth and in the succeeding weeks, changes in the anatomical structure of the heart occur to make oxygenation from the lungs possible. It is when these changes do not fully occur that some types of congenital heart diseases arise.

Blood vessels

The blood vessels – arteries and veins – form a network over the whole body. From the large aorta arising from the left ventricle of the heart the arteries become progressively smaller until they end up in the capillary bed in various tissues and organs. It is here that exchange of nutrients, oxygen and waste products occurs. The capillaries then in turn combine into larger and larger veins which eventually become the superior and inferior venae cavae, which pass their deoxygenated blood into the right atrium of the heart.

Structure of the blood vessels

Arteries (Figure 2.5):

- have a thick elastic wall to withstand the high pressures with which the blood is pumped from the heart;

- have a round discrete lumen;
- have no valves;
- are mainly placed deep in the tissues.

Veins (Figure 2.5):
- have relatively thin inelastic walls;
- have a larger more irregular lumen than arteries;
- have valves at intervals to prevent back-flow of blood;
- are placed more superficially in the tissues.

These anatomical facts relate closely to the differing functions of the arteries and veins. Table 2.1 shows the main differences in function.

Figure 2.5 Cross-section of artery and vein.

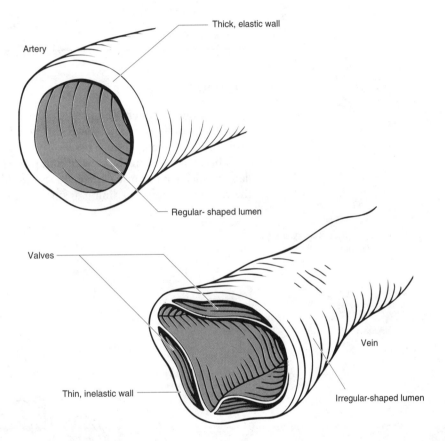

Blood pressure

Blood pressure is the pressure in the arteries, and is measured more routinely in adults rather than in children, although there are some conditions in which measurement is important in children.

Two figures are recorded (with a special instrument known as a **sphygmomanometer**). The pressure in the arteries during a contraction of the heart is known as the 'systolic' pressure; this is the upper of the two recorded readings. The pressure in the arteries during a relaxation phase of the heart cycle is known as the 'diastolic' pressure; this is the lower of the two readings.

Table 2.1

Arteries	Veins
Carry blood away from the heart	Carry blood to the heart
Carry oxygenated blood (exception being pulmonary artery)	Carry de-oxygenated blood (exception being pulmonary vein)
Blood is at high pressure	Blood is at low pressure
Blood high in nutrients and oxygen	Blood low in nutrients and oxygen
Blood low in waste products	Blood high in waste products
Arterial bleeding less common due to position	Venous bleeding more common due to position

RESPIRATORY SYSTEM

The respiratory system (Figure 2.6) consists of the air passages starting from the mouth and nose down through the trachea (windpipe) to the bronchi into the actual lung tissue.

The **nose** contains hairs which trap small particles of dust and other debris which could cause damage to the delicate lung tissue. Further down the respiratory tract the lining again has tiny hairs, known as **cilia**, which

Figure 2.6 Position of lungs in the thoracic cavity.

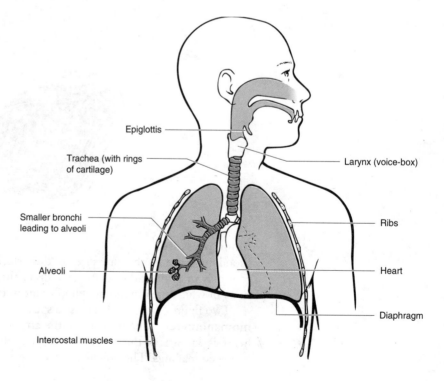

Epiglottis

Trachea (with rings of cartilage)

Larynx (voice-box)

Smaller bronchi leading to alveoli

Ribs

Alveoli

Heart

Diaphragm

Intercostal muscles

perform a similar function. These cilia are in constant motion upwards so that any contaminates that have entered the system are passed out through the mouth and nose.

The anatomical structure of the **trachea** and **bronchi** is beautifully designed with horseshoe-shaped rings of cartilage in their walls. These more rigid structures keep the air passages open during the passage of air into the lungs with the negative pressures involved in this function.

The **epiglottis** is a flap of tissue above the larynx, or voice-box, which moves during eating to stop food being taken into the air passages.

Air consists of 20% oxygen, and it is this gas which is necessary for the proper function of all the bodily tissues and organs. The remainder of the air consists of largely nitrogen, around 75%, water vapour and carbon dioxide. As air is breathed in and out, at the rate of approximately 16–20 breaths per minute, the gases pass down to tiny structures in the lung tissue, known as **alveoli**. These alveoli have a very rich blood supply and it is here that the actual gaseous exchange of oxygen and carbon dioxide takes place.

During **inspiration** (breathing in) the two groups of muscles concerned with breathing contract. The large sheet of muscle separating the thoracic and abdominal cavities – the **diaphragm** – contracts and is pulled down towards the abdomen. The contraction of the intercostal muscles, situated between the ribs, causes the ribs to be pulled upwards and outwards. Both these muscular actions cause an increase in size and volume of the thoracic cavity, but decrease the pressure inside this cavity. So a partial vacuum is made and air is sucked in. During **expiration** (breathing out) the two groups of muscles involved relax. So the size and volume of the thoracic cavity is decreased, but the pressure is increased so that air is forced out (Figure 2.7).

Between these two everyday, and involuntary, actions sufficient oxygen is passed into the alveoli for the body's needs. Only around 6% of the 20% of the oxygen available in the air is used; thus around 14% is exhaled in the breath. This is of importance when artificial respiration has to be done (Chapter 13).

The **lungs** in common with the heart, perform these functions day in, day out, at the rate of 16–20 breaths a minute (and more when exercise, emotion or illness increases the breathing rate) for a whole lifetime.

DIGESTIVE SYSTEM

This system is concerned with the ingestion, digestion and absorption of nutrients necessary to sustain all the many activities of the body. The structures of the digestive system are collectively termed the 'alimentary canal' (Figure 2.8).

Alimentary canal

Mouth and pharynx
Here food is taken in, or ingested. Mastication, teeth, tongue and cheek muscles are all involved, to reduce the food to smaller pieces. Saliva,

The human body

Figure 2.7 Mechanism of breathing.

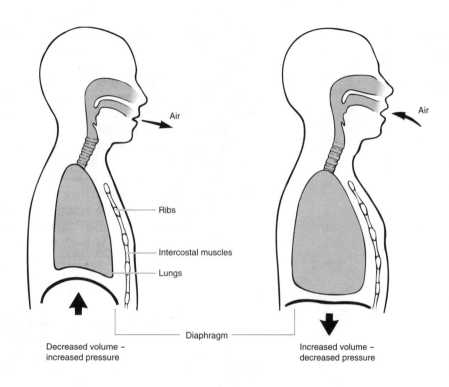

Air

Air

Ribs

Intercostal muscles

Lungs

Diaphragm

Decreased volume –
increased pressure

Increased volume –
decreased pressure

Figure 2.8 Alimentary canal.

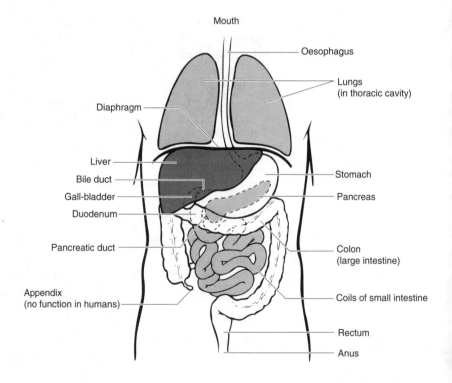

Mouth

Oesophagus

Lungs
(in thoracic cavity)

Diaphragm

Liver

Bile duct

Gall-bladder

Duodenum

Pancreatic duct

Appendix
(no function in humans)

Stomach

Pancreas

Colon
(large intestine)

Coils of small intestine

Rectum

Anus

containing the enzyme ptyalin, water and mucus, starts off the process of digestion in the mouth.

Oesophagus

This is a long tube connecting the pharyngeal region to the stomach. The masticated food is transported down this tube by 'peristalsis', the alternate contraction and relaxation of the muscles pushing the food down. Peristalsis takes place in the whole digestive tract, and is the means whereby food is passed through the alimentary tract.

Stomach

The stomach, which lies under the diaphragm in the abdominal cavity, has a number of functions:
- further breakdown of food particles;
- hydrochloric acid and water added;
- further digestive enzymes added;
- absorption of some glucose and alcohol.

Duodenum

The duodenum, leading on from the stomach, is the start of the 30 or so feet of small intestine. This part of the digestive tract also has a number of specific functions:
- receives bile from the liver;
- receives pancreatic juices, containing further specific digestive enzymes, from the pancreas.

Ileum

The ileum, the main part of the small intestine, also secretes a number of enzymes which further breakdown the food into absorbable particles. The ileum also is concerned with the absorption of the much broken-down food. On absorption from the small intestine, food is taken via the blood and lymphatics to the liver where further processing and storage is done.

Colon

The colon, or large intestine, absorbs water. The lower part of this part stores the waste products of metabolism – the faeces – until it is convenient for them to be eliminated.

Liver

The liver is a large organ situated under the right ribs. It is one of the most important organs in the body from the metabolic point of view. (In children the liver is large in relation to the other abdominal contents. This accounts for the relatively large abdomens in children of around 2 to 4 years.) The main functions of the liver can be divided into two distinct groups.

Productive functions

- **Bile** is an important substance particularly involved in the digestion of fats. Emulsification and desaturation of fats is done by bile in order that the digestive enzymes from the small intestine can proceed with further digestive processes. Bile is a yellow fluid. Excess production is stored in the gall-bladder for use when required. It consists of bile pigments, emulsifying agents and cholesterol.
- **Urea** is produced from the excess amino acids (the final breakdown products of metabolism of protein) taken in. These amino acids cannot be stored in the body (unlike carbohydrates and fats), and so have to be turned into a form which can be excreted. Urea is this end-product.
- Substances concerned with the clotting of blood – **fibrinogen** and **prothrombin** – are produced by the cells of the liver.
- Heat is produced by the liver as a result of the constant activity this important organ undertakes. Blood vessels carry this heat to the far reaches of the body. So the liver can be said to be part of the temperature control system.

Storage functions

- Glucose ingested in excess to immediate needs is stored in the liver in the form of **glycogen**. When glucose is needed by the muscles for activity, for example, this glycogen is converted to the usable form, glucose, by hormones from the pancreas and the adrenal glands.
- **Iron** is also stored in the liver. Red blood cells have a relatively short life. As they break down the iron in the haemoglobin contained in the red blood cells is stored to be used again in the manufacture of new cells in the bone marrow. (Babies have a limited store of iron in their livers at birth. By six months of age this is mainly used up. So it is important that mixed feeding – with iron-containing foods – is begun before these supplies become completely exhausted. Milk alone does not have sufficient iron content for the baby's needs at this age.)
- **Vitamin B_{12}**, a further vital ingredient in the manufacture of red blood cells, is also stored in the liver.

Functions of the liver
- Production of:
  - bile
  - urea
  - blood
  - clotting substances
  - heat
- Storage of:
  - glycogen
  - iron
  - vitamin B_{12}

Enzymes

As the food passes down the alimentary canal a series of enzymes act progressively. These enzymes are secreted:
- from the **salivary glands** in the mouth: **ptyalin** is the enzyme involved and acts on starchy foods;
- from the **stomach**: **pepsin** and **rennin** are the enzymes involved and act on protein foods; rennin acts specifically on milk protein; **hydrochloric acid** is also secreted in the stomach and aids the digestive process as well as having a role in the destruction of ingested bacteria;
- from the **pancreas** which pours its enzymes into the duodenum via the pancreatic duct: **amylase** acting on starchy foods; **lipase** which acts on the fats that have been emulsified by the bile form the liver, and **trypsinogen**;

- from the **small intestine**: three enzymes, **lactose, maltose** and **sucrose** act further on starch following on from the work done by the ptyalin form the salivary glands; **enterokinase** is another enzyme acting in conjunction with trypsinogen. This mixture of enzymes breaks down protein foods into absorbable amino acids.

Absorption

Following on from the breakdown of complex foodstuffs into simpler forms by the enzymes of the alimentary canal, absorption into the tissues via the blood and lymphatic systems is able to occur. This mainly takes place in the **ileum**, the main length of the intestines. The marvellously adapted inner surface of the ileum gives rise to an incredibly large surface area over which this exchange takes place. The interior of the ileum is covered with a network of finger-shaped **villi**. Into these villi pass tiny capillaries carrying blood and lacteals carrying lymph. It is here that glucose and amino acids pass into the capillaries and digestible fats into the lacteals. (In coeliac disease, these villi are seen to be flattened by an allergic reaction to gluten, the protein found in wheat and wheat products. As a result of this, proper absorption of food is unable to occur.)

Finally as the (much altered) food passes into the large intestine, water is absorbed leaving behind a relatively solid mass of waste material, the faeces. This is then evacuated at regular intervals via the anus.

EXCRETORY SYSTEM

Waste products are eliminated from the body in a number of ways, but the kidneys and accessory organs (bladder, ureters and urethra) are usually thought of as the main system of excretion (Figure 2.9).

Other systems involved in the removal of waste products of metabolism are:
- the lungs: carbon dioxide and water are breathed out regularly;
- the bowel: the waste end-products of digestion are eliminated regularly from the large bowel;
- the skin is also involved in various elimination processes, such as the removal of excess mineral salts, water and urea.

The **kidneys** (Figure 2.10) of which there are two, are tucked up near the lower ribs at the back of the body. As well as removing waste products the kidneys play an important role in stabilising and controlling the mineral and water content of the blood.

About 180 litres of blood passes through the kidneys every day via the renal arteries. Here it is filtered and processed. Water in excess to current needs, urea (the waste product of protein metabolism), mineral salts and other soluble substances are then formed into the urine. This collects in the 'pelvis' of the kidney and passes down the ureter to the bladder.

The **bladder** is a muscular bag which holds up to half a litre of urine, until it is convenient for it to be emptied.

Figure 2.9 Excretory system.

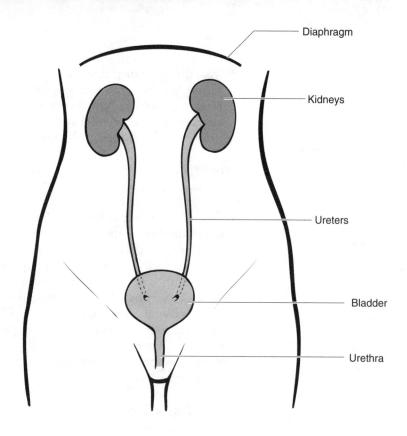

Diaphragm

Kidneys

Ureters

Bladder

Urethra

Figure 2.10 Cross-section of kidney.

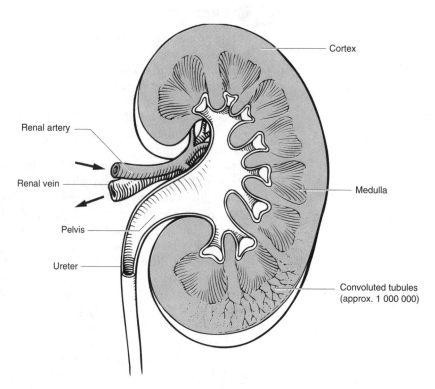

Cortex

Renal artery

Renal vein

Pelvis

Ureter

Medulla

Convoluted tubules
(approx. 1 000 000)

The kidneys are highly complex organs, consisting of a cortex around the periphery surrounding the area known as the medulla. The cortex is made up of many knots of tiny capillaries where the blood is first filtered This then passes into the convoluted (long and looped) tubules in the medulla. Here the control of water and salts is done according to the needs of the body, moment by moment.

Without the adequate functioning of the kidneys the whole metabolism of the body is compromised. Waste products build up in the blood and give rise to unpleasant, and if not treated, fatal symptoms.

The kidneys start their lifetime of work in the uterus prenatally. Small amounts of urine are passed at this time into the amniotic fluid.

ENDOCRINE SYSTEM

The endocrine system (Figure 2.11) consists of a number of glands scattered throughout the body. These glands are unique because they have no ducts in which their secretions are carried. Hence they are frequently referred to as the 'ductless glands'. Their secretions are known as 'hormones' and are passed directly into the blood stream. The effects of these secretions are felt in many different parts of the body, the blood stream providing a rapid transport system.

Endocrine, or ductless, glands pour their secretions directly into the blood stream.

The **ductless glands** of the endocrine system are specific in their actions They are, however, closely involved with the nervous and autonomic nervous systems in the control of various bodily activities.

The **pituitary gland** is situated deep in the brain tissue. This particular gland controls the functions of a number of the other ductless glands. It has been termed as the 'leader of the endocrine orchestra'!

Table 2.2 shows the specific hormones released by the pituitary gland. It can be seen that this gland has many far-reaching functions.

The **thyroid gland** is situated in the front of the neck. It is an H-shaped gland with the two main lobes on either side of the trachea. This gland also has important functions, although only one hormone, **thyroxine**, is secreted. The production of this one hormone goes through a number of complex intermediate stages. Thyroxine controls growth and development and is involved in glucose metabolism.

Table 2.2 Hormones secreted by the pituitary gland

Hormone	Function
Antidiuretic hormone (ADH)	Regulates the amount of water excreted; has an effect on the small amount of urine excreted during the night
Growth hormone	Necessary for growth during childhood; 'switches off' when growth is complete
Thyroid-stimulating hormone (TSH)	Regulates action of thyroid gland
Gonadotrophins	Regulate action of gonads – ovaries and testes
Oxytocin	Concerned with onset and continuation of labour
Prolactin	Stimulates milk production

Figure 2.11 Position of
ductless (endocrine) glands.

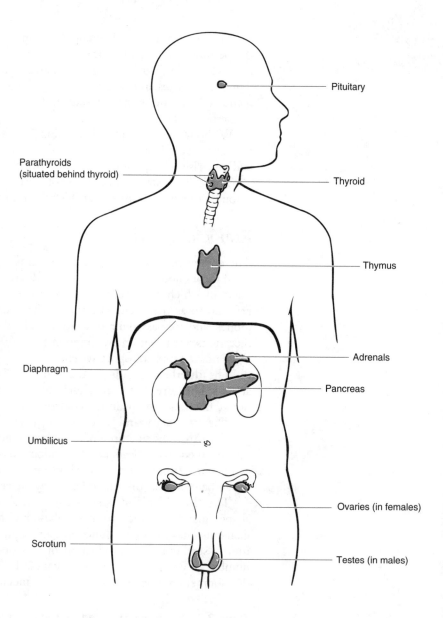

Under- or overactivity of this gland can occur. Babies can be born with an underactive thyroid gland. This causes mental delay and growth retardation if not diagnosed and treated. Tests for hypothyroidism are done routinely on all newborn babies as part of the 'heel-prick' test.

The **parathyroid glands** are four small glands situated at the back of the thyroid gland. Although they are in such close anatomical proximity, and almost share a common name, the parathyroids have quite a different function form the thyroid gland. Parathormone controls calcium and phosphate metabolism.

The **thymus gland** is an unusual gland situated in the chest, behind the sternum. It is relatively large in childhood, but practically disappears at puberty. The hormone it secretes has not been named, but it is thought to be concerned with growth, sexual maturity and also with the development of immunity in childhood.

The two **adrenal glands** are situated at the top of each kidney, but again have nothing directly to do with the excretory function of the kidney. Adrenalin is a complex substance having wide ranging effects which are intimately connected with the actions of the central nervous and autonomic nervous systems. Adrenalin affects pulse rate and volume of blood pumped by heart. It constricts blood vessels when necessary and this in turn affects the blood pressure. It also affects breathing rate.

The **pancreas** is unique amongst the glands of the body as it is both a ducted and a ductless gland. It is an elongated gland situated in the abdominal cavity behind the stomach. Digestion is aided by its secretions being poured into the small intestine via the pancreatic duct. **Insulin**, a hormone vital in the control of sugar metabolism, is secreted directly into the blood from special cells in the pancreas, known as the 'islets of Langerhans'. Insulin is also closely involved with liver function.

The **gonads** consist of the ovaries in the female and the testes in the male. There are two ovaries, situated low in the abdominal cavity. They are functionally only connected to the uterus by the Fallopian tubes. The two testes are situated in the scrotum, outside the main abdominal cavity. For proper production of sperm, these organs need a cooler temperature than would be possible to maintain inside the abdominal cavity. Hormones necessary for reproduction and sexual function are produced by the gonads (Table 2.3).

The endocrine system exerts its effects on virtually every part of the human body. Wherever rapid action is required, hormones are transferred by that excellent transport system, the blood, which permeates every living cell.

Endocrine glands
- Pituitary
- Thyroid
- Parathyroids
- Thymus
- Adrenals
- Pancreas
- Gonads: ovaries and testes

Table 2.3 Hormones secreted by the gonads

Hormone	Function
Oestrogen	Prepares the uterus for pregnancy; controls female secondary sexual characteristics
Testosterone	Controls male secondary sexual characteristics

NERVOUS SYSTEM

This is the most complex of the body's systems and exerts its effects on every part. The nervous system can be divided into a number of parts:
- the **central nervous system**, consisting of the brain and the spinal cord. Here all messages from different parts of the body are processed;
- the **sensory nerves**, arising from various organs and tissues and passing impulses to the central nervous system;

- the **motor nerves** arising from the brain and spinal cord and passing 'action' messages to the muscles, glands and other organs of the body;
- the **autonomic nervous system**, which branches throughout the body and regulates the autonomic functions of the body such as dilation of the blood vessels, heart rate and action of the digestive tract, for example; the system has two parts which act together but in an antagonistic fashion – named respectively, the 'sympathetic system' and the 'para-sympathetic system'.

Parts of the nervous system
- Central nervous system
- Sensory and motor nerves
- Autonomic nervous system
- Organs of special sense

Closely allied to the nervous system are the organs of special sense bringing in information from the external world. These organs include the eye, the ear, nose and palate and skin, all concerned with our five senses. These all provide vital information to the central nervous system alerting it to the need to take action.

Central nervous system

Brain

The brain is enclosed and protected by the strong bones of the skull. Inside this bony covering the brain also has three protective membranous layers:
- the **dura mater** which consists of thick, fibrous tissue as added protection against injury (this can be felt in young babies under the skin of the anterior fontanelle);
- the **arachnoid mater** which contains a rich network of blood vessels supplying the nervous tissue of the brain;
- the **pia mater**, a thin delicate covering which protects against infection.

Together these membranes are known as the 'meninges'. In meningitis it is these coverings to the brain that become infected and inflamed.

Between the arachnoid and the pia mater there is a space filled with a thin, colourless fluid, the **cerebrospinal fluid** (CSF). This fluid circulates in the ventricles (the open spaces in the brain) and down the spinal cord. It is this fluid that is obtained by a 'lumbar puncture' and gives information on any infection or trauma to the brain and spinal cord in certain circumstances. The CSF also acts as an extra cushion to the underlying brain when the head is banged or moved swiftly.

The brain itself consists of two **cerebral hemispheres**, which are connected in the mid-line, but the parts of which have differing functions concerned with different parts of the body.

The **cerebellum**, situated under the main part of the brain is concerned with balance and coordination.

The **brain stem**, leading into the spinal cord, is the place where control of many automatic reactions – breathing, heart rate, peristalsis – occurs in conjunction with autonomic and endocrine controls.

The **ventricles** are areas where the CSF circulates from around the brain and the spinal cord. It is abnormalities in the drainage of these ventricles that causes the condition known as 'hydrocephalus'.

Actual brain tissue consists of a mass of interwoven neurones which communicate with each other and the nerves throughout the body by electrical impulses. The chemical energy derived from food is converted into electrical energy by these highly specialized cells. Neurones are not physically connected with each other, but are separated from each other by tiny gaps known as 'synapses'. The electrical impulses jump these gaps by means of a chemical substance produced at the ends of the neurones. Acetylcholine is one of the main chemicals involved. Other chemicals – mainly sodium and potassium – are also intimately concerned with the passage of nerve impulses. Nerve impulses are extremely rapid – around 300 impulses per second being possible. Neurones are continued in both sensory and motor nerves and transmit and receive messages from the organs of special sense.

Spinal cord

The spinal cord is, like the brain, enclosed and protected by bone, the spinal column. It arises from, and is connected to, the brain. It extends the length of the vertebral column as far as the small of the back. Nerves go out from, and enter, the spinal cord at regular intervals, supplying all parts of the body. As well as passing information to and from the brain the spinal cord has the facility to produce quick automatic responses – known as 'reflex actions'.

Figure 2.12 The knee-jerk reflex.

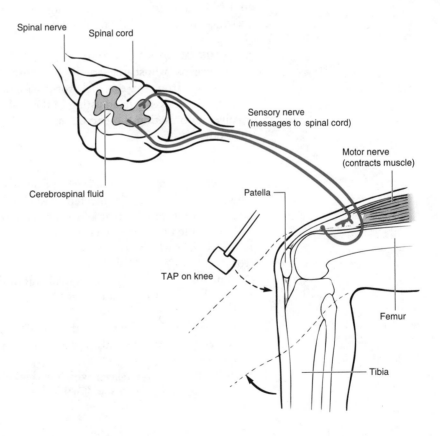

Examples of these reflex actions (vitally important for the protection and smooth running of the body) are swallowing when food touches the back of the throat. In response to this stimulus the epiglottis flops over the entry to the lungs, the soft palate is lifted up and peristalsis down the oesophagus is begun. Similarly, blinking when an object approaches the eyes and the rapid removal of a hand from a hot object are all further examples of reflex actions. The 'knee jerk' reaction is used to test reflex actions (Figure 2.12). When the tendon at the front of the knee is tapped the muscles on the front of the thigh contract and jerk the leg upwards.

Autonomic system

The autonomic system is physically closely connected with the rest of the nervous system. This system is not under voluntary control as are many of the actions associated with the central nervous system; neither are they processed through the spinal cord as are the reflex actions.

In general systems the autonomic nervous system has oversight of most of the everyday activities of the body of which we are consciously unaware. There are two main parts, the sympathetic and the parasympathetic. These two systems work antagonistically. For example, the heart rate is increased by the action of the sympathetic part, as when exercise demands a greater blood supply to the muscles. When the need for the extra oxygen, carried in the blood, is finished, the parasympathetic system takes over to slow the heart again to normal rhythm and rate.

Organs of special sense

These organs, whilst not strictly part of the nervous system, feed in the information from the external world without which the nervous system would have difficulty in adjusting to the body's differing needs. From this received information the nervous system is able to respond and motivate the body.

Eyes

The eye is structurally a miracle of adaptation to the needs of vision (Figure 2.13). Each eye, protected by the bony orbit, is a sphere controlled by a system of muscles that allow it to be moved in many directions.

The optic nerve (in each eye) passes out from the back of the eye and is the vehicle which transmits messages to the brain from the external world.

The main body of the eye is made up of three distinct layers:
- the **sclera**, the tough outer covering, which is visualized as the 'white' of the eye;
- the **choroid** which contains the blood vessels supplying nutrients and oxygen to the eye, a highly pigmented area which also acts in preventing light reflection;
- the **retina**, the inner layer which is the light-sensitive part, containing structures known as 'rods' (for black and white vision) and 'cones' (for colour vision).

Figure 2.13 Cross-section of the eye.

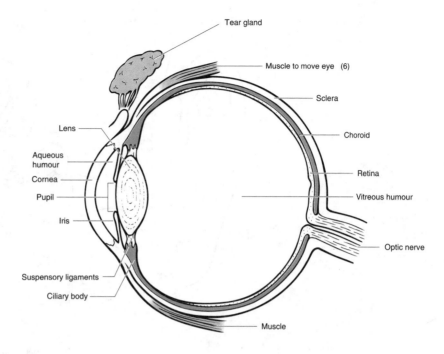

Tear gland
Muscle to move eye (6)
Sclera
Choroid
Retina
Vitreous humour
Optic nerve
Muscle
Lens
Aqueous humour
Cornea
Pupil
Iris
Suspensory ligaments
Ciliary body

Inside this sphere is the **vitreous humour**, a whitish jelly-like substance which prevents the eyeball from collapsing inwards.

At the front of the eye is the **lens** through which light rays are focused onto the retina. As objects of varying distances are regarded, this lens alters shape to accommodate the differing distances. This alteration in shape is under the control of the **ciliary body** attached to the lens by specialized ligaments.

In front of the lens is a smaller chamber filled with a transparent watery fluid known as the **aqueous humour**. The **iris** is the part of the eye giving it its distinctive colour: blue, brown, etc. The iris is a type of 'shutter' control which controls the amount of light entering the eye through the **pupil**, the black 'hole' in the middle of the iris. When a bright light is shone into the eye, the pupil constricts to prevent damage to the sensitive retina. Conversely as light dims the pupil dilates to allow more light to enter.

The whole of the front of the eye is covered by a transparent layer of tissue, the **cornea**, which is continuous with the sclera.

The **tear glands** are situated above the eye under the eyelids. This gland produces salty tears which prevent the eyeball from drying. Tears also contain an antibacterial substances helping to keep the eye infection-free.

The **eyelids** blink at regular intervals to promote the passage of tears over the eye. Tears are eventually drained away down into the nose by the tear ducts.

Figure 2.14 Structure of the ear.

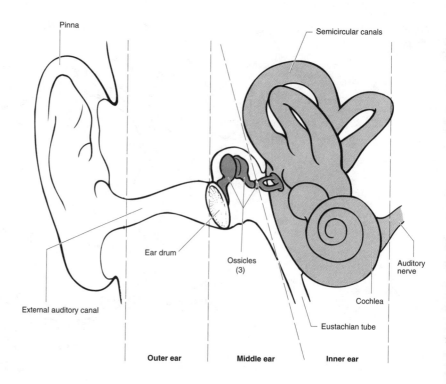

Pinna

Semicircular canals

Ear drum

Ossicles (3)

Auditory nerve

Cochlea

External auditory canal

Eustachian tube

Outer ear   **Middle ear**   **Inner ear**

Ears

The ear is a remarkably constructed organ for the purpose of hearing and balance (Figure 2.14). There are three main parts to the ear:

- **External ear**
  - The **pinna** is the part of the ear seen on the side of the head. (Animals have larger, more mobile, pinnae than humans. They are able to move this part of the ear to 'catch' the maximum of sound.)
  - From the pinna inwards the **external auditory canal** transmits the sound waves down to the **ear drum** or **tympanic membrane**. This ear drum is a tightly stretched piece of tissue which separates the external ear from the middle ear.
- **Middle ear**
  - The three **ossicles** – the stapes, the incus and the malleus – vibrate in response to the sound waves impinging on the ear drum. These ossicles are bathed in lymphatic fluid.
  - the **Eustachian tube** is a tiny canal leading from the middle ear to the back of the throat. This equalizes the pressure in the middle ear. When this is blocked by catarrh following a cold, deafness can result associated with squeaky noises in the ears.
- **Inner ear**
  - The **cochlea** is the actual organ of hearing; it is bathed in lymph fluid and connected to the auditory nerve. This nerve of hearing conveys sound messages to a specific part of the brain.
  - The **semicircular canals** are concerned with balance. Endolymph inside

these canals act on tiny hairs which give the brain information as to the body's position in space.

Sound waves pass down the external auditory canal, causing vibrations in the ear drum, and are passed on to the cochlea via the ossicles. Nerve impulses are then sent up in the auditory nerve to the auditory centre in the brain.

Organs of taste and smell

Further information regarding the outside world is sent to the brain by the **nose** (concerned with smell) and by the **tongue** and **palate** (concerned with taste).

- **Smell** (olfactory sensation) is an important part of the body's protective mechanism. Information regarding potentially dangerous situations – burning, less-than-fresh food – is sent to the brain so that appropriate avoiding actions can be taken.
- **Taste** is largely felt on the tongue, although the soft palate plays a small part. Food in the mouth stimulates various 'taste-buds' to respond to differing tastes. The front of the tongue is sensitive to salty and sweet tastes, whist the back, and underside, of the tongue is sensitive to sour and bitter tastes.

Skin

Skin is a vitally important structure from many points of view. In relation to the nervous system it is the 'organ' concerned with the sense of touch. Pain and temperature are also relayed to the brain by the skin.

Other functions of the skin include:

- Maintenance of the **shape of the body**: for example when movement takes place at a joint, the elasticity of the skin enables this to occur without the skin cracking;
- acting as a **protective covering** for the organs and tissues;
- **protects against the entry** of bacteria and fungi;
- acting as part of the general **excretory system** by removing salts and water in the sweat. These sweat glands also act as part of the temperature regulation of the body.

Structure of the skin

There are two main parts to the skin (Figure 2.15):

- The **epidermis** is the surface, and relatively thin, layer. This contains pigment which acts as a protection against ultraviolet rays. This is the layer which produces 'freckles' and the tan of sunburned skin. The surface of the epidermis is continually being worn away; the dead cells are constantly replaced by new cells lower down.
- The **dermis** is a thicker layer containing a number of important structures:
  - the **sweat glands** (over 1 000 000 in the whole body): these glands are more thickly concentrated in some parts of the body, e.g. armpits, groin; they open onto the surface of the skin by the pores;
  - the **hair follicles** from which new hair grows; tiny muscles are attached to

---

Structure of the ear
- Outer ear:
  - pinna
  - external auditory canal
  - ear drum
- Middle ear:
  - three ossicles
  - Eustachian tube
- Inner ear:
  - cochlea
  - semi-circular canals

Taste buds
- Salty and sweet tastes on front of tongue
- Sour tastes under and at back of tongue
- Bitter tastes at back of tongue

Functions of the skin
- Maintains body shape
- Protection of tissues
- Protection against bacteria
- Excretes waste products
- Helps control temperature
- Organ of touch, pain and temperature

Figure 2.15 Structure of skin.

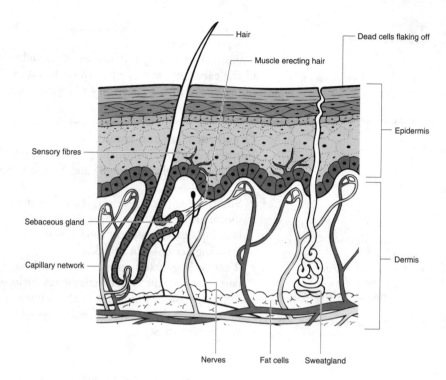

these hairs which enable the hair to stand upright, either to conserve heat (more so in animals) or when frightened;

- the **sebaceous glands,** situated near the hair follicles lubricate the hair;
- numerous small **blood capillaries** supplying the cells of the skin;
- **nerve fibres** the ends of which branch into the epidermis to react to touch and pain.

All these structures are held together in a firm, but elastic network with varying amounts of fat cells.

The skin is a sensitive indicator of many conditions. For example, in anaemia the skin is pale, in jaundice the skin is yellow and in the infectious fevers the skin shows the typical rash of the specific fever.

The skin also can be affected by bacteria, as in impetigo. Allergic reactions, such as eczema or urticaria are demonstrated in skin.

REPRODUCTIVE SYSTEM

Human beings, in common with other mammals, reproduce sexually, i.e. from the union of male and female a new being is conceived. For this to occur the male and female reproductive systems have developed quite differently from each other.

Female reproductive system

The female reproductive system (Figure 2.16) consists of:

Figure 2.16 The female reproductive system.

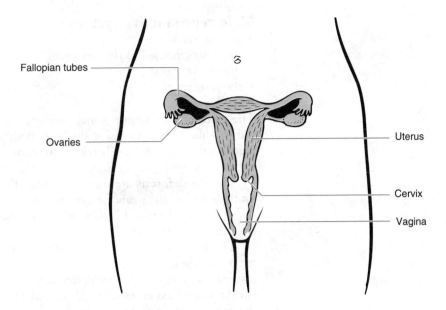

- two ovaries
- two Fallopian tubes
- the uterus (and cervix)
- the vagina.

The **ovaries** contain at birth all the special sex cells (many hundreds) needed to form ova throughout the woman's reproductive life. At puberty, hormonal influences mature some of these cells every month. The ovaries are situated low in the pelvis on either side of the uterus.

The **Fallopian tubes** have fronded ends, but are not continuous with the ovaries. As the ova are released they are guided into the tubular part of the Fallopian tube to be passed down to the uterus. Fertilization takes place in the Fallopian tubes. By the time the fertilized ovum reaches the uterus the embryo is around ten days old.

The **uterus** is a triangular-shaped, thick-walled structure. The lining is made ready by hormonal influences each month to receive a fertilized egg. If fertilization does not happen, this lining will be shed in the monthly period. If fertilization has occurred, the fertilized egg will be implanted into the wall of the uterus and the pregnancy will proceed.

The **cervix** is the structure at the base of the uterus. It is normally sealed with plug of mucus which at the time of ovulation changes its chemical composition to receive sperm. During the first stage of labour, this cervix dilates to allow the baby through into the birth canal, the vagina.

The **vagina** is the folded tube to the exterior which:
- receives the male penis during intercourse;
- accommodates the flow of blood from the uterus during menstruation;
- provides the birth canal down which the baby passes during birth.

There is no common excretory and reproductive passage in the female as there is in the male.

Male reproductive system

This consists of:

- two testes, housed in the scrotum;
- the vas deferens;
- the prostate gland;
- the penis.

The **testes** are the organs which produce the sperm. They are housed in the bag-like **scrotum** outside the main body cavity. For proper development sperm need a relatively cool temperature, and the temperature inside the body is too high.

The **vas deferens** are the coiled tubes through which the sperm pass on their way to the penis for ejaculation.

The **prostate gland** is situated at the base of the penis, and provides fluid in which the sperm swim.

The **penis** is the organ with a dual purpose, that of passage of urine from the bladder, and passage of semen (containing the sperm) during intercourse. It is usually flaccid, but during sexual arousal it becomes erect and firm by blood entering its sponge-like tissue. This enables entry into the vagina to ejaculate the semen near the cervix. Each ejaculation contains around 100 000 000 sperm, but only one will fertilize an ova.

FURTHER READING

Geraghty, P. (1988), *Caring for Children*, London: Baillière Tindall (section on anatomy and physiology).

3. PRACTICE AND SERVICES
IN CHILD CARE

OBJECTIVES

Babies
1. Know the practical skills required to care for babies, promote their healthy development and meet their nutritional needs.
2. Know how to create a safe environment for babies and young children.

Older children
1. Identify and meet physical, social and emotional needs.
2. Develop appropriate strategies for dealing with children's behaviour.
3. Provide a safe environment.

CARE OF BABIES

Human babies, unlike many other young, are completely dependent on adults for many months. They must have warmth, food, adequate rest and cleanliness if they are to survive. For healthy development, babies must also have appropriate stimuli in many aspects; they must be guarded against illness and given a sense of belonging with adequate love with encouragement throughout the early years to grow into independent adults.

Aspects of warmth

In the uterus the unborn baby is protected against changes in temperature by his mother's body and her homeostatic mechanisms. (Homeostasis is the term applied to the keeping of a constant temperature level [within narrow limits] despite how cold or hot the surrounding environment is.) As soon as the baby is born he has to control his own body temperature. There is a temperature-controlling mechanism deep in the brain tissue, but in the newborn baby this is, as yet, immature. So adequate warmth has to be provided by external means – warm rooms, adequate clothing and cot coverings. Premature, or sick, babies are especially vulnerable to temperature changes.

The temperature in which the baby lives should be ideally kept between 60 and 70°F (around 21°C). With the surrounding atmosphere within this temperature range, minimal clothing is required, e.g. a vest, an all-in-one suit and maybe a cardigan. At night when the temperature drops and rooms become colder, extra layers are necessary and cot blankets should be tucked cosily round the baby. Much heat is lost from the head, and in young and very small babies a hat is advisable at night.

Very young babies are unable to shiver, the natural way in which older children and adults attempt to raise their body temperature. It must also be remembered that very young babies are unable to move to keep warm: they are unable to pull the blankets closer around themselves if they feel cold. Movement creates warmth as can be seen by children jumping up and down to keep warm on a frosty morning.

Deposits of 'brown fat' – a specialized type of fatty tissue – found between the shoulder blades and in the small of the back are thought to play a part in the maintenance of a stable body temperature in the young baby.

Student exercise

Check the temperature in various parts of a nursery. Write down your results, and note any changes in different parts, for example near a door. Draw a plan of the best place for a baby to sleep.

Hypothermia

Babies (and elderly people) are very much at risk of hypothermia in cold winter weather.

Signs of hypothermia

- Icy arms, legs, backs and chests. Note that a baby's hands and feet can be cold when the overall body temperature is normal, so it is important to check other parts of the body.
- He may have pink cheeks and red, swollen hands.
- He will be lying quietly and not attempting to move.
- Unconsciousness can supervene and be confused with deep sleep.

Treatment

- Raise the temperature in the room.
- Remove any blankets (wrapping them more tightly will only serve to keep in the cold) and cuddle the baby close to your own warm body.
- Take him to the accident and emergency department of the nearest hospital if warmth does not return in an very short while, or contact your local doctor.

Hyperthermia is the opposite to hypothermia, and can occur if a baby is wrapped up too closely in the confines of an overheated room. (Overheating is thought to be a possible contributory factor in cot death. Further detailed information on cot deaths is to be found in Chapter 8.)

Signs that a baby is overheated is the appearance of beads of sweat on his face. Remove excess clothing and open a window to reinstate a normal body temperature.

Fresh air

Fresh air is an important ingredient in the care of babies and can usefully be considered in the context of warmth.

Oxygen is necessary for all living organisms. If a room is kept tightly enclosed with no windows open, the air can become stale and humid. Poorly ventilated rooms also mean that infection can spread more readily in the warm damp atmosphere. Rooms, therefore, should be fully ventilated at least once a day by opening doors and windows. (In very cold weather this need, of course, only be done for a very short time.) It is always advisable to have a small window open all the time, but it is important that the baby should not be lying in a draught from this. Remember he is not able to move away from a cold breeze.

An outing every day is an ideal part of every baby's routine. As well as benefiting from the fresh air, the baby is stimulated as she gets older by the new sights and sounds around her. Exceptions to this daily event are when the weather is especially cold or foggy. Prams should be robust and in a good condition to withstand rain and cold. Babies will need several layers of clothing in winter as well as a couple of loose-weave blankets when outside. Several thin layers of clothing are preferable to one thick layer. Warmth is trapped between the layers and so helps insulation. Wool, cotton or wool/cotton mix are the best materials, perhaps mixed with some man-made fibre for easier washing. In the cool spring or autumn days a hat is necessary to reduce the amount of heat lost from the baby's head. During the summer, the morning or afternoon nap can be spent outside if at all possible. Remember to keep a close eye on the baby while he is outside: 'baby-snatching' is a fact of life these days. A cat net is also a sensible precaution if there are cats in the neighbourhood. The warm, milky smell of a sleeping baby can seem a very attractive snoozing place for a wandering cat, and a heavy furry body on a baby's face is not a good idea!

Student exercise

If possible do a 'mini-survey' of mothers with young babies in your neighbourhood, and record how many mothers have a cat-net.

Clothing

Clothing is an important aspect of keeping a baby warm. Before the birth of the baby adequate clothing for the first few weeks of the baby's life should be purchased. It is advisable not to buy too many clothes of the first size. Babies grow rapidly and clothing can easily be outgrown before outworn. Also, gifts of clothing often arrive as a 'welcome' present, and the new mother can find herself overwhelmed with many items of small clothing. A minimal basic list for a new baby would include:

- six vests – 'envelope' type necks are the easiest to put on;
- six 'Babygro' type garments or dresses/rompers; Babygro or other all-in-one garments are popular: they are easy to put on and gaps around the middle do not occur; the disadvantages of these type of garments are:
  - larger sizes must always be bought in good time before the baby grows into the full extent of the garment; too tight a fit can restrict growth and active movement, important for good growth, can be diminished;
  - some are made of synthetic fibres which make the baby damp due to the lack of absorption of moisture; the material should contain at least a high proportion of natural fibres; a good compromise is some all-in-one garments and some dresses/two-piece garments at other times;
- three or four similar garments for night-time wear (it is important that clothes for night and day are different; as the baby gets older this will set the routine for night-time sleep);
- six cardigans: natural fibres or a mix are again best; avoid lacy patterns as baby's fingers can easily become caught in the holes;
- two hats or bonnets, woolly for a winter baby and sun-hats for summer babies;
- two pairs of mitts for a winter baby;
- three pairs of socks or bootees (shoes are not necessary until walking is a fact of life).

Natural fibres can be difficult to find and also need careful washing and ironing, but they do allow the skin to 'breathe' and reduce the possibility of the baby becoming damp from contained moisture. Mixture clothing, with a small proportion of wool or cotton, is the best compromise.

Student exercise

Look around various baby clothes shops and list the cost of various necessary items, Calculate how much a new parent with a first baby will need to spend on the basic essential clothing.

Nappies

Disposable or terry towelling? Most mothers opt for disposable nappies these days. Much washing and drying is saved, but the weekly shopping bill will be higher due to the need for constant replacement of these items of baby care. (However, it has been calculated that if you take into account the original cost of the terry nappies and the ongoing cost of washing powder and electricity, this extra weekly expense is not so much as may seem at first sight.)

There are two types of disposable nappies available: the all-in-one variety and ones that fit inside special plastic pants.

Advantages and disadvantages of disposable and terry nappies are listed in Table 3.1.

Table 3.1 Advantages and disadvantages of disposable and terry nappies

Disposables	Terry towelling
Advantages	Advantages
Easy to put on	Standard sized square
Complete	
Varying types and sizes available	Disadvantages
Better for travelling	Initial high cost
Keeps baby's skin drier	Can be fiddly
Time saving	Nappy/liners plastic pants also necessary
	Need to be rinsed/sterilized
Disadvantages	Have to be taken home to wash
Continuing cost (around £7 per week)	Takes time to wash/dry.
Can be difficulties with disposal	More frequent changing needed

Napping-changing

This need not be as much of a chore as may seem at first sight – not exactly a wholly pleasant task, but one in which the baby can enjoy the company of his mother or carer. Many babies find this an enjoyable time when they can kick free of the encumbrance of a nappy.

Be sure that everything is to hand before you start to change a baby's nappy – changing mat, clean nappy, baby wipes or cotton wool, baby cream, container for dirty nappy. It can be dangerous to leave an active baby alone, even for a moment, whilst you dash to find some item you have forgotten.

1. Remove the dirty nappy and place in container to deal with later.
2. Use baby wipes, cotton wool and water or baby lotion to clean nappy area. Clean carefully in the folds of the groin and round the scrotum in boys. Remember to wipe from front to back in girls so that infection from the bowel is not carried forward into the vagina.
3. Dry and apply a layer of protective cream.
4. Place the clean nappy under the baby's bottom, lifting him up by his feet to do so. Fasten by sticky tabs if using a disposable nappy, or fold and secure terry towelling nappies with a safety pin. Place the safety pin in securely and lying horizontally, so that if it comes undone it will not stick into the baby.
5. Add plastic pants if necessary.
6. Dispose of dirty nappies in container for final disposal later.

There are two main ways of folding a terry towelling nappy:

- **Triangular method.** Fold in two to make a triangle and place under the baby with the point downwards. Pull up a single thickness from the point between the baby's legs, then fold in the two sides and finally bring the lower thickness from the point between the baby's legs and secure with one pin.
- **Kite method.** Lay out the nappy in a diamond shape. Fold in the two sides and the top to make a long triangle. Then fold the bottom corner

up to around one-third of the way up. Bring lower fold up between the baby's legs. Fold in the two sides and secure with two pins.

Student exercise

Do a survey of the different types of disposable nappies available. Draw up a table showing the merits of each type.

Other equipment necessary for a new baby

Cots

A **carry-cot** is a useful piece of equipment to buy for a baby to spend most of his time in for the first few months of life. If you have a set of wheels onto which the carry-cot can be placed this will double as a pram for some time.

A **Moses basket** can be used for the first few months and has the benefits of snugness and being easy to carry.

A **cot** will become a necessity by the time the baby is around six months of age. (If a cot has been bought early this can prove useful for putting the carry-cot in at night.) It is important to choose a cot that is covered by the BSI (British Standards Institution) and carries the familiar 'kite' mark. Aspects that are covered by the kite mark include:

- The side of the cot must be 50 cm (20 in.) high, measured when the mattress is *in situ*. This will ensure that the child when standing will not be able to topple out accidentally.
- The drop-side fastener must be secure and child-proof.
- The bars of the cot must be no more than 7.6 cm (3 in.) apart. This is to prevent a child getting his head stuck between them.
- The paint must be lead-free.

Special **travel cots** which fold into a small parcel with a carrying handle are available and are of use on holiday. The travel cot can also double as a play-pen for the older baby.

Mattresses must also conform to BSI standards. They should be firm and of a recommended texture. A stretch sheet (towelling ones are good) should be placed over the mattress. Obviously the size must be suitable to fit a carry-cot or cot.

A **pillow** is not necessary or advisable for babies under one year for sleeping, but can be used during the day when the baby can be propped up when taken out, for example.

Duvets and **baby-nests** are also not recommended for young babies: they can become overheated under these coverings.

Cot blankets are best made of a wool/synthetic mix fibre. The natural fibre will allow air in so that the moisture from the baby's body does not become trapped. The synthetic element makes for ease of laundering. Cellular blankets are lightweight as well as being warm with the air being trapped between the small holes.

Safety features of cots
- Height of cot side
- Secure fastener
- Width of bars
- Lead-free paint

Prams

Prams and **buggies** are a major expensive item. With care, a type can be chosen that fulfils more than one purpose, for example as a lift-off carry-cot and later as a push-chair. Prams are also covered by British Standards:

- The height of the side of the pram should be at least 20 cm (8 in.) above the level of the top of the mattress.
- The wheels should be strong and have at least two brakes.
- The body of the pram should be made of weather-proof, non-inflammable and chemically inert material.
- There should be a hood which protects the baby fully when up.
- There should be facilities for fitting safety straps.

Safety features of prams
- Height of pram side
- Strong wheels
- At least two brakes
- Protective hood
- Safety straps

Car seat

It is vital that the baby's first journey – home from hospital – should be in a suitable car seat. Seats facing backwards, and fixed to the front seat are best for young babies. When mothers are driving they can easily keep an eye on their baby, and if an accident does occur less damage to the baby's head is done by this type of seating. Some maternity hospitals or outside firms hire such seats, as they are an expensive item to buy and are only used for a few months. After this time other types of car seats become necessary.

Student exercise

Find out from your local maternity hospital if they have any facilities available for hiring out car seats and record the price and conditions. If they have, get further details, if not obtain these details from any agencies locally who provide this service.

Play-pens

These are not vital pieces of equipment, but can be very useful when the baby is starting to move around. They should not be used for long periods of time, or just to leave an unattended baby. But to keep an active 'crawler' safe for short periods of time, while the mother is cooking or doing various household tasks, they are invaluable. A supply of toys, changed at regular intervals, will keep the occupant happy.

High chair

A high chair will be a necessary piece of equipment for use when the baby is around nine months of age. There are a number of types available with adjustable legs for use in various situations. High chairs have a large tray with rounded edges on which food and play materials can be safely placed.

Student exercise

Visit a baby equipment shop:
- List the items a new mother would need.
- List the variations and prices of a particular type of equipment, e.g. play-pens.

Feeding

Previous to birth the baby obtained all her nourishment via the placenta from her mother's blood stream. At birth this supply suddenly ceases, and the baby will need to obtain nourishment from regular feeds and process these through her own gastrointestinal tract.

Milk is the staple food for the first three to four months of life. This can be milk from the breast or a proprietary baby milk given from a bottle. Breast milk is the ideal food for a human baby, and all mothers should be encouraged to feed their babies for as long as possible, at least for the first few weeks of life.

Reasons why 'breast is best'

The constituents of breast milk are exactly right for each individual baby.

- The amount of **protein** is less in human milk than in cows' milk (which is the main source of all artificial milks): 1.5% in human milk and 3.5% in cows' milk. In human milk one of the types of protein present – **caseinogen** – is softer and so more easily digested than that in cows' milk.
- The **fat** content of cows' milk is marginally higher than in human milk and the fat in breast milk is also more easily digested by the baby.
- **Carbohydrate**, in the form of lactose, is higher in human milk. It is also thought that this lactose helps with the absorption of calcium, an mineral important for the proper formation of bones and teeth.
- **Vitamins** A, C and E are present in greater quantity in human milk.
- **Mineral** content also differs between the two milks. There is more calcium in cows' milk, but it is less readily absorbed than that in human milk.
- **Iron**, a mineral necessary for the proper formation of red blood cells, is low in both types of milk, and babies of over six months of age will need solid foods containing iron if they are not to become anaemic.
- **Water** is present in exactly the right amount to quench a baby's thirst. Breast-fed babies do not need extra drinks of water.
- **Colostrum** is the yellowish fluid secreted by the breasts late on in pregnancy, and in larger amounts for the few days following the birth of the baby. High in protein and antibodies this colostrum is of great benefit. Within two or three days the mature milk comes in and is mixed with diminishing amounts of colostrum for around ten days. After this time the milk becomes thinner, more watery-looking and often of a

bluish colour. (Mothers can become concerned with this lack of 'creamy' appearance. They can be reassured that their milk is entirely satisfactory.)

Other advantages of breast feeding
* There is virtually no chance that the milk can become contaminated. Breast-fed babies rarely suffer from gastroenteritis.
* There is no need to heat the milk. It comes at exactly the right temperature.
* Breast milk contains antibodies which help protect the baby against infection during the early days of life before immune systems are mature enough to cope for themselves.
* Breast feeding is the ideal situation to promote good bonding between mother and baby. (This does not mean to say that bottle-fed babies are denied this closeness: feeding can be a time of intimacy, however it is done.)
* Breast feeding is thought to be of value in the development of the baby's jaws and teeth. The vigorous sucking necessary to promote a good flow of breast milk helps bone and muscle development. (The rate of flow from a bottle tends to be constant with little effort on the baby's part.)
* Breast feeding is cheaper than bottle feeding.
* Breast feeding helps the uterus to return more quickly to is prepregnancy size and state.

Anatomy of the breast
The breast is made up of milk-secreting cells (or alveoli) enclosed in variable amounts of fatty tissue. (The size of the breasts is largely determined by the amount of fatty tissue present. The size of the breasts does not affect the ability to breast feed: small-breasted women are just as likely to be able to breast feed successfully as their more well-endowed sisters.)

The alveoli are arranged segmentally, around 15–20 in each breast. The milk produced by these alveoli passes into a main duct for each segment, which in turn opens onto the surface of the nipple. Immediately behind the nipple these ducts are enlarged. Milk is held in these 'reservoirs' prior to starting a feed. These reservoirs lie immediately under the areola, the darker area of skin around the nipple. When the baby sucks pressure is exerted on these reservoirs and the milk starts to flow out of the nipple. As well as this stimulation to milk production, the flow of milk is under hormonal control from the pituitary gland. These hormones initiate the 'let-down reflex' which acts on the breast to continue the flow of milk.

The small glands, known as 'Montgomery's tubercles', seen on the areola secrete a minimal amount of fluid which keeps the nipple soft and pliable.

There are a number of reasons why breast feeding is not always possible:
* Some women find the whole thought and experience of breast feeding embarrassing and distasteful. Their decision not to breast feed should be

respected and help given to settle the baby on formula milk from a bottle.

- Nipples may not be suitable for breast feeding. This fact should have been noted, and treated, during pregnancy. Inverted nipples can be improved by gentle massage around the base of the nipple and/or wearing a breast shield during pregnancy.
- Establishment of breast feeding can cause problems for the inexperienced mother who has not benefited from skilled help after the birth of her baby. (The early discharge from hospital after a birth can exacerbate these problems. Midwives have great skill in helping to establish satisfactory breast feeding. A visiting community midwife cannot have quite the same effect as a midwife who is available for most, if not all, the early days of feeding.)
- On return home, perhaps to other demanding small children and certainly the rigours of running a house, breast milk supply can easily fail unless sufficient help for everyday chores is available.
- A disabled baby can have difficulties with breast feeding. For example, abnormalities around the mouth can pose problems with sucking. Other physical problems which entail operative procedures can also upset the routine of introducing breast feeding. Expressed breast milk, to be given when practicable, is a good compromise under certain circumstances.
- Long-term serious illness in the mother can also make breast feeding impossible.
- A drowsy baby can cause a poor supply of milk. Vigorous sucking is necessary to establish, and continue, a good supply of milk.
- Excess production of milk, particularly if also associated with a sleepy baby, can cause engorgement of the breasts. Manual expression of the milk, or with the help of a breast pump, can help with this painful condition.
- Cracked nipples, caused by prolonged sucking in a less than satisfactory position, can cause failure of breast feeding. To avoid this painful condition, the nipple needs to be well back in the baby's mouth so that the sucking, pressing movements of the baby's jaw massages the areola and not the nipple itself.

Successful breast feeding

- Adequate information on, and preparation for, breast feeding during pregnancy. This will include treatment for flat or inverted nipples.
- Sympathetic, knowledgeable help in the early days in getting the baby 'latched on' to the breast because babies can take a day or two to learn the technique:
  - early introduction to the breast – within a few minutes of birth;
  - holding the baby close in a comfortable relaxed way;
  - touching her cheek with the nipple. Her mouth will open and she will turn to the breast ready to feed;

- making sure that the nipple is fully inside the baby's mouth so that the fore-milk in the reservoirs is squeezed into the mouth by the action of her jaws.
- Mothers should be relaxed and comfortable and with, if possible, no interruptions during a feed.
- Demand feeding, i.e. feeding whenever the baby wishes, will help to establish breast feeding. Within a week or two feeding will become less frequent, and feed times will gradually settle down into a roughly 4-hourly pattern.
- A breast feed ideally takes around 20 minutes – 10 minutes on each breast. It is important that both breasts are completely emptied so that engorgement does not occur.

Insufficient milk

This is a common source of worry to breast-feeding mothers. The baby is getting sufficient milk if:
- he is sleeping peacefully between feeds;
- he is gaining weight steadily;
- he is passing soft yellow stools (maybe at every feed or maybe only once or twice a week – both these variations are quite normal).

To increase a failing supply of milk:
- feed the baby more often – this will stimulate milk production as well as satisfying his needs;
- advise mothers to drink an adequate amount and to eat small nourishing meals at regular intervals;
- make sure breast-feeding mothers are getting adequate rest.

Giving 'complementary' bottles of formula milk is not the answer to a diminishing breast milk supply. In fact if this has to be done because of a screaming hungry baby, breast feeding is probably on the way out! (A bottle of formula milk left to be given if the mother has to go out is, of course, quite a different matter, and will pose no problems to the continuation of breast feeding.) Babies become used to the easier flow of milk from a bottle and be unwilling to persevere at the breast. So a vicious circle is set up with less sucking causing less milk and so on.

However, for a wide variety of reasons, breast feeding is not possible for all mothers. There should be no feelings of guilt if breast feeding has failed, or never successfully started. A bottle feed, lovingly given, will ensure that good bonding occurs.

Formula milk

All formula milk for bottle feeding is based on cows' milk (with the unusual exception of soy milk for babies who have been found to be allergic to cows' milk). The composition of the cows' milk is altered in the commercial baby milks so that it resembles as closely as possible the composition of human milk. (Doorstep, or supermarket, milk is not suitable for young babies, but can be used in an emergency if it is boiled and diluted with half as much again of boiled water.)

Equipment necessary for bottle feeding:
- six wide-necked bottles with teats;
- sterilizing equipment for bottles, based on either chemical or steam methods of sterilization; commercially available containers are large to accommodate six bottles and other equipment at one time;
- measuring jug, with a lid, for making up feeds;
- plastic knife.

Every piece of equipment that comes into contact with the milk feed must be sterilized. Feeds can be made up in the jug or straight into the bottles. The former method is probably easier and quicker, and will be described. A similar pattern needs to be followed if feeds are made up straight into the bottle.

Making up feeds

It is easiest to make up a 24-hour supply of feeds and keep them in the refrigerator until needed.

The **amount** to make will, of course, depend on the baby's appetite, but as a rough guide, a baby will need 150 ml/kg ($2\frac{1}{2}$ fl oz/lb) body weight every 24 hours. So a 4 kg baby will need 600 ml of milk every 24 hours (or a 10 lb baby will need 25 fl oz every 24 hours). It is always wise to make up a little extra in each bottle. Baby's appetites vary throughout the day as much as do adults.

Student exercise

Check on the variety of formula milks available for feeding babies and draw up a table to show the similarities and differences between the different milks available.

1. First of all, wash the hands thoroughly, and boil sufficient water in the kettle.
2. Take the measuring jug and stirrer out of the sterilizer. Shake to remove excess fluid if the chemical method of sterilization is used. Do NOT rinse any of the equipment as this will desterilize it.
3. Pour out a measured amount of water, which has been allowed to cool slightly.
4. Add the number of scoops of milk powder necessary for the amount of feed you need to make. Be sure to measure off absolutely accurately a flat scoop of powder (level the spoon off with the back of a knife).
5. Stir until all the powder is fully dissolved.
6. Remove the feeding bottles from the sterilizer; shake off any excess sterilizing fluid and do not rinse the bottles. Fill to the appropriate level for each feed. Fit the sterilized teats upside down into the neck of the bottle and secure with the rings and caps provided.
7. Put all bottles in the fridge until needed.

Giving a bottle feed

1. Warm made-up feed by standing the bottle in a jug of hot water for about five minutes. Check that the temperature of the milk is correct by shaking some of the milk onto the back of your hand. It should feel pleasantly warm and not hot or cold.

2. The person giving the feed should be sure that he or she is in a comfortable position with the baby tucked comfortably into the crook of an arm, and perhaps resting on a pillow. A time of communication, sharing and enjoyment should be the aim of feed-times, not a hurried necessary chore.

3. Gently insert the teat into the baby's mouth. Make sure that the bottle is always tilted to such an angle so that a flow of milk is maintained into the teat. If the bottom of the teat is not always covered the baby will be taking in more air than milk.

4. 'Wind' the baby about halfway through the feed. Sit him up and gently pat his back. Do not be surprised if there is no result from this – some babies never seem to feel the need to 'burp'. Others seem to suffer excessively from wind. If this is the case, try feeding in a more upright position. Enlarging the hole in the teat with a red-hot needle can also help if it is thought that the baby is having to work too hard to get the milk.

5. When he has had enough, the baby will cease to suck. Never try to force him to take more than he wants, even if there is some left in the bottle. He will only get upset and probably bring it all back anyway! Any milk left must be thrown away.

6. Finally tuck the contented baby down to sleep, after changing the nappy if this is necessary. Feeding does sometimes promote a bowel movement.

7. Rinse the used bottle, teats, jug and stirrer carefully under running water. Take especial care with the inside of the teat – it is all too easy to leave flecks of milk inside. Place all used equipment conveniently on a tray ready for the next daily session of sterilization.

Early feeding problems

Colic

This is not a condition from which all babies suffer, but when they do it can be very distressing for all the family. Babies as young as two weeks can suffer from colic. They will draw up their legs and scream with what seems to be acute tummy pain. These symptoms can last up to an hour or more, and nothing seems to relieve the spasms of pain. Many babies seem to find the evening from around 6 p.m. onwards a particularly difficult time from this point of view.

There are a number of different suggestions as to the basic **cause** of colic in young babies. It is possible that there is a lack of regular smooth movements of the intestine as it goes about its work of digestion. The movements of the gut appear to be spasmodic rather than regular, as is evidenced by the irregular attacks of pain. It is also thought possible that air is trapped in parts of the intestine due to the uncoordinated activity. It is this stretching of the gut that causes the pain. Against this latter theory is the fact that colicky babies do not appear to need winding any more than do babies without this problem.

A further theory is that the nervous control of the intestine is too immature to regulate intestinal movements. This would fit in with the fact that the colic in all but a small minority of babies ceases around the age of three to four months. (This is the reason why the condition is often termed 'three-month colic'.)

A few babies with colic are found to have a definable **intolerance to cows' milk**. This intolerance may be only a temporary problem, cows' milk being introduced into the diet again when the baby is older with no ill effects. If the colic has not disappeared by six months of age, the health visitor may advise trying the baby on some milk other than cows' milk.

Some **relief** can be obtained from the colic by giving 'gripe water', obtainable from chemists or as medicine combining a mild antacid, e.g. 'Dentinox Colic Drops'. Other actions, such as walking with the baby, rocking her, taking her out in the pram or car can distract her attention from the pain temporarily at least, and give parents some respite from a crying baby. Sharing the problem with a partner or close friend can help mothers cope with this particularly trying phase. An organization 'Cry-sis' (see Appendix) has been set up by parents who have suffered from this problem. They are available to give advice and to lend a sympathetic ear to parents having a baby with three-month colic.

Other problems of feeding include:
- difficulties in establishing breast feeding (see previous section);
- waking/crying at frequent intervals:
  - check for colic;
  - try giving smaller feeds more frequently;
  - try goat milk or soy milk if problems persist; there is little to gain in changing the type of cows' milk formula.

Weaning

Weaning is the process of getting a baby to take foods other than milk. Milk will still be a staple part of the diet for some months, but will no longer be the only source of nutrition.

It is not necessary to start weaning a baby until three months of age. Milk alone is quite sufficient until this age. But by six months all babies must be receiving food other than milk; so around four months of age is thus about the right time to start the weaning process. Most babies by this time will be needing such large quantities of milk to satisfy their appetites that it will be obvious that something else is required. Quite apart from the quantity, milk is lacking in many of the nutrients necessary for proper growth from this age on. As just one example, the iron stores in a baby's liver (laid down from the mother's intake of iron during the latter months of pregnancy) are running low at this time. As milk, of any kind, is low in iron content, this mineral, which is necessary for the proper formation of blood, must be obtained from foods other than milk.

Weaning foods

Solid food intake is started with either one of the commercially available cereal baby products (based on grain or rice) or puréed fruit or vegetables. Cereal is made up by the addition of some of the formula milk mixture until it is a rather sloppy consistency. It should be given off a spoon – a teaspoonful is quite sufficient initially – and not added to the feeding bottle. One of the aims of mixed feeding is to get the baby used to the different textures and tastes of everyday food, and also the differing techniques that are needed to be learned. Solid food has to be passed into the back of the mouth by the tongue before being swallowed – quite a different technique from just swallowing fluid milk.

Solids once a day is sufficient for the first week or two of mixed feeding. After this time another taste – perhaps a little puréed apple or mashed banana – can be added at a further feed. It is wise to allow time between offering different tastes. This will allow the new feeder to get used to one specific taste as well as ensuring that the particular food is being digested adequately.

The addition of too much solid food all at once can cause dehydration. So take it slowly and remember to offer drinks between feeds – cooled, boiled water or diluted fruit juice. Some babies will refuse all extra drinks, but they should still be offered at regular intervals, but not forced. Milk will still form a major part in the baby's diet for some months to come, and this, for the babies that refuse water or juice, is obviously sufficient fluid intake for their needs.

By around eight months of age, some part of the day's supply of milk can be offered from a trainer beaker. Some babies are particularly resistant to giving up any sucking from breast or bottle and will not accept milk from a beaker at any price; much patience and perseverance is needed to persuade them. By one year of age, however, most babies should be taking the major part of their fluid intake from a cup or beaker. The last breast or bottle feed at night is the last to be given up. It is important that this 'comfort' feed is not stopped until the baby indicates that it is no longer necessary.

Early weaning
- Start around 3–4 months
- Once a day initially
- Give from spoon
- Offer extra drinks

Student exercise

Prepare a leaflet, for a new mother, on how to wean her baby onto solid feeds in terms of what, when and how much; plus advice and examples to help her with the weaning process.

The weaning process continues with the gradual addition of a wider variety of foods until the child is eating the same meals as the rest of the family.

Exceptions to this, until several more years, are highly spiced foods, nuts and fruit with seeds or pips. All foods given must at first be puréed, and then later finely minced. Grated cheese, flaked steamed fish, mashed potato with finely grated vegetables, with yoghurt or mashed banana for a second course, are just some of the foods that can be slowly added to the diet. Later still, lumpy foods can be introduced. A deep dish containing the food, together with a spoon, can also be provided at this time, but be prepared for messy mealtimes. Be ready with another spoon to pop food into the baby's mouth as he misses his mouth yet again! Finger foods can also be given at this stage, such as rusks, fingers of toast or cheese, pieces of apple or other pip-free fruit.

By nine months of age, babies will be needing a high chair in which to sit at mealtimes. Family meals should, if at all possible, be part of the day's activities – a time when parents, older children and the newest member can all be together to get to know each other and to exchange news. This provides a useful learning experience for the new baby as he learns how to manipulate implements by watching other family members.

This weaning process can cause problems for busy mothers who have to go out to work, and for them the commercially prepared jars of baby food are a boon. (They are also of value when travelling.) There are available foods for all stages, from the completely puréed ones to foods of all kinds as 'junior' foods. It is advisable, however, to be sure that the baby gets some opportunities to eat ordinary foods. He can become very used to the flavours and textures of commercially prepared foods and be unwilling to eat family meals.

Later weaning
- Increase variety of solid feed
- Increase amount of solids
- Introduce beaker/cup
- Encourage self feeding
- 'Finger' foods

Student exercise

Draw up a couple of day's menus for:
- a child of 6 months;
- a child of 1 year.

Check with the following section (on older children's diets) that the menus are working towards a satisfactory fully mixed diet.

Rest and sleep

All babies spend a good part of their days asleep. It is a common misapprehension, however, that newborn babies sleep all the time apart from feed times. It is thought that a newborn baby is awake for around six hours out of the 24. This period of wakefulness is spread out during the day and night so that half an hour to an hour is spent awake before the baby dozes off again.

Exactly why sleep – for any of us – is necessary is largely unknown. It is considered that certain chemicals in the brain need time to rebuild before further activities are undertaken the following day. Just why some people can manage with a minimum of sleep, whilst others need a full eight hours every night, is not known.

Sleep is divided into four stages of depth – stage 1 being the lightest sleep and stage 4 the deepest. A further division is made into 'rapid eye movement' (REM) sleep and quiet sleep or non-REM sleep. REM sleep occurs in the lighter stages of sleep and is the time when dreaming occurs. As the name suggests the eyes can be seen to be moving rapidly under the eyelids during this time.

Babies at birth are unaware of the difference between night and day. They sleep on and off erratically throughout the 24 hours, and continuous sleep rarely lasts longer than three hours. By six months of age, six to eight hours can often be managed in one go. Learning to sleep through the night is one of the first lessons that new mothers will want to teach their babies! Initially, of course, feeding is necessary four hourly or thereabouts throughout both day and night. But by the time the baby is four to six months of age, a reasonable night's sleep should be possible.

To encourage night-time sleep:
- By three to four months of age, develop a definite bed-time routine: bath, change into night clothes, a last, quiet bottle or breast feed, followed by a lullaby or quiet music before putting down gently into the cot.
- Do not be tempted back into the room by quiet crying or babbling. Maybe this is just the night-time pattern of getting off to sleep, just as some adults read for a while.
- Plenty of stimulation during the day is needed: talking and playing with some time spent, if possible, in the fresh air.
- Be sure that the room is not too hot or too cold.
- Some babies need to be tucked in securely before they go to sleep, but remember to avoid any possibility that the bedcovers will fall over the baby's face later on in the night.
- Be sure to lie babies up to the age of one year on their backs or their sides (preferably on their backs). This position has markedly reduced the number of cot deaths.
- As the baby gets older a favourite toy or some other 'comforter' (a piece of blanket, for example) can help set the pattern for sleep.
- Also later on, a favourite, non-exciting, picture or story book to look at together is useful. This sets the trend for the later bedtime story.

To encourage night-time sleep:
- Bed-time routine
- Leave to babble
- Stimulation during day
- Warm room
- Securely tucked in
- Lie on back or side
- Have a 'comforter'

Own room/parent's room?

Most parents feel they need to have their very young baby in the same room as themselves, so that any crying or movement can be easily heard and attended to. It is also easier for feeding in the middle of the night.

By the time the baby is sleeping for relatively long periods of time at night, it is probably sensible to move him to another room. Putting on the light or parents preparing for bed can disturb a peacefully sleeping baby. Baby alarms are invaluable at this stage as the slightest movement can be picked up and heard. Around four to six months is a good time for this change and can coincide with the change from a Moses basket or crib to a cot.

Cot or bed?

The time to move a child from a cot to a bed is variable. It is often the child himself who decides when is the right time – 18 months to two years being the usual age range. There can be some difficulties at the start of the move to the 'big' bed. It is tempting indeed to hop in and out of bed every other minute and maybe come downstairs! A certain amount of firmness is necessary should this be happening too frequently. Stick to the usual bed-time routine and take the child quietly but firmly back to bed and tuck him in. If he sees that there are no long-term gains in getting out of bed he will soon settle.

Cleanliness

At first sight cleanliness may not seem to be in the first line as a survival necessity, and maybe it is not when compared with food, warmth and rest. Nevertheless the baby/child who is not kept clean at best will not feel at all comfortable and at worst can be prey to a host of infections which lack of cleanliness encourages. Nappy-changing (see earlier in this section), bathing and clean clothes are all part of the remit of keeping clean.

In earlier days the first event in a newborn baby's life was a bath – literally within hours of birth. Today it is thought not to be necessary to bath a baby until two or three days after the birth. The 'vernix', the greasy substance on the skin of newborn babies, protects the skin from the drying effects of the air. Remember the baby, before birth, was surrounded by fluid. Also babies readily become chilled, unless great care is taken to avoid this, on exposure to the air. It can also be quite a frightening experience to be fully immersed in water when one has only just started to breathe through previously unused lungs! Instead of complete bathing for the first few days, 'topping and tailing' can ensure that the vital parts of the baby's body are cleaned.

'Topping and tailing'

1. Fill a bowl or baby bath with warm water. Check with the back of your hand, or preferably your elbow, that the water is not too hot.
2. Have a supply of cotton wool and a soft towel nearby, together with baby cream or Vaseline.
3. Start by cleaning the baby's eyes. Dampen a small piece of cotton wool, and starting from the corner of the eye nearest the nose, wipe outwards.
4. Repeat this process with the other eye, being sure to use a separate piece of cotton wool. (This is to prevent the spread of any possible infection from one eye to the other.)
5. Again with a fresh piece of cotton wool, wipe gently over the face, remembering not to miss under the baby's chin.
6. Dry carefully with a soft towel or dry piece of cotton wool.

7. The armpit must also be washed on a regular basis. Folds of skin in this area lead to trapped moisture which, if not cleaned can become red and sore. Again, be sure to dry thoroughly.

8. The cord area – before this remnant of prenatal life drops off – also needs to be kept scrupulously clean. A little added surgical spirit is useful if this area become moist.

9. The baby's bottom needs to be kept as clean and dry as possible by frequent nappy changes and cleaning routines. Also do not forget to clean in the folds of the groins where moisture can lurk and give rise to soreness. In the nappy area a protective cream needs to be applied to prevent nappy rash.

This 'topping and tailing' procedure will need to be done once a day together with, of course, regular cleaning and changing of the nappy area.

Nappy rash

Although theoretically avoidable, rare indeed is the baby who has never had nappy rash. There are several different types of nappy rash.

Ammoniacal dermatitis. This is the commonest type of nappy rash. It is caused by bacterial enzymes in the faeces acting on the urea in the urine. Frequent changing of nappies, with scrupulous cleansing, will reduce this to a minimum. The addition of a barrier cream at each nappy change will also help. Kicking without a nappy in a warm room will also allow air to help heal the rash. (If terry towelling nappies are used, be sure that they are well-rinsed at each wash. Residual detergent can add to the problem.)

Candida infection or '**thrush**'. This rash is a bright red with scaly edges, and should be considered if a rash does not clear within a few days. Nystatin cream will clear a rash of this type. (It is important, under these conditions, to be sure that the baby does not also have thrush in her mouth.)

Seborrhoeic dermatitis is often seen in conjunction with the condition elsewhere on the baby's body, such as behind the ears, on the forehead or as 'cradle cap'. A mild hydrocortisone cream will clear this type of rash.

Types of nappy rash
- Ammoniacal dermatitis
- 'Thrush'
- Seborrhoeic dermatitis

Bathing

As the baby gets older a daily bath will be much enjoyed, and certainly by the time he is moving around and feeding himself, a daily bath is a vital necessity! For young babies, up to around two months of age, alternate days of bathing and topping and tailing are sufficient.

The secret of happy bath-times is a quiet, unhurried routine in a warm room with all the necessary equipment readily to hand.

Equipment

- Baby bath: a bath with a stand means that bathing can be done in any room in the house, wherever it is warmest during the cold winter months, otherwise the baby bath can placed inside the large bath; make sure that the bathroom is warm.
- Soft towels and cotton wool.

- Soap or baby bath liquid.
- Clean nappy and clothes.
- Barrier cream, and baby talc if used.

Method
1. Undress the baby except for her nappy.
2. Wrap her warmly in a towel and clean her face as for 'topping and tailing'.
3. Holding her over the bath and supporting her head with one hand, gently wash and rinse her hair. Pat her hair gently dry.
4. Remove the nappy and lying her on your lap or a towel gently soap all over (special care needs to be taken at this stage – soaped babies are very slippery!).
5. Gently lower her into the warm bath water, holding her firmly with one arm around her neck to hold the opposite arm.
6. With the other hand gently swish water over the baby's body to remove all the soap. This is the stage that most babies enjoy when they become used to the bathing routine.
7. Take her out of the bath and gently dry all over, taking care to dry under arms and in the groins. If talc is used, be sure the baby's body is quite dry before the talc is sprinkled. Damp talc can clog into painful lumps.
8. Add barrier cream to the nappy area.
9. Put on nappy and clean clothes.

Young babies can find bath-time tiring and, after a feed, will probably fall peacefully asleep.

Washing clothes

Clean clothing is important and washing for a baby can seem an endless chore, but with today's disposable nappies and clothes that can be happily washed in a washing machine, time spent on this aspect of baby care can be reduced to a minimum.

Healthy development

In addition to all the necessary ingredients for survival, babies need stimulus to enable them to practise all their developing skills. The chapters on development and learning all concentrate on various aspects of a stimulating life style for babies and children. Suffice it to say here that parents and full-time care-givers should be responsive to children's needs at all times within the context of the wider family. It is especially important in the early weeks and months of a baby's life to be aware of needs which, as yet, cannot be voiced.

A further ingredient which makes for healthy development is the obvious enjoyment in her baby seen by a happy and contented mother.

Protection against injury and illness

Chapter 13 gives overall information on accidents, their possible causes, both environmental and human, but, in daily life with a baby or young child, a few basic safety factors must be remembered and practised. Parents need to be aware of potential dangers around the home (a large proportion of accidents occur in the home), dangers from various bought goods and equipment and their packaging as well as dangers in the garden and out in the wider world.

Dangers in the home

Young babies

- Remember babies of four to six months will be learning to roll from their backs onto their fronts and can easily roll off a sofa, bed or other high surface when attention is momentarily diverted.
- It is dangerous – and unkind – to leave a baby alone with a propped-up bottle. She could easily choke on this, as well as missing out on much good companionship.
- Always take care to ensure that the bath water is never too hot. Check very carefully before putting water anywhere near a baby or toddler.
- Clothing needs to be loose and warm for young babies. Tight ribbons around the neck are potentially dangerous. A ribbon caught on any projection could pull tight around the baby's neck. Lacy shawls and blankets with holes in which tiny fingers can become trapped can result in the actual loss of a finger, the blood supply being cut off by the tight material.
- Parents should never drink a hot cup of tea or coffee with a baby in their arms. One unexpected kick and the scalding liquid is all over the baby.
- Night-wear should be flame resistant. Many pyjamas and night-gowns are covered by legislation, but some are not.

Toddlers

General safety aspects include the following points:

- Plastic bags must be kept well away from toddlers, who can find these common articles of packaging a fascinating toy. The flimsy plastic found covering many articles, if put over a toddler's head, can easily suffocate him.
- Never give toddlers small coins or buttons to play with. At this age they are still exploring objects with their mouths, and could easily choke on small objects. The same dangers apply also to small sweets. Peanuts, too, must never be given to any child under the age of five years – these tempting foods are just the right size to be inhaled. (Remember to clear away all such leftovers from a party the night before. A half-empty dish of salted peanuts can be tempting the following morning for the early-rising toddler. The extra salt on these type of peanuts will also do him no good.)
- Finger foods are admirable to give toddlers learning to chew, but must always be eaten under supervision. Again choking can occur if a large piece is broken off and swallowed.

- Food should always be eaten sitting down quietly. The dangerous habit of eating while walking around (so common today) can again cause toddlers to choke if they should stumble, a common event when they are still unstable on their feet.
- Cords pulling curtains shut or blinds down are a further source of potential danger if they become looped round fingers or even necks.
- Fires – open, gas or electric – must always have a sturdy guard.
- Windows must be securely locked, and furniture not placed too near the window as chairs will provide easy access to windows by an active climbing toddler.
- Glass doors provide a further source of danger to toddlers. A glass door at the bottom of a flight of stairs is in a particularly dangerous position. Toddlers, unsteady in their negotiation of stairs, can fall and bounce straight through the glass unless it is made of safety glass and specially strengthened. Patio doors, too, are hazardous. Coloured stars or strips of paper at relevant heights should be stuck on to make children – and adults – aware that the doors are there.
- Electric sockets and plugs are all items of interest to the exploring toddler. Socket covers can be life-savers by stopping small fingers from inquiring into the workings of the socket.
- Trailing wires from lamps are also a hazard. It should also go without saying that all electrical wiring in the house should be made safe.

The **kitchen** is a particularly dangerous place for toddlers (A play-pen for use when necessary cooking needs to be done is a good idea.)

- Kettles with long, hanging cords should either be avoided altogether (kettles with concertina cords are available) or pushed well out of reach.
- Hanging tablecloths under hot dishes and liquid-filled mugs should be avoided.
- Use cooker guards, or turn saucepan handles away from the edge so that youngsters are not tempted to pull them down to investigate their contents.
- A hot iron is a source of danger. Never leave a child alone – even for a moment – with a hot iron on the board. Remember, too, to store it in a safe place to cool: heat can stay in an iron for some time.
- Matches should be kept well out of reach.
- Sharp knives and scissors must be kept in a high drawer or cupboard. Remember toddlers can quickly learn to open drawers.
- Kitchen cupboards contain dangerous cleaning materials – bleach, soap powder, silver-cleaning equipment to mention just a few. These, ideally, should be stored in a locked cupboard or high on the wall.

Toys must also be careful monitored for safety. For example, the eyes on cuddly toys must be firmly fixed. Other mechanical toys for older children must have no sharp edges or lead-containing paint. Toys should be bought with the 'lion mark' of safety, and any cheap toys bought from a market stall should be very carefully checked.

Kitchen hazards
- Kettle leads
- Hanging tablecloths
- Saucepan handles
- Hot irons
- Matches
- Sharp knives
- Poisonous chemicals

Student exercise

Catalogue all the toys in a nursery or similar situation, detailing: type, use by age group, price, safety marks, condition.

The **garden**, too, can be a dangerous place:
- Red, glossy **berries** can seem tempting to a toddler. Many of these are highly poisonous. Also the **seed pods** of many common garden trees and flowers are poisonous, e.g. laburnum and lupin.
- Garden **ponds** are a hazard to toddlers. They should be netted – or done away with altogether – until children are old enough to understand the potential dangers.
- Garden sheds contain all kinds of **poisonous substances** – weed-killers, fertilizers, etc. They must all be kept on a high shelf well out of the reach of toddlers.

In the wider world, **road traffic accidents** are the single major hazard to young children.
- Never allow a young child, under the age of eight years, out in the road on his own. This includes, of course, being sure that the garden gate is shut so that he will not wander out.
- Reins are a good idea for a toddler when out in the street. With shopping to carry it is all too easy to leave go of a toddler's hand momentarily. A familiar face across the road is all that the toddler needs to run across the road in front of traffic.

Playgrounds are far better equipped these days and safe swings, slides and rocking equipment are usually available for fun. Nevertheless, there is still some unsafe, old equipment in some playgrounds. The local council should be informed of these.
- Check that swings are made of rubber or plastic and not metal or wood. Teach older youngsters never to run in front of, or behind, a swing.
- Slides should ideally be built into the side of a hill, so that the child need not climb up dangerous steps to reach the top. Be sure to have an adult available to catch young children at the bottom of a slide.
- The ground in a playground should not be of tarmac or concrete, but of soft bark, sand, gravel or some other impact-absorbent material.

As children get older they should be taught to look out for dangers themselves. Ongoing instruction into all aspects of safety from the earliest age is the best protection that can be given against accidents.

Children can be taught the Green Cross Code for traffic safety (see later in this chapter). Over the age of three years they can join the 'Tufty Club' run by ROSPA. (The local authority traffic section will give details of local availability.)

Garden hazards
- Berries, cotoneaster, bryony
- Pods, e.g. laburnum, lupin
- Ponds
- Contents of garden sheds

Playgrounds
- Swings should be of rubber or plastic
- Slides built into a bank
- Ground – impact-absorbent material
- Rocking equipment safe

Student exercise

Obtain a range of pamphlets on road safety from:
- Local District Council road safety officer;
- Local 'Tufty' clubs (Tufty has recently been joined by friends from cyberspace – Willy and Watchit).

From these design a leaflet especially suited, both in design and content, for disabled people. (For purposes of the exercise specify any special printing requirements but allow for them in your design, e.g. large print.)

Protection against illness

The only real answer to accidents is prevention – and yet more prevention.

All children must be protected against infection as far as is possible. This will include the giving of the routine babyhood immunizations against a wide variety of serious infections. (Details of immunization schedules are given in Chapter 9.)

Whilst it is impossible to protect babies and young children from many of the minor, usually upper respiratory, infections, it is wise to ask friends and relatives to stay away for a day or two if they have a particularly virulent head cold. If – or when – children do succumb to a cold or other type of infection, they must be treated adequately with recourse to medical services if any worries are felt about the child's condition.

Children are utterly dependant on adults to provide clean disease-free surroundings and food. This means clean houses and clothes and good hygienic practices when preparing food as a basic minimum.

CARE OF OLDER CHILDREN (18 MONTHS TO EIGHT YEARS)

Nutrition

By the time the growing baby reaches 18 months of age he should be eating mainly family meals with the exception, as mentioned previously, of very spicy foods, fruit with seed or pips, and nuts. The diet will need to be a balanced one with samples from all the different foods available on a regular basis. This variety in the diet is of importance in the growing years as all types of food contribute to some part of the growing and changing body.

The **amount** of food, measured in calories, needed by a growing child is comparatively high. For example, his mother needs around 2000 calories daily to keep healthy. Her son of 18 months will need around 1000 to 1200 calories daily to supply his growing needs and active body.

Types of food

Carbohydrates

These are the foods such as bread, rice, cereals and pasta. They are necessary for energy, which children in this age group should have in abundance. They also provide fibre necessary to prevent constipation. (Extra bran, sometimes used for this latter purpose, should not be given to children. This form of carbohydrate can interfere with the proper absorption of various minerals, zinc and calcium in particular, necessary for health. Other foods, fruit and vegetables, which contain a high percentage of fibre, should be sufficient to ensure regular bowel movements.) Certain vitamins and minerals necessary for health are also found in carbohydrate foods.

Sugary foods also come under the heading of carbohydrates. These foods should, however, only be given in minimal amounts. There is no doubt that sugary foods and drinks which are held in the mouth for long periods of time, such as sweets, do have a bearing on the incidence of dental decay. Sweets are best given at the end of a meal, with, if possible, a tooth cleaning session afterwards.

Protein

Protein foods are necessary for body-building and repair. They are found in meat, fish, cheese and eggs. Certain oily fish are rich in vitamins, and egg-yolk and liver are rich in iron. Milk and milk-products also contain a certain, although limited, amount of protein.

These foods are known as first-class protein, but second-class protein is also to be found in pulses, beans, peas and lentils for example. Mothers who are bringing up their babies on a vegetarian diet will need to provide adequate amounts of proteins for healthy growth. (Nuts are also a very good source of second-class protein, but whole nuts are dangerous to give to children under the age of five years. Peanut butter, however, can be used, as long as the child is not allergic to peanuts. Allergy to peanuts is a very real danger for some susceptible children.)

Fats

These form the third major class of foods. They can be divided into two major groups: saturated and unsaturated fats. Research has indicated that too much saturated fat in the diet is linked to heart disease in later life. This type of fat is found in red meat and dairy products. These foods should not be omitted altogether from a child's diet – certainly not the dairy products – but sunflower oil for cooking, poultry and fish could be used to replace saturated fats.

Whole milk is necessary for children under five years of age. This is needed for energy and adequate growth. Skimmed or semiskimmed milk is not satisfactory for this age group. Yoghurt and cheese should be included in the daily diet of children. Protein is available in these foods for body-building as well as calcium and vitamin A for healthy bones and teeth.

Fresh fruit and vegetables

These are a vital part of every child's diet. As well as having a high fibre content, fruit and vegetables contain valuable vitamins, for example vitamin C in citrus fruits and green leafy vegetables for resistance to infection

Types of foods needed daily
- Carbohydrates
- Proteins
- Fats
- Fruit and vegetables, for vitamins

and tissue growth. Vitamin A is also important for healthy skin and good eyesight. This vitamin is found in highly coloured fruit and vegetables such as carrots, tomatoes and green vegetables. The vitamin content of vegetables can be largely lost by prolonged cooking or storage. So raw vegetables, carrots or celery sticks, and fresh fruit are a vital part of the daily diet. Cooked vegetables should be fresh and cooked for a minimum of time. Steaming or microwaving will retain more vitamins than boiling.

Good eating habits

These are learned in childhood. So **now** is the time to teach children a few basic rules.

- **Eat regular meals** and do not 'graze' all day long. Children in the 2–5-year-age group need three main meals a day interspersed by a snack mid-morning and mid-afternoon and a drink at bedtime. The snacks should only be small so as not to spoil the appetite for the main meals. A piece of fruit along with a drink is one of the most suitable foods to give as a snack, with perhaps a plain biscuit as a treat.
- **Eat a wide variety of foods** so that all the constituents of a balanced diet are taken daily. New tastes will probably be rejected initially, but with persistence and the giving of small amounts they will eventually be accepted. (Occasionally, of course, a child will really dislike – as we all do – a certain food, and this should not be forced, under these circumstances.)

Good eating habits
- Regular meals
- Wide variety of foods
- Not to develop a sweet tooth
- No extra salt.

- **Do not to develop a taste for sweet sugary foods**. If a 'sweet tooth' has been developed, it can be difficult to alter. So only allow sweets and sugary drinks as a treat.
- **Do not add extra salt** to food. Again, this has been thought to be a possible factor in later health problems such as high blood pressure. Also, too much salt can make young children dehydrated.

The amount eaten at any given meal should be decided by the child. Never force a child to eat any more than is wanted. Portions should be small: children can always ask for a second helping if they want, rather than face an overloaded plate. If the adults in the house eat their main meal in the evening, it is better that a portion should be saved and refrigerated until the next day. Children's nutritional needs are best served by a main meal in the middle of the day.

Drinks should be freely available, especially in hot weather. These should be fruit juice (perhaps mixed with fizzy mineral water if desired) or plain water rather than sweet sugary squashes.

A typical day's menu for a 2-year-old child could be:
- Early morning drink
  - fruit juice or milk, if wanted
- Breakfast
  - cereal with milk
  - boiled egg
  - toast
  - milk to drink

or
- porridge
- toast and jam
- milk to drink
- Mid-morning
  - milk or fruit juice
- Dinner
  - fish
  - vegetables
  - apple
  - fruit juice or water

  or
  - meat
  - vegetables
  - milk jelly
  - fruit juice or water
- Mid-afternoon
  - fruit juice with plain biscuit
- Tea
  - sandwiches (cheese; ham)
  - banana
  - milk to drink

  or
  - salad with grated cheese
  - wholemeal bread
  - milk to drink
- Bedtime drink
  - milk or hot chocolate

Student exercise

Write up a further typical day's menus for a 2-year-old for a busy mother with a part-time job and older children to feed. Be sure that your menu contains a balanced diet.

Student exercise

Record one particular child's food intake over a week and comment on:
- the balance of the diet;
- the foods disliked;
- any optional food offered and its nutritional value.

Fussy eaters
Many children go through a stage when they will not eat. Between two and four years is the most usual age for this to take place. Life is exciting and busy and the youngster finds eating rather a boring occupation which

keeps him from exploring his environment, and when he finds out that he can gain attention from this refusal to eat, it all adds to the enjoyment. Food is tipped onto the floor or totally ignored, and mouths are firmly shut against all blandishments to eat. The concerned parents become more and more worried, and irritated.

There are ways of dealing with this phase.

- Do not show concern, however difficult this may be.
- Remove the refused food, allowing the child to go and play and **do not offer anything further to eat until the next meal**. Odd biscuits or other snacks to 'make up' for the missed dinner will create a pattern that will be repeated again and again at each meal.
- Check with the health visitor that the child is still growing satisfactorily by measuring height and weight. If these parameters and general development is proceeding satisfactorily parents can be reassured that sufficient food is being taken.
- Drinks can be filling, so do not offer a large drink immediately before a meal. Whilst children of this age should be drinking at least one pint of whole milk a day, this should not be given at a time when other foods may be refused following the drink.

Fortunately most fussy eaters will improve in a spectacular fashion once schooldays arrive. The sight of other children tucking into meals is a potent encouragement to follow suit.

(It must be remembered, however, that often the first signs of an infection is a falling-off of appetite. Under these circumstances subsequent signs and symptoms will point to the true cause of the lack of appetite. In a previously fussy eater an infection can tip him over into a more permanent refusal of food. So care needs to be taken, once the illness is over, to tempt back a jaded appetite with small helpings of favourite food, but still at regular mealtimes.)

Fussy eaters
- Do not show concern
- Give no snacks
- Check height and weight
- Check for signs of infection

Special diets

At some time or other, nursery nurses may have children in their charge who need a special diet. These can be divided into two quite separate groups:

- those children who need a special diet for some medical reason, e.g. diabetes, cystic fibrosis or coeliac disease; these diets will be discussed further in Chapter 10;
- those children who eat a special diet for religious or philosophical reasons:
  - Muslim children who do not eat pork or dishes containing pork and strict Muslims who do not eat any meat that has not been ritually killed;
  - Hindu children brought up in the strict Hindu faith who are strict vegetarians; less strict observers eat meat as long as it is not beef;
  - Sikh children who do not eat beef;
  - Orthodox Jews who do not eat pork in any form; other meat has to be slaughtered and prepared in a special way by a 'kosher' butcher. Foods made with dairy products are not eaten at the same meal as meat-type foods;

- vegetarians whose diets vary widely, some families abstaining only from all meat, but eating eggs, fish and cheese, others who are 'vegans' who do not eat any animal products at all; the latter children, if the parents insist that they also conform to a strict vegan diet, can be at risk of not obtaining sufficient protein for growth; insufficient supplies of iron and vitamin B_{12} are also a problem and synthetic supplies need to be given to maintain health.

Toilet training

Toilet training is probably the most anxiety-provoking aspect of child care to many mothers, and maybe to their children if expectations are unrealistic! At birth babies have no control over bladder or bowel, those organs which eliminate the waste products of metabolism form the body. In babyhood, the emptying of bladder and bowel is a reflex action. Even if the baby who is passing a motion does go quiet or red in the face, this is not a sign that he has any conscious control. The nerves supplying bladder and bowel need to be mature before any conscious control is possible. This usually occurs at any time between the ages of 18 months and two years. (Parents anxious for their baby to acquire control can save a dirty nappy or two by holding their baby out over a potty immediately after a feed. This can have a fair degree of success, but does not mean that the baby is toilet trained, only that the mother is aware of her baby's probable reflex actions.)

The best time to start day-time toilet training is when it becomes obvious that the child is himself becoming aware that the bladder and/or bowel need emptying. There are various signals for this:

- A dry nappy may have been noted for longer than has been the case previously, and then maybe a sudden soaking as conscious control suddenly fails!
- A child may come a tell a parent or care-giver that she has had a bowel motion. Praise her for telling, and do not grumble because it was too late. Encourage her to say just before she needs to go; when she does, drop everything and take her to the lavatory.
- If there is a potty conveniently available he may even manage to use it himself.
- She may say she no longer wants a nappy.

When this stage is reached, continue the good work by:

- putting her into trainer pants, and taking her to the potty or lavatory on a regular basis;
- making sure that the potty, or child's seat on the lavatory, is safe and that she feels secure and comfortable;
- encouraging older children to be available to help; there is nothing like imitating an older brother or sister in 'grown-up' ways;
- being sure to give praise when she is successful, but never grumbling if she does not get to the lavatory in time.

If the child is ready, i.e. the nervous control has reached a sufficient stage of maturity, toilet training can take a very short time, one to two weeks. If, however, training is begun before the signs that a child is ready, many months can pass before full reliability is gained.

It is more usual for bowel control to be attained before bladder control, but this is not always the case. Some children are reluctant to 'let go' of a motion, and can continue to dirty a night-time nappy for some time. Again, no grumbling about this, just praise when the toilet is used.

Night-time control of the bladder will come later, around three years or even later. Most children are dry at night by the time they reach primary school age, but there is a proportion of children who do not attain this goal until much later (see Chapter 8 for enuresis).

Problems that can occur with toilet training are listed below.
- The arrival of a new baby, a move of house or some other event that upsets the even tenor of the toddler's day can cause a relapse to occur. If this does happen, go back a few stages, even as far as using nappies again, and patiently persevere in the same encouraging way.
- If it seems that urine is being passed very frequently or if it is cloudy or contains blood, medical advice should be obtained. An infection is the most likely cause of these symptoms.
- The change from the potty to the large lavatory (with a child-size seat attached or a small stool available for boys who may feel happier passing urine standing up) can be upsetting unless handled carefully. Even such normal events as the flushing noise of the lavatory can cause alarm.
- If the child has had an infection previously, of any kind, precarious bladder control can be temporarily lost.
- 'Toddler diarrhoea', more common in boys than in girls around the ages of two to four years, can pose a problem. This diarrhoea is not caused by an infection, but by the hurrying through the intestine of the contents, owing to the immaturity of the nervous control of the bowel. Remind the child to use the lavatory regularly if toddler diarrhoea is a problem. Be reassuring and sympathetic if an accident does happen. Check with the general practitioner that there is no infection.

Discussion

List the possible reasons why toilet training has not been successful for a child with whom you are familiar. As a group consider the findings of each of the group members and develop a strategy for coping with these difficulties. Summarize and note the findings plus any of your own comments.

Exercise

All children need adequate opportunity to exercise their growing bodies. They have a natural liking for activity, but need space and encouragement to fulfil this. A child who is strapped in a pram or high chair, or confined to a play-pen for long periods of time will eventually lose the desire to move around actively.

As soon as a baby begins to crawl at eight to ten months, allow a gradually increasing time to explore the immediate environment. (These are the days when safety precautions need to be extra secure. Remember that furniture in these early days must be sturdy enough to give a newly standing child full support.)

Later, toys for pushing and pulling, balls to toddle after will all encourage mobility. Later still, tricycles, paddling pools, sandpits all give stimulation to try different activities and to stretch growing muscles. Toys do not need to be sophisticated or expensive. Just as much fun can be obtained from a cardboard box, a saucepan lid, a clothes peg or a wooden spoon as from an expensive toy. The different textures of water, sand, dough and mud will all be being readily absorbed into the child's mind as part of the learning process during these play activities. Again, good preventative care against a multitude of possible accidents must be a prime consideration for the care-giver.

Social contacts

Until the age of around two years, the baby's family and family friends are all the social contact he needs. The mother or permanent care-giver will be the person he is most dependent upon during these early months.

After two years of age, children enjoy meeting other children of a similar age. As yet, combined play will not take place but they will enjoy playing alongside another child, watching and imitating.

Within a short year the developing child will be ready to join in play with children of a similar age. A small group is advisable at first, as too many active noisy children can put a shy child off all social contact for a while. This is the age when attendance at a playgroup or nursery is valuable. The parent or care-giver should not, however, abandon the child immediately on the first day. Stay to see he is well settled before leaving, then say goodbye and depart quickly. Remember to reassure him that you will be back to collect him in a short while.

Be sure to tell the person in charge of any special words the child has for needing to use the toilet. An accident on the first day, due to lack of communication, can be upsetting.

Student exercise

Watch a group of children playing at a playgroup or in a garden. Note and record:
• each child's favourite activities;
• how they are sharing with other children.
Then comment on the amount of participation needed from the adult in charge.

Moral development is perhaps a more difficult concept to evaluate. Essentially it is the development of a sense of 'right' and 'wrong' that a child learns throughout his learning years. Different norms of this aspect of development are seen in different cultures and even in different groups amongst the same society. Children will relate to the ideas of the society in which they find themselves. A 'conscience' is acquired over the years, so that a child becomes aware of what is acceptable to a particular society and what is not. (It does not mean, of course, that the dictates of conscience will always be followed!)

Moral development has been extensively studied by psychologists: Freud, Skinner, Piaget and many others.

Nursery nurses should endeavour to stabilize the moral dilemmas that children in their care meet daily within the context of the child's home moral code. A nursery must also have an ethos of its own to which staff must work. Parents will choose nurseries which have similar moral standards to their own.

Safety

This again is a wide aspect of child care in the active growing years. From the hesitant wobbly steps of the 18-month-old child to the comparatively sophisticated skills of the 8-year-old is a long step, and all along the way there are potential dangers. Safety in the home has been discussed earlier in this chapter.

There are, however, three further major aspects of safety that need to be considered – sporting safety, safety in the nursery and road safety.

Sports safety

As children mature and become more and more involved in the many activities associated with school, sport of all kinds will play a part. Running, jumping and skipping are all part of the growing process, but it is when children mix actively with their peers that complaints of aching limbs at night can occur. Usually this is only the result of excess use of muscles. A warm bath and a night's rest is usually all that is required to cure this. It is when the pain continues the next day or if an ankle is swollen that further investigations for possible sprains or strains are necessary. Vigorous football can result in pulled muscles and too vigorous activity on gymnastic equipment can cause similar problems. Staff should be on the look out for such overuse of young muscles. Children with some, albeit minor, physical disability can be especially prone to such injuries. Under these circumstances sporting activities must be geared to abilities.

Nursery safety

Workers in nurseries, where children spend a large part of their days, have an enormous responsibility to keep their charges safe at all times. The nursery must be at all times clean, safe and tidy, especially in the kitchen and toileting areas.

Other important considerations are:
• Floor coverings must be:

- easy to keep clean;
- have no frayed edges;
- not be slippery.
- Furniture must be:
  - the right size;
  - easy to clean;
  - have no sharp edges or potential splintering parts;
  - kept in good condition and replaced when necessary (this applies also to outside play furniture).
- Doors and windows should be secured to prevent being blown shut onto small fingers. Windows should have a locking device. Fire doors must always be kept shut.
- All toys and equipment must be safe and preferably have a British Standard mark. Again, they must be replaced when worn or damaged. Large items, both indoors and out, must be stored safely.
- Safety equipment – smoke alarms, stair gates, fire-guards, safety film on large areas of glass – must be all available and checked regularly.
- Disposable nappies, unwanted food and other waste must be disposed of carefully and quickly.
- Dangerous cleaning equipment must be kept in a locked cupboard.
- First aid boxes must be readily available and contents checked on a regular basis.
- Emergency procedures for fire and other dangers must be clearly understood by all staff. Procedures should be written down and displayed in a readily visible place. Any injury to children must be dealt with quickly and competently, and the child's parents informed as soon as possible.
- If the nursery caters for children with special needs, it may be necessary for specialized safety equipment to be available. For example, extra help with feeding or toileting may be required.

Safety features in a nursery
- Floor coverings
- Furniture
- Doors and windows
- Toys and equipment
- Safety features, e.g. smoke alarms
- Special care for special needs children

Student exercise

In small groups compose a video using different scenarios, e.g. kitchen, playroom, lounge, playgrounds to simulate various hazards. Get the other groups to evaluate the video.

Student exercise

Draw a plan of your place of work experience showing doors, windows, kitchen, toilets. Note any potential fire hazards. Make notes on, or draw into the plan, places where safety equipment is kept, notices shown, escape routes and 'gathering' points. Include a full list of all safety equipment.

Student exercise

Keep a diary or log book of activities over a period of time with particular reference to action taken to ensure a safe environment. Include, if possible, video and/or tape recordings together with relevant photographs with explanations alongside.

All nursery placements have to be registered by the local authority, and stringent requirements must be satisfied. Safety standards are high on the list of these requirements.

Road safety

Road traffic accidents are the single most common hazard to children outside the home. Children are more at risk than adults because:
- their small size makes perception of distance and height incomplete;
- they are unable to judge speed – difficult enough for an adult, but impossible for a child;
- instruction in road safety is not remembered for any length of time.

Adults should set a good example on road safety by:
- crossing roads correctly;
- teaching children why and how they are crossing the road in this particular way.

Children under the age of eight years are not safe to cross busy roads.

Road accidents to children show an increase at around the age of five years when school starts. Independence is just beginning, but speed and distance are difficult concepts.

The Green Cross Code should be taught from an early age:
1. Find a safe place to cross such as a pelican crossing (green man), zebra crossing, lollipop lady, traffic lights.
2. Stand on pavement near kerb.
3. Look and listen all around.
4. If traffic coming let it pass.
5. Look around again.
6. If no traffic, walk – not run – straight across the road.
7. Look and listen all the way across.

Safety under all circumstances is a vital part of child care. Fatalities and permanent disability can be the result if good care is not taken.

Children under the age of 10 years should not be allowed to ride a bicycle on busy roads, and then only after passing a Proficiency Test. They should wear fluorescent belts or other clothing.

FURTHER READING

Brain, J. and Martin, M.D. (1989), *Child Care and Health*, Cheltenham: Stanley Thornes.

Francis, D. (1986), *Nutrition for Children*, Oxford: Blackwell Scientific.

—— *Present Day Practice in Infant Feeding*, London: HMSO.

Illingworth, R. and C. (1984), *Babies and Young Children*, Edinburgh: Churchill Livingstone.

Leach, P. (1988), *Baby and Child Care*, London: Penguin.

Luben, J. (1986), *Cot Deaths*, London: Thorsons.

Poskitt, E.M.E. (1988), *Practical Paediatric Nutrition*, London: Butterworth.

CHILD DEVELOPMENT

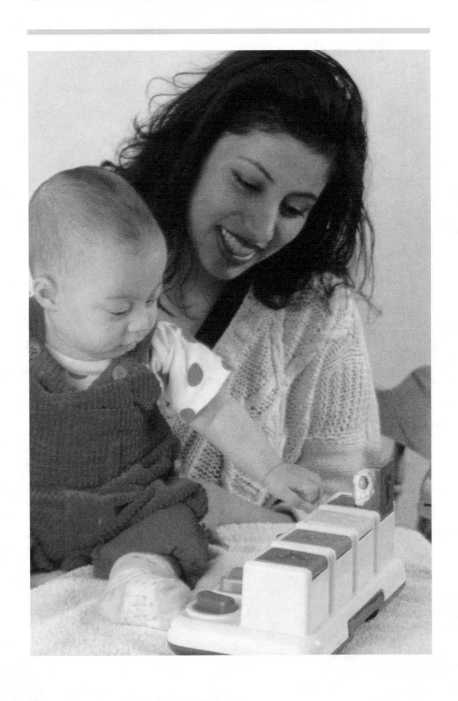

4. EARLY DEVELOPMENT UP TO SIX WEEKS

OBJECTIVES

1. **Understand prenatal growth and development.**
2. **Recognize the importance of prenatal, and immediate post-natal, care.**
3. **Acquire an in-depth understanding of child development up to six weeks.**

CONCEPTION

This is the term applied to the fusing of a female sex cell (an ovum) with a male sex cell (a sperm). In other words fertilization of the ovum or egg cell has occurred, and a new baby has started on the long journey to adulthood.

There is an optimum time during the **menstrual cycle** when fertilization can take place. The average length of a menstrual cycle is 28 days, but this varies from woman to woman. Some women have a short cycle of 21 days; others have a longer cycle of anything up to 35 days, whilst others have a completely irregular cycle. Taking an average 28-day cycle, **ovulation** (the release of an ovum from one or other of the ovaries) occurs about half way through the cycle on the 14th or 15th day. So, if sexual intercourse has occurred without contraceptive measures being taken, fertilization of the ovum is possible around this time.

There are physical changes which can alert women to their time of ovulation and so enhance their chances of becoming pregnant if intercourse is planned around this time:

- there is a slight rise in body temperature;
- vaginal secretions become clear;
- some women are aware of ovulation by pain or discomfort in their lower abdomen.

More than one ovum can be released from the ovaries during a cycle. If both or more of these ova are fertilized (and there are millions of sperm available to do this) more than one baby can be conceived.

The ovum released from one or other of the ovaries (all the ova available for reproductive purposes are present in a female baby at birth) passes straight into the funnel-like ends of the Fallopian tube. It is here that **fertilization** actually takes place. This fertilized egg – a potential new human being – travels slowly down the Fallopian tube to the uterus, the lining of which is being prepared for **implantation**.

During this time – around four to five days – the fused male and female cells have started dividing and multiplying. By the time the uterus is reached the new baby will be a round ball of cells with the potential for differentiation into firstly the placenta (or after-birth) and later into the many complex structures of a human baby.

All these complicated, and incredible, events are under the control of hormones. **Hormones** are chemical substances secreted by the **endocrine glands** of the body. The hormones produced by the ovaries and involved in the reproductive cycle are:

* **oestrogen** responsible for the development and function of the female sex organs;
* **progesterone** which alerts the uterus to prepare for the fertilized ovum. Throughout the menstrual cycle and pregnancy, oestrogen and progesterone act closely together. (Oestrogen and progesterone, in varying combinations, are the basis for the chemical method of contraception – the 'pill'.)

A further group of hormones – **chorionic gonadotrophins** – are produced by the placenta once this has been formed. These hormones act by controlling the amounts of oestrogen and progesterone necessary throughout pregnancy. The measurement of the amount of one of these hormones is the basis for the home-testing kit for pregnancy.

Two further hormones are secreted later in pregnancy and immediately after birth. These are:

* **oxytocin**, the hormone which stimulates the contractions in the uterus when the baby is due to be born and made in the hypothalamus (a specific part of the brain) but stored in the posterior part of the pituitary gland (another endocrine gland situated deep in the brain tissue);
* **prolactin**, again from the pituitary gland, which stimulates the production of milk.

PRENATAL GROWTH AND DEVELOPMENT

From the fusion of two microscopic cells a fully developed and functioning human being will be formed in just nine months. All the systems and organs necessary for an independent life will be in place and in working order. The length of a pregnancy is, on average, 40 weeks – between 38 and 42 weeks being within normal limits. As it is impossible to know the exact date of conception, the expected date of delivery (EDD) can be roughly calculated by adding one week to the first day of the last period and then subtracting three months. This is only a rough guide and more accurate predictions can be made later in pregnancy by the use of ultrasonic scans which will show the size and maturity of the baby.

During the first **six weeks** of pregnancy the mass of cells which have arisen from the fusion of the sperm and the ovum will become more and more differentiated. By six weeks after conception the embryo is firmly attached by the placenta to the wall of the uterus. The embryo lies in a sac called the amnion and is surrounded by fluid known as the **amniotic fluid**. This fluid acts as a shock absorber protecting the developing baby. The thick muscular walls of the uterus also fulfil this protecting role.

At this stage the baby is about 1 cm in length. The head can be distinguished from the body, and rudimentary limb buds are beginning to appear. The central nervous system is established, and the heart, liver and kidneys are formed.

By **12 weeks** of pregnancy, the baby is fully recognisable as a human being, with a well-differentiated head with eyes, ears, mouth, nose and chin. Growth will have increased ten-fold, so that the baby is now 10 cm (4 in.) long and will weigh around 55 g (2 oz).

He is able to swallow, frown and move his head from side to side, although his mother is not, as yet, able to feel these minute movements. Fingers and toes with formed nails can be seen on arms and legs, and the heart can be seen to be beating rapidly on ultrasonic scanning.

All the main systems and organs of the body are fully formed by this stage of pregnancy. After this time the main activity is growth and further development of detail for life in the outside world.

By **week 20** of pregnancy the fast developing baby will weigh around 350 g ($\frac{3}{4}$ lb). He will not as yet be capable of independent life outside the womb. Finer details of development will be proceeding and his whole body will have a fluffy covering of fine hair, known as laguno. The heart beat can be heard with a fetal stethoscope through the mother's abdomen.

From the mother's point of view around this time she will become aware of the new life within her uterus. Little fluttery movements – initially put down to indigestion! – will be the new son or daughter flexing muscles and moving fingers and toes.

At **28 weeks** development is practically complete. The next 12 weeks or so will be spent by the baby growing larger and stronger. By now the weight will be over 1000 g (around $2\frac{1}{2}$ lb) and the baby could sustain life outside the womb – with specialist help. As the length increases, the uterus becomes a tight fit, so the baby will be lying with a curved back, bent head, knees bent and arms crossed over the chest.

By around **32 weeks** the 'head-down', or vertex position, will be attained by most babies. This is the best possible position for birth. A few babies are born 'bottom first' – a breech birth – and even fewer adopt a more unusual position for birth. Most, if not all, of these unusual positions will need to be born by caesarian section.

From this time until birth at, or around, **40 weeks** of pregnancy, the main activity will be growth.

FUNCTIONS OF THE PLACENTA

This organ is unique to pregnancy. It is formed in the very early days of pregnancy when the fused sex cells (busily dividing) are implanted into the wall of the uterus. The placenta is a large disc-shaped fleshy structure which, when fully grown (at around 12 weeks of pregnancy), weighs about 500 g (1 lb) and has a diameter of 15 cm (6 in.).

The placenta has a multitude of blood vessels which intertwine with the highly vascular walls of the uterus. Although the mother's and fetal blood lie in close proximity, they never directly mix. Nutrients and oxygen, vital for growth and development, are diffused from the mother's blood stream into her baby's blood stream. Carbon dioxide and other waste products of metabolism are passed the other way – from baby to mother – to be excreted from the mother's body.

Whilst the placenta also exerts a protective function against noxious substances from the outside world, some viruses and chemicals can be passed to the baby via this organ. An example is the rubella virus and cytomegalovirus which, if the mother contracts one of these viral infections, can damage the developing baby. Chemicals too, such as alcohol, smoke from cigarettes and some drugs, can also be passed across the placental barrier to affect the unborn baby. Mothers who drink alcohol to excess during pregnancy can give birth to a baby with the fetal alcohol syndrome. Smoking in pregnancy can restrict the unborn baby's growth. Certain anticonvulsant drugs taken by the mother to control her illness can also have effects on the unborn baby. Drugs necessary to the mother's health and well-being have to be very carefully monitored during pregnancy because of these possible effects on the unborn child.

On the good side, however, antibodies to various infections can also pass to the baby. These will protect her from these infections during the early days of life. (The mother must have suffered from the specific disease herself, of course, before any antibodies can be transferred to her baby.)

Functions of the placenta
- Convey oxygen to baby
- Convey nutrients to baby
- Remove waste products
- Antibodies passed to baby

POSSIBLE PROBLEMS IN EARLY PREGNANCY

Ectopic pregnancy

Fertilization of the ovum occurs high up in the Fallopian tube. During the seven-day journey to the uterus these fused cells are actively dividing. On rare occasions, implantation of this tiny mass of cells occurs within the Fallopian tube. The placenta grows and the baby begins development in this restricted unhealthy environment. When a certain size is reached – usually when the pregnancy has lasted around six weeks – the Fallopian tube ruptures, being no longer big enough to contain a developing baby. This causes acute abdominal pain as the contents of the Fallopian tube are spread inside the abdominal cavity. The expectant mother will be in urgent need of medical attention. Surgical removal of the Fallopian tube pregnancy is necessary along with treatment to counteract shock.

Miscarriage

This is the term applied to the expulsion from the uterus of an early embryo. It is thought that as many as 20% of pregnancies end in a miscarriage, some occurring so early that the woman is not even aware that she is pregnant. The most common cause of this early expulsion of the embryo is some genetic fault.

A common time for a miscarriage to occur is around the third month of pregnancy. This is the stage at which the placenta becomes fully mature and takes over the main hormonal control of the pregnancy.

Pain and vaginal bleeding are the signs of a miscarriage. Many miscarriages are completed with no further problems, but sometimes surgical help is needed to control the bleeding and make sure that all the products of conception are removed.

Termination of pregnancy

A pregnancy can be terminated artificially before the end of the 24th week. There are two main groups of legal reasons for this drastic step to be taken.

- If, as a result of specific antenatal tests, the baby is found to be developing abnormally (an example would be if a woman were found to be carrying a Down's syndrome baby; she, and her partner, would be asked if they wished the pregnancy to be terminated – a hard, and difficult, decision to make); other serious or life-threatening conditions in the baby such as spina bifida, grossly malformed limbs or serious heart defects, as visualized on ultrasonic scanning, would also be considered reasons for termination.
- If two doctors agree that continuation of the pregnancy would worsen an existing physical, mental or emotional problem in the mother.

Premature birth

The World Health Organisation's definition of a premature birth is one where the weight of the baby at birth is $2500\,\text{g}$ ($5\frac{1}{2}$ lb) or less. About 10% of all births are premature by this definition. A number of notable people were premature babies, Winston Churchill being one example.

Premature babies are small and weak at birth and will have difficulties with the control of their body temperatures as well as problems with breathing and sucking. They will need specialized care for days, or even weeks and months. Warmth, extra oxygen and nasogastric feeding for a time may all be necessary before these tiny babies are able to survive on their own.

Some babies who are born with a normal birth weight can also need specialized care for a while before they are able to survive unaided. Examples of this include some babies born to mothers who have diabetes, or mothers who have had toxaemia of pregnancy. Such babies are termed 'immature' rather than 'premature'.

Twins and multiple births

A twin pregnancy usually proceeds smoothly, but there is obviously an extra strain on the mother's resources as she copes with the demands of two growing babies instead of the usual one. So it is relatively common for these babies to be born early.

Twin pregnancies can arise in two different ways:

- One sperm fertilizes one ovum, but in the very early stages of development a split occurs and two separate babies continue to develop. There is frequently only one placenta under these circumstances although this is not always the case. As these two babies have the same genetic make-up – there being only one ovum and one sperm involved – they will be identical twins.
- Two ova will be released in one cycle and will be fertilized by two sperms. So again two babies will begin development. In these circumstances, the twins will not be identical. (See Figure 4.1.)

The chances of having twins is around one in 100. If there is a history of twins in the family the chances are higher.

Figure 4.1 Genetics of the formation of identical and non-identical twins.

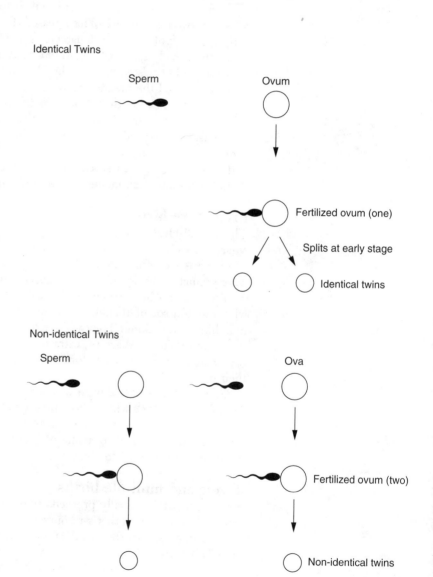

Identical Twins

Sperm   Ovum

Fertilized ovum (one)

Splits at early stage

Identical twins

Non-identical Twins

Sperm   Ova

Fertilized ovum (two)

Non-identical twins

With fertility techniques multiple births are occurring with greater frequency.

SIGNS OF PREGNANCY

Menstruation cessation

Menstruation ceases when a pregnancy has begun. By the time the monthly period is missed in a woman with an average 28-day cycle, the pregnancy is already around two weeks under way. Occasionally one period, usually less in amount of bleeding, can occur after conception. Women with very irregular periods can be much further advanced into pregnancy by the time they are aware of a missed period than those women who have a regular cycle.

Morning sickness

Morning – or occasionally evening – nausea and/or vomiting can occur in some women during the first three months of pregnancy. This is due to hormonal changes that are taking place at this time. Small frequent meals rather than larger less frequent ones can help, and a drink and dry biscuit before getting up in the mornings also works for some women.

Some unfortunate expectant mothers continue to feel nauseated throughout pregnancy. If much vomiting occurs, weight can be lost and the whole nine months be a misery. Fortunately this is rare.

Tiredness

Tiredness can be overwhelming during the first few weeks of pregnancy, and can be one of the first definite signs that a pregnancy has begun. When you think of all the major activities that are taking place in the uterus, these feelings are hardly unexpected! If at all possible extra rest – and at least, a good night's sleep – will do much to alleviate this fatigue and incidentally can also help to reduce nausea.

Frequency

Frequency of the need to pass urine can be an early feature of pregnancy. This is due both to the effects of hormonal changes on muscle tone and to the pressure on the bladder of the enlarging uterus.

Breast changes

Breasts will become fuller and tingling feelings occur as pregnancy advances. The areola (the area immediately round the nipple) will enlarge and become darker in colour, especially in darker-skinned women.

Food cravings

Some women find that they have cravings for certain articles of food such as carrots, cherries or even more unusual foods such as lobster or mangoes.

Signs of pregnancy
- Menstruation ceases
- Early morning nausea
- Fatigue
- Frequency
- Breast changes
- Odd tastes and cravings
- Chemical tests

Tea, coffee and/or alcohol can be disliked to an extreme extent. These odd appetite quirks are commonest during the early months.

Tests

Chemical tests on urine will become positive around the fifth day after conception.

ANTENATAL CARE

Historically antenatal care of pregnant women began in an organized way soon after the First World War. At this time maternal mortality during, and immediately after, childbirth was high. This was in spite of a good deal of improvement in the general standards of living of many people.

Antenatal care is a first class example of how preventative measures can help to avoid later problems. The aim is to monitor the course of each and every pregnancy. Adverse events can thus be anticipated and, if not preventable altogether, effects on both mother and baby can be minimized. An example of this is the regular monitoring of the maternal blood pressure. If, at any time during the pregnancy, but more usually towards the end, this rises to an unacceptable level, steps can be taken to lower it. (A raised blood pressure, together with other signs and symptoms – swelling of ankles and hands and protein in the urine – indicate that **pre-eclamptic toxaemia** is occurring. This is a condition unique to pregnancy, and is dangerous to both mother and baby.)

In today's society, women expecting their first baby rarely have the support of an extended family. Pregnancy is not an illness, but nevertheless there are enormous demands, both physical and emotional, on women during these nine months. Worries and fears about labour itself, as well as the later care of a totally dependent human being are natural responses in anyone contemplating the birth of a first baby. So an important part of antenatal care is to give clear, concise and accurate information on the many aspects of pregnancy, labour and care of the new member of the family. Excellent antenatal classes, to which prospective fathers are welcome, help to build emotional bonds for the new family as well as encouraging partners to work together in the care of the baby.

Student exercise

Prepare a leaflet summarizing all the antenatal classes for mothers and fathers in your locality giving details as to time, place and the content of the preparation classes. Prepare a second leaflet incorporating your suggestions for any improvements, e.g. different languages, more convenient times.

In the UK, most women are booked in for antenatal care following their first visit to their general practitioners to have the suspected pregnancy confirmed. Antenatal clinics are run by nurses and doctors with a special interest in the care of the expectant mother. In many cases antenatal care is shared between general practitioners and the maternity hospital. The first visit to the clinic will be the longest. A baseline of specific measurements is needed with which to compare and contrast future measurements, e.g. weight gain, blood pressure readings and other physical parameters. Subsequent visits will be at monthly intervals until the 30th week of pregnancy. After this time antenatal checks are fortnightly until the 36th week. At this time the obstetrician in overall charge will review the pregnancy to date, and detailed arrangements will then be made for the birth. Following this, weekly visits are the norm until the baby is born or it is felt that labour needs to be instigated.

Student exercise

Prepare a questionnaire to find out how many mothers in your neighbourhood (with children up to two years of age) attended antenatal clinics. Design the questionnaire to ask:
• where they attended;
• when they first attended;
• if they thought it worthwhile;
• whether they learnt much about labour and the care of the newborn baby.
Then analyse the results and from this present the information in graphical form, e.g. pie charts.

What happens at the first antenatal check
• General **physical health** is assessed. Important questions need to be asked about any previous illness, any problems during previous pregnancies (if this is relevant) and any family history that might have a bearing on the development of the expected baby, such as any possible inherited disease in members of the immediate family. This latter information is valuable when monitoring any future problems that may occur.
• **Heart and lung function** of the expectant mother are checked to be sure that these vital systems are healthy and strong enough to cope easily with the extra demands of pregnancy.
• **Blood-pressure** is measured for two main reasons:
  • A high blood pressure (which is unusual in the child-bearing years) can be an indicator of disease in the cardiovascular system. If this is found to be the case, further investigations are necessary and treatment given.
  • The normal level of blood pressure for each individual woman needs to be known at the start of pregnancy so that a baseline against which subsequent readings throughout pregnancy can be measured.
• **Height and weight** are measured. The weight figure will again give a baseline against which to measure the weight gained during pregnancy. By the end of pregnancy, most women will have gained between 6.4 and 9.6 kg ($1-1\frac{1}{2}$ stones). This extra weight is due to:

- the baby;
- the placenta, umbilical cord and amniotic fluid surrounding the baby;
- the greatly enlarged uterus with its thick muscular wall protecting the baby.
- An initial **blood test** is done for a number of factors:
  - The **blood group** is determined. This is necessary in case an emergency blood transfusion is necessary. Briefly, blood groups are either A, AB, B, or O. If incompatible blood is transfused, life-threatening coagulation can occur.
  - The **Rhesus (Rh) factor** is also determined. About 85% of people have this in their blood. Under these circumstances they are termed Rh-positive. The remaining 15% of people do not have this factor, and are so termed Rh-negative. Whether this factor is present or not is determined genetically, as with the inheritance of the other blood groups. Problems due to different Rh factors between mother and baby can cause problems in pregnancy. If a Rh-negative mother conceives a Rh-positive baby (this latter Rh factor being inherited from the father), her blood can be sensitized by the baby she is carrying and antibodies produced. No ill effects are seen in the first pregnancy, but any subsequent pregnancies are at risk from the antibodies produced due to the sensitization of the first pregnancy. These subsequent babies can be extremely ill (sometimes fatally so) with anaemia and jaundice. This problem can be avoided by giving an injection to the mother immediately after the birth of the first baby which will 'mop up' the antibodies. So a fresh start is given to any future pregnancies. If the father is Rh negative as well as the mother there will, of course, be no problems.
  - **Haemoglobin estimation**. This blood test measures the amount of haemoglobin (the oxygen-carrying substance in the red blood cells). If this is low, the expectant mother will be anaemic, and be feeling tired, lethargic and looking pale. A deficiency of iron is the most usual reason for anaemia and so extra iron, together with folic acid, needs to be taken to cure this type of anaemia.
  - **Immunity against rubella** (German measles). An attack of rubella during the first three months of pregnancy can have devastating effects on the unborn baby – deafness, blindness, mental retardation and heart defects are all possible problems that can be encountered. If an expectant mother is found to be non-immune, no action is possible to protect the current pregnancy. (So it is vitally important that all pregnant women should avoid contact with rubella. If contact has occurred, medical advice is necessary to consider whether termination of the pregnancy should be considered.) Following the birth of the baby, an unprotected mother is given immunization against rubella to protect future pregnancies. In the UK and other western countries, the incidence of the birth of 'rubella babies' has fallen dramatically due to immunization programmes given during childhood before the reproductive years are reached.
- **Urine** is tested for:
  - **Protein** (albumen). The presence of this substance in the urine can point to a bladder or kidney infection. This will need to be treated early in pregnancy before greater demands on the women's renal system in later pregnancy occurs. (Later in pregnancy, too, a test for albumen in the urine is important as this is a sign of toxaemia of pregnancy.)
  - **Sugar**. If there is found to be excess sugar excreted in the urine, further tests for possible diabetes will be needed. It is unusual for this condition to be first diagnosed by a urine check during the early stages of pregnancy, as the disease will usually have shown itself earlier.

Blood is tested for:
- Group
- Rh factor
- Haemoglobin
- Immunity to rubella

- **Vaginal examination** is often done at the first antenatal visit. Information regarding the age of the pregnancy can be obtained by this 'internal' examination. Also, any vaginal infections, such as 'thrush', can be found and treated. A cervical smear can also be done to detect any warning signs of cancer of the cervix – rare in this age group, but nevertheless important to eliminate.
- **Teeth** can be more prone to decay during pregnancy as well as gum disease. The old wives' tale of 'a tooth lost for every baby' has no basis in fact, but nevertheless dental health is important at this time. (In the UK dental treatment is free during pregnancy and for one year following the birth of the baby).
- **Varicose veins** can appear for the first time during pregnancy, or existing veins can worsen as pregnancy progresses due to the extra weight of the developing baby. Advice about resting with the feet up whenever possible, and wearing support tights or stockings is given
- At this first visit, advice on **diet** is given (no need to 'eat for two'!). Regular nourishing meals will do much to make for a healthy mother and a healthy baby.
- **Good posture**, even at this early stage, needs to be practised. As the weight of the uterus increases so does the tendency to stand with hollow back and protruding tummy. Much back-ache can be avoided by practising good posture throughout pregnancy.

Other checks include routine measurements, along with certain other specific tests.

Later antenatal checks

Weight, blood pressure measurement and urine testing will be a regular part of all antenatal checks. In addition:

- Examination of the increasing **size of the uterus** by feeling this through the abdominal wall becomes an important part of the estimation of the size of the growing baby. Later in pregnancy the baby's position and size can also be estimated by this means.
- **Ultrasonic scan**, usually done routinely at 16 weeks of pregnancy and also, if necessary, at other times, gives information on the size and position of both the placenta and the baby. (Ultrasound is a device whereby high frequency sound waves are bounced off structures inside the human body giving pictures of shape, size and position on monitor screens.)
- From about the 20th week of pregnancy onward the **fetal heart beat** (beating rapidly at between 120 and 160 beats per minute) can be heard through the mother's abdomen via a special short, funnel-shaped stereoscope, known as a fetal stethoscope.

Three further tests may be found to be necessary during the course of the pregnancy:

- The triple test for the presence of a **Down's syndrome baby**. This is a blood test which checks the levels of three substances in the mother's blood: human chorionic gonadotrophins (HCG), oestriol and αfetoprotein. The results of this test, together with account taken of the mother's age and any relevant family history gives information as to the likelihood of a Down's syndrome baby. If the results indicate that this might be a possibility, an amniocentesis is arranged, if this is in accordance with the wishes of the parents. (Ultrasonic examination can also gives clues as to the likelihood of a Down's syndrome baby if a specific measurement at the back of the baby's neck is above a certain level.)

- **Amniocentesis**. This is a test which involves the withdrawal of some of the amniotic fluid from the uterus through the mother's abdominal wall under a local anaesthetic. The fluid thus obtained contains some of the baby's cells which can then be examined for any chromosomal disorders, including Down's syndrome. This test is carried out at around 16 weeks of pregnancy.
- **Chorionic villus sampling**. This test involves the removal of a tiny piece of the placenta, which is then examined for certain genetically determined disorders. This test is carried out at 11 weeks of pregnancy. (Both of the latter tests carry a small risk of inducing a miscarriage. If either test proves positive for a baby with a genetically inherited disorder, the difficult decision whether or not to terminate the pregnancy will need to be made by the parents.)

THE BIRTH

Home or hospital?

The pattern of where babies are born has changed markedly since about 1950. Before 1950 the vast majority of babies were born at home, with a midwife and, if necessary, a doctor, attending the birth. By the end of the 1950s, however, 65% of all births were taking place in hospital; by the end of the 1980s 99% of babies were born in hospital.

The main reason for this relatively rapid change has been the view of doctors and some midwives that the safest place for a baby to be born is **in hospital**. In hospital:

- trained staff are available throughout the 24 hours (more babies are born between midnight and 6 a.m. than at any other time during the 24 hours);
- monitoring equipment is available to check the progress of labour and the baby's vital functions;
- facilities for emergency help are immediately available, e.g. theatres for caesarian sections, staff for forceps deliveries, blood for blood transfusions;
- nurses and midwives are always present to help with after care of mother and baby throughout the 24 hours;
- mothers are free from other domestic responsibilities.

There are certain other circumstances which make a hospital delivery preferable:

- mothers expecting their first babies;

- mothers who already have needed a previous caesarean section;
- women who are Rh-negative;
- women who have certain medical conditions, such as high blood press- ure or diabetes (in both these conditions the baby can be at risk during and immediately after delivery);
- mothers whose homes are unsuitable for delivery;
- when labour starts prematurely.

However, in recent years, more couples have been requesting **home births** for a number of reasons:

- the family can be involved in the birth of the new member;
- there is less likelihood of infection;
- there are no problems with visiting, long journeys sometimes being involved;
- the care of other children is not so difficult to arrange.

Often this has been difficult to arrange as fewer doctors are prepared to be responsible for delivery at home. A good compromise would seem to be the system worked in many areas of the country. The actual birth takes place in hospital, but mother and baby are discharged home within 24 hours or less (if all is well with both mother and baby) to the care of the community midwife and the general practitioner.

Role play

You have been asked, by a diabetes clinic, to give a talk to some first time mothers-to-be who are very keen on a home delivery. The clinic has asked you because they know that, as a nursery nurse, you have experience of both kinds of delivery. They would like you to explain the advantages and disadvantages of each but because of their concern for the mothers, they would like you to persuade the mothers that a hospital delivery is safest for them and their babies.

Prepare a set of foils for the overhead projector (OHP) taking especial care to make them lively, interesting and informative to use in your 10-minute presentation and design supporting leaflets to hand out afterwards.

Present the talk to some of your colleagues representing the rather disbelieving and somewhat disgruntled mothers-to-be who may well ask 'difficult' questions.

People involved in birth and the care of mothers and babies

- **Midwife**. This is a nurse who has had further training in care of women during pregnancy and labour. Around 75% of all babies are delivered by a midwife. They can work in the maternity departments of hospitals or in the community. Most of the routine antenatal care is done by mid- wives. The community midwives are also responsible for the care of mother and baby for 10 days after delivery.
- **General practitioner**. This is a doctor who has pursued further train-

ing in general practice. A number also have a special interest in obstetrics.

- **Obstetrician**. This is a doctor who has specialized in the care of pregnant women and childbirth. Their work is almost entirely in hospital, at antenatal clinics and when complications of pregnancy or labour arise needing a caesarean section or a forceps or breech delivery. (Their work also often includes the care of women of all ages with diseases of the reproductive system. This part of the work is termed 'gynaecology'.)
- **Paediatrician**. This is a doctor who has specialized in the care of children. They have the care of the newborn baby as well as all children up to the age of 16 years. They will be in attendance at all difficult births to resuscitate the baby if necessary.
- **Health Visitor**. This is a nurse who has undertaken extra training for the care of people in the community. A large part of the work involves the care of babies and young children.

Labour

'Labour' is a good term to describe the actual process of giving birth. It is hard work, and mothers need to exert much muscular effort to deliver their babies.

Labour is divided into three stages:

- Stage 1 is the time when the cervix (the neck of the uterus, or womb) is dilating to allow the baby out of the uterus down the vagina into the outside world. This is the longest stage of labour for the majority of women, and can take anything from 2 to 12 hours – or more.
- Stage 2 is the actual passage of the baby out of the cosiness of the uterus into the harsh light of day.
- Stage 3 is the expulsion of the placenta from the uterus.

Signs that labour has started

- **Contractions** of the uterus become more regular and frequent. During the latter weeks of pregnancy, the uterus will have been contracting at irregular intervals. When labour begins the contractions will be stronger, and come initially about every 20 minutes. The time between these contractions will gradually decrease until at the end of the first stage of labour, they will be occurring every two or three minutes.
- A '**show**' of blood from the vagina means that the plug of mucus sealing the cervix has been expelled, which in turn means that the cervix has started to dilate.
- The '**waters**' – the bag of amniotic fluid surrounding the baby – will break. This allows the baby's head to come into closed contact with the cervix. This will help in the dilation process.

(The description below is of a normal head-down – vertex – delivery.)

First stage

This is the longest, most trying and potentially the most painful stage of labour. Every woman has her own unique way of passing this time – some prefer to walk around, others to lie on their backs or side whilst others find it easier to crouch or kneel as the contractions intensify. There is no one way better than any other. It is helpful to have someone with the expectant mother during this – sometimes long – time. Her partner, relative or friend can all be of comfort at this time.

Pain relief

There are several types of pain relief available to be used during the first stage of labour:

- 'Gas-and-oxygen' can be breathed in through a mask or tube into the mouth as the contractions become strong during the latter half of the first stage of labour.
- **Pethidine** – a strong analgesic drug – can be given by injection if the mother becomes very distressed.
- **Epidural anaesthesia** can be given for total relief of pain during childbirth. This is a local anaesthetic injected into the lower part of the back. If a mother wishes for this type of pain relief during labour this will have to be discussed beforehand so that an anaesthetist is available to perform the block.
- **Relaxation and breathing techniques**, learned at antenatal classes, can do much to reduce the discomfort.

Second stage

This is the stage when the baby is travelling down the birth canal, the cervix now being fully dilated. The mother at this time will feel the irresistible desire to 'push down' with each contraction. The midwife will be encouraging her to use each contraction to the full by her added muscular effort, and then to relax between contractions.

The largest part of the baby to be born is his head. If the vaginal opening is too tight to allow the baby's head through without tearing the mother, a cut is made to enlarge this opening. This is known as an episiotomy, and will need to be stitched up after the birth.

Once the head is born the rest of his body will follow amazingly quickly. As the head is born, the midwife will clear away any mucus from the mouth so that the first breath can be taken.

Third stage

This is the time when the placenta is expelled from the uterus. Up to 20 minutes can elapse between the birth of the baby and the delivery of the placenta – or 'after-birth' as it is sometimes sensibly termed. This time can be happily used to acquaint mother and baby, and start the 'bonding' process so essential to good mothering.

As the placenta is pushed out the mother will feel one more – much less painful – contraction, and the fleshy organ that has nourished the baby for nine long months will be expelled.

Sometimes other types of birth are necessary. These include:

- **Forceps-aided delivery**. This can be necessary when the contractions of the uterus are too weak to push the baby out of the uterus, or if either mother or baby are showing signs of distress. In the latter circumstance it is advisable for the baby to be born as quickly as possible. An instrument – rather like a large pair of sugar tongs – is placed on either side of the baby's head, and the doctor will then ease the baby into the world. Either a general, local or epidural anaesthetic is necessary for most cases of forceps deliveries.

- A **breech birth** is one where the baby is born bottom – or breech – first instead of the more usual head first position. Forceps may again be needed to delivery the baby's head.
- A **caesarean section** (done either under general anaesthesia or local anaesthesia by an epidural) in which the baby is born by cutting into the woman's abdomen and uterus. This method of delivery will need to be performed if:
  - the pelvis is too small to allow the baby's head to be born normally;
  - if the placenta is placed awkwardly over the cervix (under these conditions uncontrollable bleeding would occur once the cervix started to dilate);
  - when it is thought advisable that babies in the breech position should be born by caesarean section.

Types of birth
- Normal vertex delivery
- Forceps-aided delivery
- Breech birth
- Caesarean section

As soon as the baby is born, an assessment of his or her condition is made by the midwife. Certain features are noted and given a score. This system of assessment is known as the **Apgar Score** after Dr Virginia Apgar, the American doctor by whom this was devised. The features noted at 1 minute, 5 minutes and 10 minutes are shown in the Table 4.1. (The first two features are the most important). In a perfectly healthy baby, the score will be 10.

Table 4.1 Apgar scores

Feature	Score 0	Score 1	Score 2
Heart rate	Absent	Below 100 beats per minute	Above 100 beats per minute
Respiration	Absent	Irregular, slow, weak	Lusty cry
Muscle tone	Limp	Poor, some movement	Strong movement
Reflex irritability (Stimulation of the toe)	No response	Slight withdrawal	Vigorous withdrawal
Colour	Blue, pale	Pink body, blue hands and feet	Completely pink

If the final added scores are:
- below 7 at 1 minute;
- below 8 at 5 minutes;
- less than 9 at 10 minutes,

special care for the baby will need to be considered. For example, a baby who scored:

- 2 on 'heart rate';
- 2 on 'respiration';
- 1 on 'muscle tone';
- 1 on 'reflex irritability';
- 2 on 'colour' at 1 minute after birth – all adding up to 8

would be thought to be healthy, even though the score at 1 minute is not the maximum of 10. (When scored again at 5 minutes it is probable that the score will have risen to 10.)

This scoring system has to be modified slightly for dark-skinned babies. At birth, the colour of the skin of these babies can look a greyish colour, so the mucus membranes – inside the mouth and under the eyes – need to be examined to see if the baby is in a satisfactory condition.

POSTNATAL PERIOD

Needs of the mother in the immediate postnatal period

In spite of the enormous physical effort necessary for birth, most mothers recover quickly from their immediate exhaustion. The excitement of welcoming a new member of the family overrides all other feelings.

Sometimes around the third day after delivery, mothers will feel out-of-sorts and depressed. The excitement is calming down and life – never to be the same again – seems one long round of feeding, bathing and changing nappies. This common event is known as 'baby blues'. It is due to:

- changes in the pattern of hormone secretion now that the pregnancy is over. It can take a while for the usual pattern to be re-established. This change is mirrored in the time that menstruation starts again after the birth of a baby. This can be as long as six months, particularly if the mother is breast feeding. Other women will start menstruating again within a month or two. (It is possible to become pregnant again before periods return, so adequate contraceptive measures need to be taken if another pregnancy is not wanted.)

'Baby blues' due to:
- Hormonal changes
- Fatigue
- 'Let down' feelings

- Continuing fatigue due to disturbed nights and hectic days looking after the needs of a new baby as well as, perhaps, the needs of other children.
- The 'let-down' feelings that normally occur once any exciting event is over and general routine begins again.

In the vast majority of new mothers these feelings improve within a week or two especially if she realizes that this is common and will pass. It will help if she can talk to someone knowledgeable about the needs of new mothers, or to someone who has recently experienced the same problem. Adequate rest is also vital for a rapid recovery.

Occasionally these depressive feelings can persist and worsen, and the new mother can suffer from a full-blown **depressive illness**. She may feel deep feelings of inadequacy in looking after her baby, even though the new son or daughter was a much wanted child. This type of mental illness can occur in any woman after childbirth, even the most happy and carefree. Urgent medical attention is necessary under these circumstances.

Postnatal exercises

These are exercises which help muscles stretched by pregnancy to return to normal. After a birth, the muscles of the abdomen are slack and floppy. Also the muscles of the pelvic floor – which again have been stretched during the birth – need to be toned. Advice on the type of exercises to do is given by midwives and health visitors. These exercises should be done – gently at first but regularly. After a surprisingly short time, most mothers will regain their figures again.

Postnatal examination

This takes place, either at the general practitioner's surgery or at the hospital, six weeks after the birth of the baby. The mother's general health is checked, her uterus is examined to be sure that it has returned to its normal size, any problems can be discussed and contraceptive advice given.

Documentation

Necessary documentation following the birth of a baby include:

- **Notification** of the birth to the Local Health Authority, within 36 hours, will be done by the midwife attending the birth.
- **Registration** of the birth to the local Registrar of Births, Marriages and Deaths will need to be done, within six weeks, by the parents. To do this either parent will need to visit the Registrar's office; their address can be found in the local telephone directory. The name under which the child is to be brought up is recorded.
- A **medical card** is given at the time of registration. This will need to be taken to the family doctor so that the baby is registered into the National Health Service for treatment if necessary at any later date.
- Later, following on from the health visitor's visit, a **Personal Child Health Record Card** is given to the mother. On this card, both the mother and the professionals concerned with the care of the child keep a record of the baby's growth, development progress, dates of immunization and any illness, teething and all the many other aspects of child care. This record is of immense value if the parents move to another part of the country or abroad. A written record of past events in the baby's life is extremely helpful if there any problems of health or development at a later date.

Documentation
- Birth notification to Health Authority
- Registration of birth to Registrar
- Medical card
- Personal Child Health Record Card

Student exercise

Arrange a group visit to, or by, your local Registrar of Births, Marriages and Deaths. Ask particularly for the information required on the various forms used for when:

- the parents of a baby are not married to each other;
- the father is unknown or
- re-registration at a later date when the father's details can be added;

• a child born in the UK of foreign nationals.

Summarize and record this information, preferably with a copy of the forms.

THE NEW BABY

However many new babies one has seen, it always comes as a surprise to find how small they are! Even though a baby may be of an average size – weight 3.5 kg; length 50 cm; head circumference 35 cm (7.7 lb; 20 in.; 14 in. respectively) – she will still seem tiny.

The **umbilical cord** will still be attached to the navel. This will drop off between one week and 10 days, leaving the typical umbilical scar as a reminder of prenatal dependence.

The amount of **hair** on the head will vary from baby to baby. Many babies are born with a shock of dark hair, lose this within a few weeks and mothers can be surprised to find it replaced with hair of quite a different colour. Other babies have less hair, but this will often remain the same colour throughout their lives.

There are two **fontanelles** – or 'soft spots' – on a newborn baby's head (Figure 4.2). These are the places where the flat plates of the bony skull join. This plays an important part in the 'moulding' of the baby's head during the journey down the birth canal. The fontanelle, in the midline, towards the front of the baby's head – the anterior fontanelle – can be seen to pulsate at times. This is due to the beating of an artery immediately below the surface and is quite normal. The anterior fontanelle will gradually become smaller as the baby develops, and will eventually close completely between the ages of one year and 18 months. This fontanelle can give valuable information in the early days of life. Normally the surface of the fontanelle is flat to the bone of the head. If the baby is dehydrated for any reason, because of a fever or just plain thirst for example, the level of the fontanelle will be sunken below the surface of the bones of the skull. In other conditions, such as hydrocephalus for example, the fontanelle will be full and taut.

The posterior fontanelle is much smaller and lies in the midline behind the anterior fontanelle. This will close within a few weeks of birth.

Both fontanelles are covered with a thick, tough membrane, so there need be no fear of damaging the baby's brain when washing her head.

Many babies have blue **eyes** at birth except those babies with dark skins who have dark eyes right from birth. Often eye colour will change during the first few weeks of life and the adult colour will be that inherited from parents.

The baby's **skin** at birth is covered with a greasy, greyish substance known as 'vernix'. This protects the skin during prenatal life when the baby is immersed in the amniotic fluid. Some authorities consider the vernix to act also as a protection against infection in the early days after birth and so delay washing the baby for a few days.

Jaundice, a yellow coloration of the skin, can develop in some babies

Figure 4.2 The top of a baby's head.

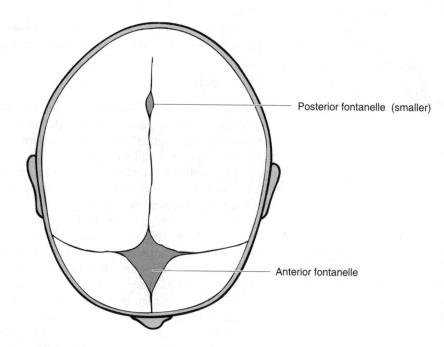

Posterior fontanelle (smaller)

Anterior fontanelle

(up to 50%) around the second or third day of life. This is due to the breakdown of some of the haemoglobin in the red blood cells. This will normally clear within three or four days without any special treatment. Close watch needs to be kept, however, on the level of jaundice in case it persists or worsens. If this is the case, confirmatory blood tests as to the actual level of jaundice will be needed, and treatment given – usually phototherapy – if results are above normal limits.

Small **red marks** on the baby's eyelids, back of the neck or middle of the forehead may be much in evidence in the immediate few days after birth. These are often termed 'stork bites' in deference to the old wives' tale of these areas being the places where the stork carried the baby! No treatment is necessary as these marks will gradually fade in the first few months of life.

What the new baby can do

Although completely dependent on others for supporting his life, there are many things that a new baby can do. Arms, legs and body can **move**. Although the movements are small in range and seemingly purposeless, it is a method of flexing small muscles which, until recently, have been tightly confined within the confines of the uterus.

Newborn babies will **sneeze, yawn and hiccup** – all practice for learning to control the newly acquired process of breathing.

They will spend much of their time **asleep**, but will wake to **feed** and to **cry**. Crying also helps to open up those new lungs.

Babies can **see** from birth, although they are short-sighted, focusing on objects only 20 cm (8 in.) or so away. Vague shapes, blurred images, movement and changes in the intensity of light are the main visual stimuli of which the newborn baby is aware. His mother's face, as she bends to attend to his needs or feeds him is a source of great interest. It is thought that within a few days of birth the baby is able to recognize his mother's face. Within a week or so, she will be gazing intently at his face during feed times. Also within a few days, the baby will turn his head towards a brightly lit window, and shut his eyes tightly when the sun or a sudden visual object comes directly into his path of vision.

Hearing, too, is present at birth. Sudden noises will cause the newborn baby to jump, and even the interesting activity of feeding will cease at a sudden loud bang. Crying babies will often quieten at the sound of a soothing voice and quiet, rhythmical sounds, such as sung lullabies, will often induce sleep in a crying baby. Held close in the crook of someone's left arm, near to a heart beat, babies will also often quieten. The rhythmical beat has, until birth, been part of the baby's environment from the first moment that awareness of sound existed.

Newborn babies are also sensitive to **touch**. They are comforted by being held securely in someone's arms, and will cry if a sudden blast of cold air impinges on their body, or if the bath water is too cold.

Taste and **smell** are the other two of the five senses that are present in the newborn baby. Unpleasant tastes or smells will cause tiny heads to be turned away. Breast-fed babies frequently turn their faces towards their mother's breasts, and smell is thought to exert an influence on this movement.

New babies can:
- Move
- Sneeze and yawn
- Sleep
- Feed
- Cry
- See
- Hear
- Taste
- Smell

Reflexes

There are several reflexes present in the baby at birth. (Reflex actions are ones which occur involuntarily in response to certain stimuli.) These reflexes are consistent in all newborn babies. If they are not present, or if they persist longer than is usual, further neurological investigation is necessary. The first two reflexes are important for survival.

- The **sucking reflex** is present from birth, and even before birth babies can be seen on ultrasonic scan to have their thumbs in their mouths. When anything is put into a newborn baby's mouth, she will automatically make sucking motions.
- The **rooting reflex** is also connected with feeding. If a newborn baby's cheek is gently touched, for example, by the nipple of the mother's breast, her head will turn automatically towards the stimulus.
- The **'walking' reflex** occurs when a baby is held upright and his feet placed on a firm surface. He will then automatically take steps forwards. This reflex will disappear long before he begins to walk in reality, and the purpose of this reflex is unclear.
- The **grasp reflex** is again present from birth. Tiny fingers will curl themselves around an offered finger and clasp it tightly.
- The **'startle' or Moro reflex**. When a baby's head is suddenly released, for a few centimetres only, from a firm grasp, the baby will throw wide

Reflexes in the newborn
- Sucking
- Rooting
- Grasp
- Walking
- Startle, or Moro

his arms, maybe cry and then bring his arms together as if trying to hold onto someone. This can again be thought of as a rudimentary survival reflex.

Most of these reflexes will have disappeared by the time the baby is three months old. After this age, much of the baby's movements will be conditioned by what he has learned.

Basic needs of the newborn

Shelter and warmth

After the close protection of the womb with all necessary oxygen and nutrients supplied, the world must seem a cold, alien place. Oxygen has to be obtained by one's own efforts of breathing. Food, even when offered on a regular basis has to be imbibed, metabolized, absorbed and the waste products excreted. Body temperature, too, has to be stabilized. Newborn babies have poor control over their own body temperature for the first few months of life. (This is especially so when the baby is born prematurely.) Normal body temperature is between the narrow range of 36 °C and 37.5 °C. Small variations can occur during the night and day.

Tiny babies cannot move to warm themselves, so suitable clothing is an important aspect of baby care in the early days of life.

Room temperature should ideally be kept as constant as possible for the first few months of life. An ideal temperature range is between 16 and 20 °C.

Food

Food is a further basic necessity and must be given at frequent, regular intervals. Breast milk is the ideal food for babies, but there are many excellent substitutes available on the market (see Chapter 3).

Sleep

Newborn babies spend around 20 hours out of the 24 hours asleep. At birth the pattern of sleep is quite irregular, but as the weeks go by a routine of sleep as well as of feeding becomes established.

The sleeping position of young babies is of importance as regards cot death. This is the tragic event when a young child (usually between the ages of one month and seven months) is found dead in the cot quite unexpectedly and suddenly. Young babies should always be put down to sleep on their backs with their heads turned to one side. (Since this advice was given, the incidence of cot deaths has markedly decreased.)

Love and attention

Even very young babies, who seem not to respond in any way, need plenty of affection. A crying baby cuddled snugly in loving arms will eventually quieten unless there is pain or discomfort causing the crying. All babies cry. It is the only way they have of communication in the early days. As the new mother gets to know her baby better, she will be able to understand what she is trying to tell her. She may be trying to tell her that she is:

- **hungry**. There is no point withholding a feed until the clock says that it is time the baby should be fed. We all feel hungry, and not hungry, to different degrees at different times, and babies are no exception.
- **thirsty**. Milk is not an especially good thirst quencher. In hot weather in particular babies can get thirsty. Plain boiled, and cooled, water or diluted fruit juice can soothe a hot crying baby.
- **uncomfortable**, possibly due merely to a dirty nappy. Some babies do seem especially susceptible to the unpleasant feelings of a dirty, or wet, nappy. So a quick change, with its concomitant helpings of love and attention, can often soothe a crying baby.
- **in pain**. He may be in pain, perhaps from colicky tummy ache. This type of crying often occurs at a set time of the day , between 6 and 9 p.m. seems to be the commonest time. This usually lasts until around three months of age and is often referred to as 'three-month colic'. Lying the baby on his tummy, or offering anticolic drops are all worth trying. If a baby cries constantly, or whimpers quietly continuously, for no obvious reason, it is wise to seek medical advice.
- **lonely or bored**. Slightly older babies will cry because they are lonely and want to be involved in the activities going on around them. A little extra attention at these times will usually stop the crying. Young babies will not be 'spoilt' by their mothers or carers picking them up and giving them attention for a while. Later on this can happen, but not in the very early days of life.

Crying babies may be:
- Hungry
- Thirsty
- Uncomfortable
- In pain
- Lonely or bored

Special tests soon after birth

As well as a routine all-over physical check for any obvious congenital defects by a paediatrician soon after birth, there are two special tests carried out between the seventh and tenth day of the baby's life. These are done on a small amount of blood obtained by a 'heel-prick'.

- **PKU test**. This test is done to exclude the presence of a condition – phenylketonuria – in which the baby is unable to metabolize the amino acid phenylalanine. The basic cause of this failure is the absence or deficiency of a specific enzyme. If this is the case serious developmental anomalies will occur and the child will have a mental disability. Treatment is by a diet from which phenylalanine is excluded.
- **Thyroid function test**. On the same sample of blood, tests are done for adequate thyroid function. If the function of this endocrine gland is low, normal growth and development will be affected. Treatment is by giving routine thyroxine treatment.

Development assessments

Six weeks is the age at which mothers in the UK are offered a developmental check. (If mothers, midwives, health visitors or doctors are worried about the baby's health or development before this time, these will, of course, be looked into.)

Developmental assessments at various ages were slow to develop when compared with the routine checks on weight which had been done for many years. Whilst this routine measurement did give information on a baby's physical growth, and hence well-being, it was a very inaccurate and brief pointer as to what babies can do at specific ages.

The development of tests of skills at various ages took several years to finalise and meant the examination of hundreds of children. From these results, guidelines of developmental progress at each age were drawn up. For example, most babies are smiling by the age of six weeks, most children have a few words at their command by one year of age and most children are walking by the age of 18 months; but it must again be emphasized that there is no definite hard-and-fast rule of 'pass' or 'fail' on developmental testing. Rather there is a range of 'normality'.

The purpose of developmental tests is to determine as early as possible problems in any of the developmental areas. Once these are found help can be given to overcome these, often temporary, difficulties.

It is always necessary to understand the normal before the abnormal can be recognized.

Discussion

Collect background information about the parent's attitude to and opinions about, developmental checks. Pool this information in a group discussion and afterwards write a summary in the form of a table showing the advantages and disadvantage of such checks with comments on the parent's opinions.

Development at six weeks

For ease of recording, and also as an aide-mémoire, development is divided into four main areas. Each of these areas cannot, of course, be tested strictly in rotation (babies and children have no idea of developmental areas!). So observations will need to be made over a specific length of time. Nursery nurses and other professionals caring for children over a long period of time are in an ideal situation for such observations. If these are then recorded, any difficulties with certain tests can be checked again in a few days' time or discussed with other people also having the care of the child.

Motor development (i.e. the big wide-ranging movements of the body)

- When lying on her back (supine):
  - arms and legs are partly flexed. Arms are bent at the elbows so that the baby's hands are up beside her face – almost in a 'boxing' position!
  - arms and legs move freely and symmetrically. At this early age there is no difference in the amount of movement on each side of the body as there is later in childhood when 'handedness' is established. It is important to note

whether any limb appears stiffer in movement than the others. Children with even a minor degree of cerebral palsy will show a difference in the amount and range of movement of the affected limb or limbs.

- When lying on her tummy (prone):
  - knees are drawn up intermittently under the abdomen, almost as if she is trying to crawl. At this early age, of course, the baby has not sufficient muscular power to move, but the basic movements are already in place.
  - chin is lifted off the floor or bed briefly, only to fall down again immediately due to insufficient muscular power and control. 'Floppy' babies – such as Down's syndrome babies – with poor muscular control (hypotonia) will be unable to perform this movement.
- When in a sitting supported position:
  - the back is rounded in a C-curve. To check on this the baby is gently pulled, by her hands, into the sitting position from lying on her back. A hand should be held behind the head to control this – at this age – top-heavy part. The spine will be rounded as the baby is momentarily held in this position, the muscles again not being strong enough to straighten her back.
  - head is held up intermittently. This mimics the raising of the head from the bed when the baby is lying on her tummy.
- The reflexes which can be elicited in the newborn period are still all present, with perhaps the exception of the 'grasp' reflex. Many of these reflexes will disappear within the next six weeks by the time the baby is three months old.

Vision and fine movement

- The baby's gaze is fixed on an object or face. This is particularly notice-able at feed-times, when the baby will be searching his mother's face as she feeds him with breast or bottle.
- When an object, e.g. a dangling toy, is held in front of the baby's face, at a distance of around 25 cm (10 in.), he will follow it from the midline to the side and back again when it is slowly moved.
- Similarly a moving person within his range of vision will be followed visually. At this age babies will be beginning to recognize their mothers, and will focus on her as she comes into view.
- If an object approaches too near the baby's face he will blink in a rudimentary attempt to protect his eyes.
- The eyes of babies of this age will still squint at times, particularly when he is tired. This is quite normal at this age. Squinting should occur only rarely after the age of three months, and should certainly have ceased by the time six months of age is reached.

Student exercise

Design a toy suitable for testing a young baby's vision. Remember to consider, in your design, the relevance of colour, size and shape, and the lack of auditory stimuli.

Hearing and speech

When spoken to, babies of six weeks will quieten if they have not been left to cry for too long a period of time.

- Attempts at cooing and gurgling will also be heard when 6-week-old babies are spoken to directly, especially by a familiar person.
- Sudden loud noises will cause a 'startle' reaction in the baby – arms and legs flung wide if the noise is near and very loud. His eyes will also move in the direction of the sound. (It is important to remember that deaf babies also vocalize in a reflex type of way at this age. Clues as to possible deafness can be gained when they do not 'startle' at loud noises.)

Social behaviour

- This is the age when mothers and carers are rewarded with a truly social smile in response to their speech. Some babies smile earlier than this – at around four weeks – but most frequently the 'smile' at this age is due to wind!
- When picked up and cuddled after a bout of crying babies of this age will usually quieten unless they are hungry, in pain or uncomfortable.
- Sucking and swallowing are now well controlled, and feeds will be taken with gusto in normal healthy babies.

All future developmental tests follow the same basic pattern, and, as with the centile charts for growth, give a complete picture of the individual child's development over time. This continuing record of steady progress is of far more value than individual measurements.

Student exercise

Visit a child health clinic and watch a six-week assessment being done. Write a report of your visit explaining what you found especially interesting and unusual, and why.

FURTHER READING

Brain, J. and Martin, M.D. (1989), *Child Care and Health*, Cheltenham: Stanley Thornes.

Gray, P. (1987), *Crying Baby*, London: Wisebuy Publications.

Hall, D. (1989), *Health for All Children*, Oxford: Oxford Medical Publishers.

Hilton, T. (ed.) (1993), *The Great Ormond Street Book of Baby and Child Care*, London: Bodley Head.

5. LATER DEVELOPMENT

UP TO EIGHT YEARS

OBJECTIVES

1. Understand factors relevant to developmental variations.
2. Acquire an in-depth understanding of child development in the first eight years of life.
3. Recognize important aspects of human development post-childhood.

UNDERSTANDING DEVELOPMENTAL VARIATION

Before looking at the detailed development of children a various ages, we shall take a look at the reasons why every child – and indeed every individual – is different.

Every person in the world is quite unique. (Even so-called identical twins – developed from the fusion of one egg and one sperm – have minor variations identifiable at birth. As they grow so will different characteristics appear in response to their reactions to environmental factors.)

There are three main factors which have an effect on a child's development:

- genetic factors;
- environmental factors;
- possible health problems during the childhood years.

Genetic factors

The study of genetics has taken a vast leap forward in the 1980s and 1990s. New information on the mode of inheritance of characteristics – both mental and physical – are reported weekly, along with genetic information about the inheritance of various diseases. Work is continuing in many centres throughout the world on the 'mapping' of the genes for various conditions on the chromosomes. As a result of this work, genetic treatment of various diseases is becoming a possibility.

Every cell in the human body consists of two basic parts – a nucleus and the cytoplasm surrounding this important structure. The genetic material is held on the chromosomes (literally 'coloured bodies', named due to the certain stains they take up), which in turn are in the nuclei of the cells. There are 46 chromosomes (23 matched pairs) in each cell. The one exception to this is in the sex cells – the sperm and the ovum. These latter cells contain only 23 chromosomes. So at the fusion of a sperm and an ovum the whole complement of 46 chromosomes is again made up to form the new individual. In this new individual 23 chromosomes are the exact copy of the chromosomes in the child's father (from the sperm) and 23 from the mother (in the ovum).

It is on these chromosomes that the genes are placed – many thousands of them. Each gene contains information necessary for the growth and development of the new individual. Typical information contained in the genes includes eye colour, blood group, body shape, maximum height that can be attained as well as a host of other information, including certain inherited diseases and the potential for other conditions.

The **sex** of the new baby is determined by one particular pair of chromosomes – the sex chromosomes (Figure 5.1). A female has two X chromosomes (denoted as XX) and a male has one X chromosome and one Y chromosome (denoted as XY). So every ovum will have an X chromosome, whilst a sperm can contain either an X chromosome or a Y chromosome. Depending on which sperm fertilizes an ovum, either a girl (XX) or a boy (XY) will result. So it can be seen that it is the male partner who determines the sex of the child.

Figure 5.1 How the sex of a baby is determined.

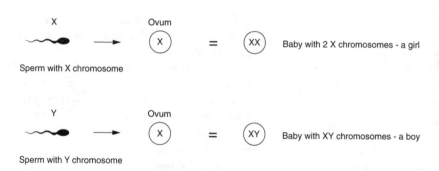

As the genes from the male and the female pair off, certain genes will be stronger or weaker for different characteristics. These are known as 'dominant' or 'recessive' genes respectively. An example can be found in the inheritance of eye colour. If a child's father has blue eyes and her mother brown eyes, she will have brown eyes as the gene for brown eyes is dominant over the gene for blue eyes. However, in the child's genetic make-up, the gene for blue eyes still remains. In other words she is a 'carrier' for blue eyes. So her children in turn may have blue eyes, depending on the genetic make-up of the father.

Certain inherited diseases have as their basis the dominance or recessiveness of the gene, or genes, involved in the disease. In a **dominant mode of inheritance** (Figure 5.2), one or other of the parents will be affected by the condition. Each of their children will stand a 50% chance of inheriting the condition. The inherited condition neurofibromotosis is an example of this mode of inheritance.

In a **recessive mode of inheritance** (Figure 5.3), it is only if both

Figure 5.2 The dominant mode of inheritance.

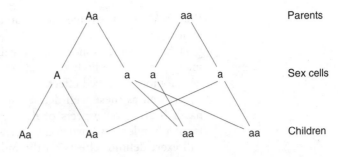

A = Dominant gene of dominant condition   2 children with condition
a = Normal gene   2 children without condition

Figure 5.3 The recessive mode of inheritance.

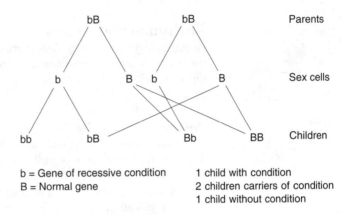

b = Gene of recessive condition   1 child with condition
B = Normal gene   2 children carriers of condition
                                   1 child without condition

parents are carriers of the defective gene that the baby born to the couple will stand a one in four chance of having the condition. (Under these circumstances also each child will stand a 50% – or two in one chance – of being a carrier for the condition.) It is in this way that the disease cystic fibrosis is inherited.

To further complicate the picture (and genetics is very complex) some conditions are 'sex-linked'. These conditions are only apparent in the male but are carried by the female. Each son will have an equal chance of inheriting the faulty gene. Haemophilia is one such well-known condition that is inherited in a sex-linked manner.

As well as these disorders attributable to the genes carried on the chromosomes, certain other conditions are caused by a fault in the chromosomes themselves. This can be due to either a numerical, or a structural, fault in a particular chromosome. The best known and documented **numerical chromosomal fault** is that resulting in Down's syndrome. Here, an extra chromosome is present, so that the chromosomal make-up of a Down's syndrome child is of 47 chromosomes instead of the usual 46. **Structural faults** can also occur in chromosomes. For example, part of a specific chromosome can be missing. The fragile X syndrome and the

Prader–Willi syndrome are examples of this type of chromosomal abnormality.

Chromosome abnormalities will produce wide-ranging effects on many parts of the body of an affected person. Single gene problems will have a more localized effect.

As well as these well-defined specific effects **genetic predisposition** has a bearing on aspects of development. Certain predispositions – or familial tendencies – when interactive with outside environmental factors will exert definite effects on the individual concerned. This is known as **multifactorial inheritance.**

So there can be seen to be a number of ways in which inheritance can have an effect on development as well as on a child's physical characteristics.

Environmental factors

As previously briefly discussed, there are many aspects of a child's environment which exert an effect on development. These effects are, of course, quite outside the ability of the children to control even if they were aware of them.

Position in the family

This single chance event will, without doubt, exert an effect on the child. The experience of an **only child** is quite different to that of a boy or girl born into a large family. The only child will:

- be more in the company of adults rather than other individuals nearer in age. This can mean that experiences can be very different than children who have the day-to-day company of other children. The attitude of the parents to their only child will also need to be considered.
- be likely to have more possessions to call his own. Money spent on toys, clothes and educational activities will be entirely his and not shared.
- have more privacy. Not for the only child a shared bedroom, but one entirely to herself to behave in as she pleases. This in later childhood when it becomes necessary to share can cause difficulties.
- have no cut-and-thrust of sibling rivalry. All parenting energies will be theirs alone.
- have no responsibility in later childhood for looking after younger brothers or sisters. The effects of this may well be felt much later in life when they become a parent. Skills in caring for younger children, however rudimentary, can be imprinted early in life and come to the surface much later when necessary.

There are both advantages and disadvantages in being an only child. Nevertheless this chance of birth will undoubtedly have some effect on the child's development and later personality.

Psychological research has come up with some personality traits in children of differing family position. These are by no means cut and dried for every child , but merely tendencies that have been noted when a large number of children have been studied with regard to their position in the family.

- **Only children** tend to always relate better to adults than to their own age group.
- **First children** often do better academically than their younger brothers and sisters, but are more prone to emotional problems.
- **Second children** tend to pursue more unconventional careers, and have an easier-going attitude to life than first-born children.
- Being the **middle child** of three can also have a special effect. For this child there is none of the status or responsibility of being the oldest – or only – child, nor yet any of the 'perks', or excuses for unusual behaviour, often accorded to the youngest of the family. There is more chance that this child will exhibit difficult or unusual behaviour in an attempt to establish a position for himself in the family. How this is done will depend very much upon the personality of the child – some middle children being quiet and withdrawn or, at the opposite extreme, exhibiting downright bad behaviour.
- **Twins** (or triplets or members of a larger group of simultaneous births) can also exhibit different developmental characteristics. The development of language in twins, for example, is often slower than in singleton children. Twins often have a language of their own and communicate on a daily basis to each other alone – they see little need to learn the language of the everyday world!
- **Stepchildren** in today's climate of divorce and remarriage can also exert profound effects on the development of the children concerned. Without doubt divorce and separation does have an effect on children of all ages, as recent research has shown. Remarriage with, in many cases, the coming together of two groups of similarly aged children can mean yet a further adjustment to be made. The way in which parents handle the needs of the children in these reconstituted families will have much to do with the success of the settling down process. There is a National Stepfamily Association which can give advice (see Appendix).

Whilst discussing the effects on development of different family positions it must be remembered that the arrival of a new baby can also temporarily upset smooth ongoing development. Unless carefully handled, this event can be seen as the 'arrival of a rival'! Behaviour patterns can alter, and the hitherto placid child can become difficult and demanding, with temper tantrums high on the daily agenda. Skills previously learned can also appear to be forgotten. For example, a 3-year-old who was previously dry during the day can revert to wetting again.

Adequate preparation before the birth of the baby, around the actual birth date and the subsequent introduction to the new brother or sister will do much to reduce problems to a minimum.

Children are adaptable and resilient young people, but nevertheless different developmental profiles can be seen against the changing family backgrounds.

Student exercise

In your place of work experience, or in a clinic or nursery you visit, find out which children, noting their gender, are only children or the middle one of three children. From this information, and using a spreadsheet package, print a pie chart showing the numbers as percentages of the total number of children. Record the ways in which children from different family backgrounds relate to other children. Prepare a guideline, that could be given to a playgroup helper, on how a diffident withdrawn child can be encouraged to play.

Discussion

A study team is required to produce a working paper for professional child carers to help children come to terms with traumatic situations involving their parents. As a member of the team, prepare by reading various articles on the subject, noting the essence of the article and details about it, e.g. title, author, date, source. The team then meets to consider the traumatic effects on children of:
- quarrelling parents;
- divorcing or divorced parents;
- belonging to a new re-constituted family;
- the significance of these effects on the child's development.

From this discussion the team then goes on to produce the working paper.

Economic factors

Closely involved with the position of the child in the family are economic factors. Children cost money, and even with the two incomes of many families today, money worries are still paramount.

Working mothers

Working mothers are commonplace today but in the mid-twentieth century this state was almost unheard of for mothers with young children. Children as young as eight weeks will need to be taken to a child-minder or crèche each day whilst both parents work outside the home. Whilst this is not necessarily disadvantageous, the child's development will proceed along different lines than if he, or she, were at home with their natural mothers all day during the early years.

The need for adequately trained child-minders and nursery staff is highlighted by this social change. They will bear a large part of the responsibility for providing a suitable environment for the children in their care to develop their full potential.

For many families, mortgage repayments or high rents will mean little money available for extra possessions, toys, clothes or excursions. Budgeting and balancing the needs of all members of the family can be hard, and especially so if there are a number of children in the family all with different and expensive needs.

Nutrition

Diet is of vital importance in the growing years, and here again economic factors will play a part. Quick, starchy 'fill-up' food is cheaper than the ingredients of a balanced diet, and many families can be forced into this situation by economic factors. Whilst malnutrition has to be extreme to exert an immediately noticeable effect on development, lack of a reasonable breakfast, for example, can cause school-age children to be tired and unable to benefit fully from their lessons.

Housing

Economic factors can also have a bearing on housing. Buying or renting a house or flat is one of the largest drains on a family's income. Many children will have the disadvantage of living in damp, overcrowded conditions with little room for play in the early years. Experience of the outside world is limited if the outlook is only the four walls of a single room. This will undoubtedly have an effect on the child's development.

Home environment

Home environment this important aspect has close links with economic and family size factors, as well as where the child spends a large part of his waking hours. Into this equation, too, will come the ability of the parents to make the home – however needy in the goods of the world – a happy, safe, welcoming place in which to develop.

Cultural background

This has a profound effect on development. In the UK there is a wide range of cultural practices all having their effects on the children who spend much of their time together in crèches, nurseries or schools.

Educational expectations of parents

Education does not begin at school age, but from the very early weeks of life. The way parents interact with their young baby is an educative process in itself. As the baby grows into a toddler, the toys bought for him are all part of his education. Later attendance at playgroup or nursery school is an excellent preparation for later formal schooling.

All these preschool activities will need the cooperation of the parents, both to initiate them and to ensure that their child obtains the maximum benefit. Much time and effort is needed to take children back and forward from the many educational activities that are available.

Financial considerations, proximity of facilities and travel arrangements all play a part in the preschool educative process. A few parents will not see any benefit in these preschool activities. For them education begins at four or five years of age when attendance at primary school is mandatory. But with encouragement from health professionals concerned with the care of the preschool child they can often be persuaded of the benefits to their child.

Student exercise

You are visiting a family who have two children aged two and three years of age. You arrive in the middle of an argument between the mother and the father about whether or not to send the 3-year-old to a local nursery school. The father insists that it is not necessary: 'I never went to play school – and look at me!' The mother is insistent that the 3-year-old will benefit. Write up a list of the various points that could be made to help the family resolve their differences, with reasons for your choice.

Health

Health during childhood can have an effect on development. As well as congenital conditions present since birth, serious infections during the early years of childhood can also hinder development. Even comparatively minor illnesses such as one of the infectious diseases of childhood or repeated respiratory infections can have temporary effects. Also any hospital admission necessary for various health problems can exert a temporary delaying effect on development.

Depending on the type and severity, congenital conditions can have severe and long-lasting effects. Children with severe defects from birth will need much loving care and attention, possibly for many years, to be sure development proceeds as far as is possible within the bounds of their disability.

Many of the illnesses contracted in later childhood – with a few serious exceptions – give rise to a temporary halt in development. Children are resilient and will soon make up lost ground.

Congenital conditions

These are conditions with which a baby is born. They can be genetically inherited conditions such a haemophilia or cystic fibrosis. Illness of the mother during her pregnancy can cause her baby to be born with a physical or a mental problem. An attack of rubella during pregnancy in a woman who is not immune to this infection is probably the most well-known example of this. (Fortunately today this form of congenital problem is rare due to widespread immunization against this infection.) Other viral illnesses during pregnancy, such as toxoplasmosis or a severe attack of influenza, can also damage the unborn baby. Good antenatal care is vital for monitoring the health of women and their babies during the nine months of pregnancy.

Illness during the early years of childhood

The vast majority of illness in previously healthy children are the many and varied types of infection. These infections are all a necessary part of growing-up. It is only by acquiring, and overcoming, infection with the viruses and bacteria that continually surround us that immunity is built up.

Many of the previously inevitable infections of childhood, such as measles, mumps, rubella or whooping cough, are now relatively infrequent owing to the routine immunization programmes for all young children. Of the previously common infections of childhood only chickenpox is still seen with any degree of frequency. This is usually only a mild disease in children (but often more serious when an adult is affected) and development is rarely slowed as a result of the illness.

Other more serious infections, such as meningitis, can affect development adversely. In the very worst scenario this infection can cause brain damage with permanent cessation or regression of development. With less severe infections there can be a temporary halt in development, but on recovery the child will soon catch up on skills again.

Immunization against one particular form of meningitis – caused by the *Haemophilus influenzae* bacteria (HiB) – is given routinely early in babyhood. Children under the age of four years are particularly susceptible to meningitis caused by this particular organism. This infection is only one of the organisms that can cause meningitis, so the possibility of meningitis due to other organisms must always be remembered when a child is unwell.

Admission to hospital

This is always a worrying occurrence for parents, not least because it usually mean serious health problems.

The very earliest effects of hospitalization can occur when a baby – born prematurely or sick – needs intensive care in a neonatal unit. This environment, with the added probability of uncomfortable or even painful interventions, is far removed from the warmth and comfort of prenatal existence. It is also not the environment that a mother would choose for her newborn baby. Little opportunity is available for cuddles and speech stimulation to cement the bonding process of mother and baby. Problems can be counteracted by:

- involving parents as far as is possible in the care of their infant;
- providing, again as far as is possible, a homely environment with toys, patterned sheets and other comforting stimuli;
- keeping a continuity of nursing staff involved in the care of the baby since babies as young as ten days old can be seen to benefit from care being given by the same person.

Much care will need to be taken when the baby returns home to ensure good bonding. If hospitalization is necessary later on in childhood, it is important that adequate preparation of the child before admission is sensitively given. (This, of course, will not be possible if the admission is an emergency one due to an accident or sudden illness. Under these conditions even greater care will be needed by all staff concerned to be sure that the child feels as secure as possible in the strange environment.)

There are a number of useful books available on hospitals that mothers can look at with their child who has to be admitted to hospital for a routine surgical procedure, for example. 'Acting out' medical and nursing roles with a young friend can also be helpful for an older child.

Many paediatric wards encourage pre-admission visits so that the child can relate to the staff who will be caring for him and get to know general lay-out of the ward. (Information on admission to hospital is also taken as a kind of 'road-show' into playgroups and nursery schools by play therapists attached to hospital wards or child development centres.)

It is a rule rather than an exception that mothers are admitted together with their child to hospital. Providing care can be organized for any other children in the family, parents are encouraged to stay and help in the care of their child throughout the time they are in hospital. Visiting times are also extensive so that other members of the family can keep in touch. The young patient will feel far less isolated if he can hear at first hand from brothers or sisters of events at home. If an anaesthetic is necessary for any procedure parents are encouraged to be with their child right up until the time he loses consciousness.

All-in-all, hospital admission for a child should not be such a frightening event as for children in bygone days. In spite of this, however, hospitalization can lead to a temporary halt in development. (It is hard to distinguish, of course, between the effects of the original illness and the hospitalization process.)

Long stay hospitalization for serious chronic disease will have different, potentially more damaging, effects. Under these conditions hospital staff, parents and other carers will need to work closely together to minimize these effects.

Student exercise

Find out as much as you can about facilities for children in your local hospital and how much parents are integrated into the care of their child whilst in hospital. (If possible try and get one of the paediatricians or nurses to talk to the group.) Also get copies of any leaflets available for parents to read prior to their child's admission from the local hospital and any others that you can find. Prepare a suitable booklet, incorporating your ideas, for the family of a child going into hospital including a list of books which will help a 3–4-year-old child understand what will happen to him in hospital.

UNDERSTANDING CHILD DEVELOPMENT

Child development is ongoing, and generally proceeds smoothly along definite lines, unless events decree otherwise, but for the sake of convenience, and so that a certain degree of standardization can be reached, development is checked out at certain predetermined ages. At these times most children will be developmentally in line with the criteria laid down for each specific age. By these specific checks any weakness in a particular area of development is discovered and help given to the child to remedy this. (It is often found that at rechecking the particular skill a week or two later, the child has already taken the necessary developmental leap on his own!)

The ages at which routine checks are generally done are:

- nine months;
- two and half years;
- four and a half to five years.

At each of these ages, the four main areas of development (as already described for the routine six-week check) are assessed. Physical reviews of height, weight and overview of general health are also done at these times. Of course, if there are thought to be any developmental or physical problems at times other then these specific ones, further investigations will need to be done.

For ease of description, these areas – physical skills, vision and associated fine movements, hearing and speech, and social and emotional development – will be discussed separately over the span of the early years. It must be remembered, however, that all development is proceeding in parallel.

Before this we shall look at the rate of actual physical growth that can be expected over these first actively growing and developing years of life.

Weight gain is at its greatest during the first six months of life, when a weight increase of 150–180 g (5–6 oz) a week is the norm. Never again will a child routinely put on so much weight. By one year the average weight gain is around 60–90 g (2–3 oz) per week. (As a rough rule-of-thumb guide to weight gain, a baby will double her birth weight by six months, and treble it by one year.) During the second year, only 28–57 g (1–2 oz) are gained weekly. After this age weight is measured at less frequent intervals.

Height increases along the same lines as does weight. Gain in height is often a more reliable indicator of normal growth than weight gain, which can be more dependant on episodes of ill-health with associated loss of appetite.

Height can vary greatly in children of the same chronological age, and is dependant on many factors which include:

- **Genetic factors**. Short parents will usually have short children, and tall parents tall children. (Final adult height can be roughly predicted from centile charts as well as from simple arithmetical calculations, described elsewhere.) Other genetic factors will also exert their effect on height. For example, children with Down's syndrome or Turner's syndrome will always be shorter than normal.
- **Hormonal effects** such as untreated defective thyroid function or growth hormone deficiency.

- **Gross malnutrition** can affect height although, of course, lack of weight gain will be obvious much sooner under these circumstances.
- Similarly, **long-term illness** will affect height. Short periods of illness will not have this effect, in fact children who have had an acute infection often appear to have shot upwards during the course of their illness.
- Children under **severe stress** can also show a slowing of upward growth. This measurement can provide one clue – along with other signs – of the possibility of child abuse.

The centile charts, recorded over the years, give valuable information regarding the rate of growth (both weight and height). As long as this rate is proceeding along the initial line (be it the 25th, 50th or 90th centile) there need be no worries regarding physical growth. It is when one of these measurements – weight or height – deviates over a number of months from the previous pattern that there is need for concern. Advice from a paediatrician should then be sought so that any problems can be sorted out and treated. (The Child Growth Foundation [see Appendix] also gives general and specific advice and help on growth problems.)

Differences in height from their peers can have psychological effects on children, and adults caring for children should be aware of this. Effects are probably more obvious on short children, but remember also that tall children can feel out of place. It can be all too easy to overestimate a tall child's abilities and conversely underestimate those of a short child. (Perhaps the problems that can be experienced by tall children are less obvious, but they are often expected to be more 'grown-up' than their developmental age.) It is important to remember to check on both chronological age and developmental levels when assessing each individual child's abilities.

Student exercise

Measure the height and weight of two or three children in a nursery. (Remember to get permission to do this.) Plot the results on a centile chart and predict how tall each child will be at the age of eight years.

Finally, two further facts in the study of physical growth is the difference in **body proportions** which occur as the child grows. The most obvious is the difference in the head size proportional to the rest of the body as evidenced by looking at a newborn baby and at an 8-year-old child. The head of a newborn baby is one-quarter of his length whilst at eight years the head is only one-eighth of the full height.

Similarly **leg development** varies as the child grows older. When he begins to walk at around 18 months he is very definitely bow-legged. At three to five years this alters so that at this age children often appear to be knock-kneed. By eight years legs in the vast majority of children are quite straight. These – quite normal – aspects of growth can be a great source of worry to parents.

Development of physical abilities

As with all aspects of development there is no one particular d
even month when certain skills will be attained. Each child is u
will develop according to his or her own particular pattern. Neve
is usual for children to gain most skills within a week or two of the average'
age of attainment.

The newborn baby, as we have seen, is able to move his limbs, body and
head. These movements are reflex in character (automatic movement is
response to certain stimuli), the baby having very little voluntary control
over these movements. Over the first few months of life these reflexes
disappear and definite voluntary – although as yet uncoordinated – movements begin to take their place. Large wide-ranging movements using the
bigger muscles of the body occur before the finer movements of hands and
feet. This virtually means that control of the back and head muscles must
occur before limbs come under voluntary control.

Three months

By three months of age the baby will have:

- a fair degree of control of his head. When pulled up into a sitting
  position, his head will not lag behind as it did in the newborn period.
  Nevertheless control is still precarious as is seen by a definite 'wobble'
  when the head is unsupported for any length of time.
- the ability to move his head briefly in either direction. This is directly
  due to the strengthening of the muscles around his shoulders and
  neck.
- the ability to lift his head momentarily up from the floor if he is laid
  prone on his tummy. He will also be attempting to push himself up with
  his arms, but, as yet, having limited success with this task.
- the ability to take a little of the weight of his body on his legs when held
  in the upright position.

Much interest in **hand movements** is noticeable at this age. Babies will
spend much of their waking time in examining closely the movements of
their own hands. If an object is placed deliberately into her hands at this
age, she will grasp this for a few minutes only and then loosen it. Contrast
this with the firm and continuing 'grasp reflex' of the newborn. Uncoordinated swinging with the hands at various objects are also a noticeable
feature at this age.

Six months

At six months of age and the baby is able to:

- raise her head to look around when lying on her back;
- have complete head control when in a sitting position and be able to
  quite deliberately turn her head to look around;
- lift both head and chest off the ground on raised arms;
- sit upright with the support of cushions in pram or chair;
- enjoy taking weight on her legs when bounced up and down.

Within a very few weeks she will be able to roll over from her back onto her front. Dangers can arise at this stage as rolling off beds or settee is a distinct possibility.

One year
At one year he will:
- be sitting unsupported for relatively long periods of time. He is also able to stretch out sideways for toys without falling over in the attempt.
- probably be crawling with great rapidity. Some babies, however, miss out on this crawling stage altogether and get up and walk straight away from a sitting position. Others shuffle around on their bottoms – again with great rapidity – before walking. Yet others are walking with one hand being held at this age.

Walking is an attained skill having a very variable time span. Some children are walking at nine months whilst others are still firmly sitting down or crawling only at 15 months. There is no cause for concern about late walkers; in fact this skill does often seem to follow a family pattern if previous generations were walking late. If, however, there is no attempt to walk at 18 months of age, it is advisable to seek advice.

Hand movements will have improved greatly and a 'pincer' grip – holding objects between finger and thumb – will have developed. Objects will also be dropped voluntarily onto the floor. (These two aspects of hand control can be seen from around nine months onwards.) Pointing at a desired object is also much in evidence at this age.

Two years
By two years of age the child:
- can kick at a ball without falling over;
- can walk up and down stairs with two feet to each step;
- is able to feed herself and to drink from a cup;
- is able to put on her own shoes and certain other articles of clothing;
- is able to climb on furniture to look out of the window;
- can reach an object on a high table.

Hand control has developed enormously and the child is now able to practise many fine movements with her hands, such as unwrapping sweets, picking up a pin, pulling down door handles and unscrewing lids. With a pencil she will be scribbling in circles and is able to build a tower of six bricks.

All these extra skills mean, of course, that extra special care needs to be taken to ensure that accidents do not occur as a result of climbing or opening doors and jars, for example.

Three years
At three years of age a child can:
- walk upstairs with one foot on each step, but will still need two feet on each stair coming down;

- stand on one foot, but still find the concept of hopping difficult;
- thread beads and build a tower of eight bricks.

Five years

By five years of age physical skills have again increased enormously. Most children can dress and undress without help, can eat skilfully with a knife and fork, can run and jump with ease, swing on a swing and enjoy to the full all the activities of a playground.

By this time **handedness** will have developed: children are seen to be either right-handed or left-handed. Many will have decided which hand will be their dominant one by the age of three and some even earlier.

Student exercise

Draw up a table showing the relationship of hand control to age, from birth to five years of age. (Check the validity of your table by observations on children in a nursery.)

Most children are right-handed, but around 10% of boys and slightly fewer girls will be left-handed. An even smaller number can use either hand with equal ease and so are said to be ambidextrous.

In a predominantly right-handed world, left-handers can have problems in later life with certain pieces of equipment and sports gear designed for right-handed people. It is unwise, however, to attempt to force a child, who is showing a definite predilection for his left hand, to draw and write with the other hand. It is preferable to show him techniques to help in adapting his left-handedness to a right-handed world. Writing can pose problems initially, and teachers should be made aware of their new pupil's hand preference when school is begun. (The Left Centre [see Appendix] can give advice for left-handed children.)

Student exercise

Observe at your place of work experience the different ages at which children attain a certain skill. Note how each skill is preceded by an earlier developmental stage. Summarize and tabulate this information.

Along with this general development of physical skills, height and weight are also increasing along a steady line. Other physical changes, such as the eruption of teeth, and abilities, such as toileting, have also been under way and been successfully accomplished by the time the child is five years old.

Anatomical development

Teeth

Most babies are born without teeth, although very occasionally a baby is born with one or two teeth already erupted. The teeth, both first and second set, are already present in the jaw at birth. They then erupt in a definite pattern mainly during the first two years of life. The first set – the 'milk' teeth – are 20 in number. They usually begin to erupt around the age of six months. The pattern is usually that the two teeth in the middle of the lower jaw erupt first, followed a few weeks later by the two teeth in the middle of the upper jaw. As with everything there are exceptions to this pattern, some children cutting teeth either side of the midline first. In spite of a number of old wives' tales about this, no problems with either teeth or jaw will result from this different pattern of eruption. The remainder of the teeth erupt over the next two and a half years, ending with the back premolar teeth at around two and a half to three years. Figure 5.4 shows the normal timing of eruption together with the names of each specific tooth.

Figure 5.4 First set of teeth – the milk teeth.

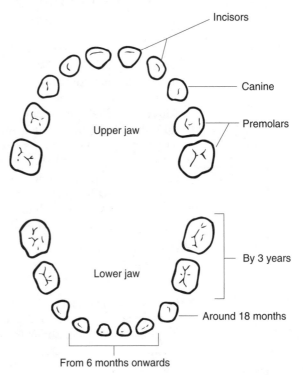

At around five to six years of age these milk teeth will begin to loosen and fall out. They will be replaced within a very short time by the permanent set of teeth. These will be in the same positions as the milk teeth with the addition of three large molar teeth on each side of both jaws, making up 32 in all. Normally the first teeth of the permanent set to appear are the first molars – often referred to as the 6-year-old molars.

Teething problems

Much is written about and handed down from generation to generation regarding the problems associated with teething. But it must be remembered that teething is a perfectly natural process, and many babies cut their teeth with no difficulties whatsoever. There are, however, a few signs and symptoms that can alert parents to the eruption of a new tooth:

- an **increase in dribbling** is often noticed;
- a **red flush** on one cheek on the side of the jaw where a new tooth is coming through;
- babies **chewing on their hands** more frequently when they are teething;
- **gums red and swollen** just prior to the eruption of a tooth;
- the baby will **dislike the feel of a spoon** in his mouth.

(NB It must be noted that teething does NOT cause bronchitis, diarrhoea, convulsions, a rash or any other illness. These conditions may, of course, coexist with the onset of teething, but they must be diagnosed and treated appropriately, and not just put down to 'teething'.)

Help for teething includes letting the baby chew on hard crusts or a teething ring, plenty of love and attention and a mild analgesic at night if the child seems to be in pain. If the pain appears to be severe, medical help should be obtained, but this is rare.

Care of teeth

It is never too early to begin to care for children's teeth. As soon as a tooth has erupted, it can be cleaned with a cotton bud. This will gradually accustom the child to tooth cleaning. From the age of around one year a small toothbrush is needed, and teeth should be brushed regularly. As they mature children should be taught how to brush teeth properly – up-and-down as well as making sure that the backs of the teeth are cleaned adequately.

Sweet, sticky foods should be reduced to a minimum. The end of a meal is a good time to allow a sweet, and this can then be followed by tooth cleaning. The worst scenario is a constant supply of sweets or sweet drinks throughout the day. Sugary substances continually in the mouth react with the bacteria that are always present and attack the enamel causing decay.

The pros and cons of fluoride rumble on through the years, but it has been conclusively proved that fluoride does help to protect the teeth against decay. If the normal water supply is low in fluoride (and this does vary in different parts of the country) fluoride drops or tablets can be given to good effect. Brushing the teeth with a fluoride toothpaste also helps protect against decay. Special coatings are also now available in dental surgeries which virtually eliminate decay.

Visits to the dentist can usefully begin from the age of three years onwards. This will ensure that the child becomes used to having her teeth examined. Treatment today is very child-orientated, and children are rarely frightened by a visit to the dentist if this aspect of health care is carefully handled. Ongoing dental visits throughout childhood are necessary to ensure that as well as controlling decay, teeth erupt correctly and in a straight manner. Overcrowded, or crooked teeth, will need to be treated orthodontically.

Eyes

Development of vision

The development of vision and the ability to perform fine hand movements are closely associated. The **newborn baby** is able to see, but can probably only distinguish light, darkness and vague shapes and patterns. He will also be aware of movement around him. His range of definitive vision is only around 20–25 cm (8–10 in.) so that objects – and his mother's face – will need to be within this distance for him to be visually aware. When mothers breast, or bottle, feed their babies, her face will be at just the right distance to be within her baby's focus. The baby's usual attention span at this early stage will be very short – a few seconds only – but as the weeks progress, he will be seen gazing intently at his mother's face during feed times. As the weeks and months progress he will take more interest in shapes and patterns than plain solid objects.

At this age – and up to around three months – a baby's eyes can be seen to squint at times. This is a normal finding during these early days, but should be checked if it persists after three to four months of age.

By **three months** the focusing range has increased, although objects and people the other side of the room will not be seen clearly. The baby will be able – and willing – to move his eyes in response to people or objects coming within his range of vision. When awake, he will also spend much time examining the movements of his own hands.

By **six months** of age the baby will be responding visually to movements across the room. She will be moving her head to different positions to see what is happening around her.

By **one year** rapidly moving objects can be tracked with the eyes, and familiar people will be recognized as they come into the room.

By **two and a half years** of age children are visually competent, and are beginning to show an awareness of colour. This facility in distinguishing colour gradually improves over the succeeding years.

By **five years** of age at least four or five colours can be competently distinguished. At this time it is possible to check broadly for defects in colour vision, although further improvement in colour detection will continue over the next two years.

Student exercise

Use a computer package to design a mobile for:
* a 3-month-old baby;
* a 2-year-old child.

Place emphasis on the differences requirements in each of these models.

Potential problems associated with visual development

- **Blindness**. This tragic event is fortunately rare: about one in 10 000 babies are born with no vision, and approximately three or four in 10 000 have some partial visual loss. It is important that the lack of vision, and its severity, should be diagnosed as soon as possible. For some types of blindness, such as congenital cataracts (clouding of the lens of the eye), help can be given to save some vision. Some babies with severe defective vision will have other developmental and physical abnormalities as part of a recognizable syndrome. It is also important that this is recognized so that early help can be given.

  Absent or reduced vision will have knock-on effects on other fields of development. Blind children are unable to use vision to watch and imitate or reach out for objects in their immediate environment; they are unable to move around so readily when crawling and walking. These children and their parents will need much help and encouragement throughout the growing years. (See Chapter 10 for further information.)

- **Squints**. A squinting eye is a normal phenomenon up to the age of three months. After this time, and certainly by the age of six months, babies that are still squinting (often referred to as a 'turn' or 'cast' in the eye) should be referred to an ophthalmologist.

There are a number of different types of squints:

- a turning inwards of one eye – a 'convergent' squint;
- a turning outward of one eye – a 'divergent' squint;
- vertical or oblique squints in which one or both eyes are tilted upwards or obliquely;
- alternating squints where both eyes alternate in moving into a squinting position. Here only one eye at a time is used to make eye contact at any one time. (This type of squint can be difficult to treat.)

The first two types of squints are most commonly seen. Treatment consists of:

- orthoptic exercises;
- wearing of appropriate glasses;
- 'patching' of the 'good' eye;
- surgery.

A mixture of all four methods is often used.

If a squint is not treated, vision will eventually be lost in this eye due to lack of use. This condition is known as 'amblyopia' and is irreversible if left for untreated too long.

- **Colour vision defects**. Colour blindness is an hereditary condition which affects around 8–10% of boys. Girls are very rarely affected, only about 0.4% being the reported figure. The most usual type of colour defect is the inability to distinguish between red and green. This can obviously give rise to difficulties during schooldays unless the problem is recognized. Also, later, careers must be chosen carefully.

Student exercise

Prepare a handout for the parents of a red/green colour blind child showing:
- possible difficulties and ways that they can be overcome, during school days;
- the careers from which people with a colour vision problem are precluded.

(Your local careers officer will be able to help.)

- **Short and long sight**. Short sight is when near objects are seen clearly whilst objects at a distance appear blurred. Long sight is the opposite; near objects are blurred whilst distant ones are clear.

  Short sight is the most common of these minor abnormalities of vision, and children can develop short sight fairly rapidly particularly between the ages of six and 10 years. This can give rise to problems with seeing objects the other side of the classroom clearly unless the condition is accurately diagnosed and appropriate glasses prescribed.

  Long sight – although less common – can cause the child to be labelled lazy, when in reality he is having difficulty in seeing his written work clearly. Here again, appropriate glasses will overcome this problem.

  There appears to be a familial tendency for both long and short sight.

- **Astigmatism**. This is the condition that occurs when the lens of the eye is not completely smooth. Objects will look crooked or out of shape when viewed through the misshapen part of the lens.

Children with an astigmatism will often be seen to be looking at objects with their head tilted to one side in an endeavour to straighten out the visual image. Spectacles will be necessary in severe cases to correct the misalignment of the lens.

Potential visual problems
- Blindness
- Squint
- Colour vision defect
- Long/short sight
- Astigmatism

Hearing

Hearing and speech are closely linked, normal speech being dependent on normal hearing.

As with vision it is vitally important that any hearing difficulties are discovered early in life so that immediate and appropriate help can be given.

Babies are thought to be able to hear before birth, and this is borne out by the experience of many mothers. They are aware that sudden loud noises cause their babies to startle and move rapidly. Soft rhythmical music can also be successful in soothing an overactive baby – when his mother needs some sleep, for example!

A **newborn baby** can certainly hear. He is soothed by his mother's quiet voice and will also be quietened by soft rhythmical sounds such as quietly sung lullabies. He will startle at banging doors and other sudden loud noises.

It must be remembered that prenatally the unborn baby was subjected to a barrage of sounds (his mother's rhythmical heart beat, the gurglings of her digestive processes, her regular breathing as well as many external noises that will filter through to the uterus). So, in one sense, perfect quiet is an unnatural situation for the newborn baby.

By **three months** of age, the baby will quieten at the sound of his mother's voice even though she is outside his range of vision.

By **seven months** of age formal testing of hearing is possible, the baby being able to discriminate sounds of differing frequencies as they are presented to each ear in turn. (The giving of these tests is an art that has to be learned carefully. The baby must not be able to obtain any clues – by vision or smell – that someone is standing behind him. Even a faint perfume can alert him to the tester and cause him to turn his head, not in response to the sound but to see what it is that smells so nice. Also the level of sound given must always be consistent.)

There are other, more sophisticated tests of hearing which can be done if there is any doubt following a simple routine test or, of course, if the mother is concerned about her baby's hearing or if there is a strong family history of deafness.

By **one year** the child will respond to his or her own name as well as other words that are recognized.

It is vitally important for the development of speech that any deafness – of any degree of severity – is recognized. Deafness can be due to a number of causes, and can be complete or partial, permanent or temporary. (For further details on deafness, see Chapter 10.)

Student exercise

Make arrangements to attend a Child Health Clinic when hearing tests are being done. Make notes on:
- the different frequencies of sounds that are being used;
- the way in which the results of the test are recorded;
- what action is taken if there is thought to be a hearing problem.

Speech
Speech is an all-important aspect of human existence. By speech thoughts and ideas are communicated, actions planned, problems solved and help given.

Assuming that hearing is normal, speech development follows a definitive pattern in every child. As with all developmental stages, the timing of each stage varies from child to child, and each stage is attained within a certain time period. It is when a particular stage is not reached within the usual time limit that further investigation is needed.

Prespeech methods of communication

From the very early days of life babies try to communicate. They have a number of ways of expressing their needs, and parents soon become adept at interpreting these.

- **Crying**. From the moment of birth onwards babies cry. This act initially expands the lungs and makes the lifelong exchange of oxygen and carbon dioxide through these organs possible. (Before birth, of course, the lungs were not involved in this process, the baby gaining oxygen from the mother's blood via the placenta.) As the weeks progress, the crying becomes more selective. Mothers will soon be able to distinguish between the hungry cry, the cry of pain and the 'I'm lonely' cry as well as the small whimperings of a baby about to drop off to sleep.
- **Vocalizations**. Gurgling and cooing become more obvious ways of expressing pleasure and comfort over the succeeding weeks. These vocalizations all play a part in the practice of formalizing words.
- **Facial** expressions. From around six weeks on, babies will be smiling in response to adult speech and actions. Expressions of sadness, bewilderment and contentment pass fleetingly across a baby's face as he becomes more and more aware of cause and effect between his actions and what is happening to his body.
- **Eye contact**. From very early days babies study their mother's face intently as they are fed.
- **Gesture**. Later, as more control is gained over hands, more and more use is made of gesture – pulling away, pushing and later, pointing at desired objects.

Many of these methods of communication will be used throughout life. They will eventually form part of an individual's 'body language' and used in everyday communication skills.

Speech development

This is probably the developmental profile in which there is the greatest variation in timing. Some children will be well ahead in talking whilst others are seen to romp ahead with other – usually more physical – aspects of development. As a general rule – although, as ever, there are always exceptions – girls learn to speak earlier than boys do.

There are a number of reasons why the development of speech can be delayed.

- There can be a familial tendency to be later than usual in acquiring speech, as indeed can occur in any aspect of child development.
- Deafness can be an important cause of speech delay. It is important to remember that profoundly deaf babies will initially coo, gurgle and babble. It is when the normal pattern of speech development ceases at the babbling stage that possible deafness, if not already diagnosed , must be investigated.
- Damage to, or lack of normal development of, parts of the body concerned with speech and communication will cause problems. For example, a child with cerebral palsy will have difficulty in controlling the

Later d

muscles necessary for speech; a child with a cleft palate a will also have initial problems with the acquisition of clear specialized help is given.

- Lack of stimulation in talking to babies from the very earlies – the baby who is never spoken to and whose babblings are never replied to – will not encourage a baby to improve his communication skills. It is vitally important for the proper development of speech that babies and young children are encouraged to talk – and be talked to – at every possible opportunity. Some young mothers need encouragement to talk to their babies when, as yet, there is no response forthcoming. They feel shy at appearing to talk to themselves!

Delayed speech can be due to:

- Familial tendency
- Deafness
- Lack of normal development
- Lack of stimulation
- Emotional problems
- Cultural differences
- More than one language spoken

- Emotional problems, such as fear or excessive shyness, can also give rise to speech delay. Regrettably, child abuse must never be forgotten as a possible cause of speech delay.
- Other serious conditions, such as autism, can also be possible causes.
- Cultural factors can at times also give rise to speech delay or confusion. Children growing up in households where two languages are in everyday use can initially have some speech delay. Usually within a year or two, however, children living under these circumstances will be found to be fluent in both languages.

Mostly, normal patterns of speech development will be seen:

- **Newborn babies** communicate by crying. As previously described, different types of cry for differing circumstances will become apparent over the first few weeks and months of life.
- By **three months** the baby is beginning to exert control over the facial and lip muscles that are necessary for speech. He will be gurgling and using sounds that are the beginnings of babble. He is also aware of communicating with his carers, and will be beginning to try to make imitative noises.
- By **nine months** communication skills will have improved dramatically, and she will be chuckling and laughing during play – and also shouting or screaming when frustrated! She is learning – fast – that certain sounds have desired responses. It is important for parents and carers, at this stage of speech and language development, to respond to attempts at communication so that speech patterns are reinforced. Also at this age, many babies are using repetitive sounds such as 'mum-mum', 'dad-dad', although probably without definite meaning at this age.
- By **one year** many familiar words are understood – the names of family members, everyday objects around the house connected with day-to-day activities. Simple commands, accompanied by appropriate movements and gestures, such as 'Wave bye-bye', 'Clap your hands', will be understood and happily followed. At this age frequent use of words and associated actions will do much to extend understanding of language and expressive speech.
- At **18 months** of age words are being added almost daily to the child's vocabulary. Around 20 words are used with the correct meaning and many more are understood. She will be talking to herself almost contin-

ually, mainly in a repetitive babble, but with an increasing number of recognizable words. This is the age when nursery rhymes with their repetitively tuneful sounds are popular and also of value in the development of speech. Picture books, with an adult pointing out objects relevant to the story, are also much enjoyed. A further useful activity is naming and pointing out various parts of the body: mouth, nose, ears etc.

- By **two years** there is a vocabulary of around 50 words, spoken with meaning. Two or more words are being joined together to make basic sentences as, for example 'Daddy go walk', 'Dog bark'. It is obvious at this age that the child's communication skills are extending beyond speech into the realm of language. (Speech and language are two entirely different concepts – speech being the physical utterance of stylized sounds, whilst language involves thought, ideas and cognitive development.) For good language development a consistent learning environment is vital. Talking about everyday activities, looking at books, pointing out unusual scenes and objects on daily walks are all important parts of the acquisition of good basic language skills. During this year vocabulary will extend markedly, and basic concepts of self-will become obvious as pronouns are used in their correct context. Much conversation is dependant on the word 'I', but other people are correctly denoted as 'you', 'she', etc.
- The **third to the fourth year** will show tremendous leaps in speech and language. Longer sentences with correct grammatical structure will be used, and by five years around 2000 words are being used and many situations are being verbalized. By the time the child attends nursery school, he will be able to make known his needs in a verbal way.

Student exercise

Talk to children of different ages at differing stages of speech and language development. Tape record these conversations and in the form of a written report for a junior colleague discuss the differences noticeable, both with different age groups and with different children of the same age.

Common minor problems
- **Articulation** (or 'pronunciation') refers to the actual physical sounding of the words. As children learn to speak they will naturally make many mistakes in this aspect of speech production. Only with continual practice and also the maturation and gradually acquired control of the muscles associated with speech, will words become clear. Common errors are:
  - substitution of 'w' for 'r' as in 'wed' for 'red';
  - substitution of 'f' for 'th' as in 'fink' for 'think';
  - substitution of 'l' for 'y' as in 'lellow' for 'yellow'.

These difficulties will, in most cases, sort themselves out so that by the time the child starts school articulation is generally clear and understandable. (Occasionally certain substitutions persist throughout life – particularly mispronunciation of the letter 'r'. Listen to the radio and note the number of broadcasters that have this difficulty!)

- **Stammering** is the frequent repetition of certain words or parts of words, allied with difficulties in proceeding with the sentence once started. This is a relatively common finding in children around the age of three years. At this age children are eager to put their thoughts into words and, as yet, verbal ability lags behind thought, and so stammering results as words are stumbled over.

  This stage is generally passed through quite quickly. If, however, parents or carers make an issue of the stammering and are continually correcting the child, he or she will become anxious, and a persistent stammer can be the result. If this occurs the help of a speech therapist should be enlisted to overcome the problem.

Social and emotional development

Social development is the learning of skills enabling an individual to live happily and successfully alongside other members of the community.

Tiny babies are completely egocentric – the world revolves around them and their needs. This, of course, is necessary in the early days for survival, but as the weeks and months pass, socialization skills appear in a regular pattern, as with all other aspects of development.

Emotional development is closely allied to social development, each being to some extent dependent on the other. For normal emotional development the child needs to:

- feel a sense of **belonging** – the feeling that he is an important and necessary member of his group in the early days of life.
- feel **loved** by parents and other family members and later by a wider group of play mates and school fellows.
- have a sense of **achievement**. This will obviously come later when skills are being attained. It is important that parents and carers should recognise achievement goals by taking an interest in all aspects of the child's daily life. For example the 'works of art' all children bring home from school and playgroup must be fully admired and given pride of place until replaced by a further offering.
- feel the **approval** of her social group. Parents should be careful to praise good efforts rather than praise the actual outcome. It must be seen that it is the trying that matters and not what is finally achieved.

Later in life it is important that the child's emotional development is continued by the acquisition of **independence** – the managing of his own life. Closely connected with this will come **self-esteem**, not pride, but the confidence to know and to use his best abilities and qualities.

Emotional development continues for many years, arguably throughout the whole of life. It is dependent upon both outside environmental factors and the child's personality or 'temperament'. (For further discussion on this aspect see Chapter 6.)

Social development proceeds along a more readily visible pattern that does emotional development:

- The **newborn baby** needs social contact right from the day of birth initially as a means of survival so that his basic needs of shelter, food, warmth and love are met. Within a very few weeks, babies will cry for no other apparent reason than that they are lonely.

- By **six weeks** babies will be smiling, crying and vocalizing in response to stimuli, both internal and external attachment to his mother – or other full-time carer – is becoming obvious. It is this interaction between parent and child that is the basis for future socialization skills. It appears that it is the quality of this interaction that is important rather than the length of time this interaction takes place. The responses given to the baby, as he attempts to communicate during the routine tasks of feeding, changing and bathing, all set the scene in the development of a positive and social relationship. At this age many babies will be 'talking back' in response to their care-giver's voice.

- By **nine months** of age, hearing and 'speech' will be so advanced that babies will be responding in a very positive way. Parents will be aware as to the wishes of their baby as he shouts and verbalizes to obtain their attention. This is the age when strangers are viewed with a certain degree of suspicion. It is wise to make sure that a familiar adult is nearby when there are comparative strangers around, for example when a grandparent visits who has not been seen for some months.

- By **one year** the child will respond readily to his own name, and will realize that he is an independent person in his own right. Familiar adults are, however, still important to him.

- At **18 months** adult actions are copied and this is the age of 'helping' with common tasks around the house. Distrust of strangers will have lessened. Yet again it appears that it is the 'quality time' that is spent with the child which is important for developing social relationships. Studies, both in kibbutzim and in other situations of child care, have suggested that it is the working parent – who only sees the child for perhaps two hours per day and so will devote all attention on the child for this time – who has most effect on social development.

- By **2 years** the clash between the child's developing independence and her need for security and reassurance can result in **temper tantrums**. Frustration at not being able to get her own way, or being unable to verbalize needs adequately will lead to a temper tantrum – screaming, kicking, lying on the floor and generally in the most public of places! Calmness and a degree of firmness is the best way to deal with this stage which will generally burn itself out as the child matures. (Ideally avoidance of situations known to provoke a tantrum is the best course to follow.) At this age the child likes to be near other children and pursuing the same or similar activities, but not to join in their play. This is known as 'parallel play' and differs from the 'solitary play' of the 1-year-old.

- At **three years** playgroup or nursery school will extend the child's social contacts. He will begin by looking on at other children, but will take a little time to join in with play.
- By **four years** of age most children will be playing in a group and joining together in a wide range of activities. Cooperation with peers alternates with arguments about activities and play materials.

  The imagination of the 4-year-old is very vivid, and long, often imaginary, stories are told when the child returns home. In some very imaginative children, imaginary playmates can appear. This can cause some problems if parents do not fully understand the imaginary nature of some of the episodes described.
- By **five years** of age, the child will understand fully the need to share and to have rules to adhere to when a game is played. They will happily join in cooperative play, such as doing crossword puzzles or games where 'turns' are to be taken.
- From **five to eight years** social skills gradually progress into the norm for the culture in which the child lives.

Learning to live together in both the family and the wider world is an ongoing social skill, and the very best ways to learn these social skills is from the adults having the day-to-day care of the child – a responsible task.

Student exercise

Choose one child at your place of work experience, and determine the developmental stage he or she has reached. Write a report on your findings suitable for presentation to a case conference covering:
- where you think the child's strengths lie;
- any weaknesses which could be helped by extra attention.

Child development is a fascinating subject covering all aspects of human activity. Each individual child develops skills at his, or her, own pace, but in accordance with an overall step-by-step pattern. When the developmental age of a child is assessed, **all** areas of development must be considered together as well as the many outside influences that can have an effect. Both strengths and weaknesses must be fully understood before individual care plans can be made for each child.

DEVELOPMENTAL ASPECTS POST-CHILDHOOD

Life is a continually changing pattern and, after the childhood years when most rapid change occurs, there are still landmarks occurring in everyone's life. These include:
- puberty;
- adolescence;
- parenthood;
- menopause.

Social play development
- Solitary play – around 1 year
- Parallel play – around 2 years
- Looking-on play – around 3 years
- Sharing play – around 4 years
- Cooperative play – around 5 years

The experiences and learning activities of the early years will all exert their effect on each stage, as well as the multitude of external factors that play a part.

Puberty

Puberty is that time of life when the boy or girl becomes sexually mature, and so able to reproduce. The age at which this occurs varies, but between 11 and 14 years is the usual timing. At around this time the secondary sexual characteristics will appear. In girls, breast development, pubic and axillary hair, the onset of menstruation and general rounding of body shape will occur. Boys will show growth of pubic, axillary – and a little later, facial – hair. The penis and scrotum will enlarge and general musculature will strengthen. Ejaculation of semen will also occur at night – the so-called 'wet dreams' of puberty.

Subtle mental and psychological changes also occur at this time. The sexes will become aware of each other – girls often being in advance of boys in this awareness. Careers will need to be chosen, and it is important that stereotyping does not occur at this age.

Adolescence

This is defined as that period of life between childhood and full adult independence. This can be a turbulent time for some youngsters, whilst others glide through the potential minefields of adolescence with relatively few problems.

Today's social climate can make adolescence a particularly stressful time, with family breakdown, strong peer and media pressures to conform to the current social norm, and the ever-present threat of drug, solvent and alcohol abuse.

Parents need courage, sensitivity and a slackening (but not total relinquishing) of guidelines to help their near-adult children through these potentially difficult years. Trust between the generations, built up over the years of childhood, is the very best inheritance any adolescent can have.

Parenthood

This will follow in the normal course of events. Often families are postponed until around the late twenties or early thirties due to both sexes concentrating on careers. Arguments both for and against this later child-bearing can be put forward. Whilst it is good to be young when children are energetic and demanding of parental energies, maturity brings added experience of life in general and, theoretically at least, better child-raising skills.

Preparation for parenthood should receive more recognition than is the norm, as the demands of babies and young children are frequently underestimated. Today's smaller families mean that children no longer have the care of younger brothers and sisters as part of the learning process. So when, later in life, a totally dependant newcomer arrives, the rapid learning of totally new skills will be necessary.

Teenage pregnancy has been an increasing part of the social scene in recent years. Many unmarried teenage mothers will now care for their babies themselves rather than put them out for adoption as was the norm in bygone days. Problems can arise and be severe for both young mothers and their children. Mothers will miss out on educational facilities and so be ill-prepared to find well-paid jobs in a difficult economic climate. They will also often feel isolated from their peer group, as the demands of their baby will preclude them from many activities.

From the child's point of view there can be development problems. Children of young unsupported mothers have been found to suffer developmental delay more frequently than other children with more conventional backgrounds. Behavioural and emotional problems are also seen to occur more often. This in turn can lead to episodes of child abuse due to multifactorial causes.

The number of **one-parent families** has also increased dramatically in recent years. It is estimated that there are around 1 million one-parent families in the UK. Again, economic and social pressures will be the lot of these families in many cases. Difficulties with child care when the parent has to go out to full-time work can be extremely burdensome financially – if, indeed, suitable care can be found at all. As well as divorce – the commonest cause for one-parent families – one-parent families can arise from death of a parent or desertion as well as children born outside marriage. (The proportion of one-parent-mother families to one-parent-father families is 6 to 1.) The effect on the children of living in a one-parent family depends very much on both economic circumstances and the reason for the situation. Children who have been exposed to much emotional stress before an acrimonious divorce will be more affected than the child whose parent has died but who still has a secure home.

Menopause

The menopause is the next 'life event' after the child-bearing years. In women this is a more definitive stage than in men. Menstruation will cease and further pregnancies are impossible after two years without menstruation. Various physical characteristics accompany the menopause: breasts often become less firm, body shape subtly alters with extra weight being distributed around hips and waist. Some women also suffer unpleasant feelings of heat – 'hot flushes' (sometimes so severe as to prevent sleep) – or crawling sensations under the skin. Others can feel irritable and tired, have a decreased libido and often have difficulties in concentration. Hormone replacement therapy (HRT), for women who are suitable for this form of treatment, can help enormously. There are also women who have virtually no problems at the menopause.

With later child-bearing years, the menopause in the mother can often clash with the turbulent adolescent years of her children, together with perhaps the care of ageing parents. A difficult scenario with which to deal for anyone!

Men tend not to have such a definite pattern in the middle years of life.

Libido tends to persist until later in life, and children can be fathered until well into the seventies. Skin will lose its elasticity – as in women – and body configuration often alters to the typical 'paunch' of middle age. Adverse physical symptoms are rarely complained of.

The way in which these post-childhood 'life events' are handled have their basis in the learning years. Ideally children will learn from their parents the best way to live through the difficult – and easy – times.

FURTHER READING

I Have Two Homes, London: Dinosaur (Harper Collins).

Davenport, G.C. (1994), *An Introduction to Child Development*, London: Collins.

Minett, P.M. (1994), *Child Care and Development*, London: John Murray.

Paul, D. (1990), *Living Left-handed*, London: Dextral Books.

Paul, D., *The Left-handed Helpline*, London: Dextral Books.

Polnay, L., and Hull, D. (1985), *Community Paediatrics*, Edinburgh: Churchill Livingstone.

6. SOCIOLOGICAL AND PSYCHOLOGICAL ASPECTS OF DEVELOPMENT

There are many aspects to child development. The straight genetic and physical aspects are perhaps the easiest to understand. To a certain extent they can be quantified and measured. It is the added effects of environment and personality and the way these influences act on each child that decide the kind of adult the young child will eventually become. In many ways, sociological factors (where in the world a child is born, the type of home he finds himself in, the colour of his skin, or, indeed, which sex the child is) can have as much effect as the genetic lines; these features are as much a game of chance as is genetic inheritance. None of us can choose the place of our birth, for example, any more than we can choose our parents.

Psychology is the study of how all these various factors act on (in our case) the developing child; how one particular child will behave under given circumstances; how and maybe why the next child will behave differently. The *Shorter Oxford English Dictionary* defines psychology as: 'the science of the nature, function and phenomena of the human . . . mind'. A further definition (from *Essential Psychology* by G.C. Davenport) is: 'Psychology is the study of human (and other animal) behaviour and human experience'.

An interface between psychology and other aspects of child development can be seen right from the early days of life. For example, even young babies react in different ways to the same type of stimulus. These differing reactions continue throughout life, but they are especially important in the early years when characters are being moulded and different reactions to various life events are being learned.

For ease of explanation, the psychological effects on child development will be discussed in three main sections:
- social and emotional development and effects on personality;
- cognition and language development;
- perception, memory and learning.

Psychology is the study of human behaviour and experience.

SOCIAL, EMOTIONAL AND PERSONALITY DEVELOPMENT

OBJECTIVES

1. **Evaluate theories of attachment and understand the effects of deprivation on emotional development.**
2. **Know the theories of social, emotional and personality development and link these to behaviour at different ages.**
3. **Evaluate the influence of the child's behaviour on relationships with caring adults and family dynamics.**

Attachment and bonding

Psychologists have long discussed which has the greatest effect on the development of a child's personality and behaviour: 'nature' or 'nurture'.

Nature means the genetic inheritance the child has gained from his parents. Most parents will be able to see, at some time during the growing years, likeness to either parent, grandparents or even more distant relatives such as aunts, uncles, cousins, etc. Physical characteristics will, of course, be much in evidence, but also personality traits will be noticeable. Some babies are difficult from the very day of birth – slow feeders, much crying, difficult sleep patterns, for example. Even the best, most placid of mothers can find herself with a difficult baby and she can often think back to someone else in the family who has similar problems. Fortunately such early difficulties are comparatively rare, about 10% of babies being the accepted figure. Most babies are contented, sleep well and only cry when they are hungry, in pain or lonely.

Nurture refers to the effect that the wide variety of social events that the young baby experiences will have on her subsequent personality and behaviour patterns. Psychologists holding this particular view are termed 'behaviourists'; B.F. Skinner was a well-known behaviourist (see the section in this chapter on Learning).

The effects of the society, culture and standards of acceptable behaviour, dress and attitudes will, of course, all have a significant effect on the child's personality. This 'nature versus nurture' debate has occasioned much psychological research, particularly in the area of child development. How best can the child be helped to attain his full genetic potential is one of the most important queries which arise. Early attachment – or 'bonding' – is the starting point for the study of the effects of outside influences on the baby.

It has been found that newborn babies prefer, and respond to, human faces rather than inanimate objects. Within a very few weeks they are smiling at a human face but not to an inanimate object such as a toy or a mobile. A few months on and the baby is able to distinguish between his mother – or permanent care-giver – and a stranger. By six to nine months the baby will have formed definite attachments; as is seen by the wariness – or even definite dislike – of strangers at this age.

Dr John Bowlby, a child psychiatrist, was an exponent of the need for attachment to the mother, or mother-substitute, for all children. He postulated that if there was any disruption of this bond, adverse effects might be seen on later personality and behavioural development. He based these findings initially on the research he had undertaken in the late 1940s into children who had no regular care-giver (in those days this was usually the mother). Not all children were damaged by a lack of attachment, but Bowlby thought unsatisfactory bonding could be a contributory factor to later personality problems in around 40% of cases. He considered that children up to the age of five years should not be separated from their mothers, or mother substitute, for any length of time.

Behaviourists are psychologists who consider outside effects to be the most important in the development of a child's personality.

Dr John Bowlby was a child psychiatrist working in the late 1940s. His book Child Care and the Growth of Love, published in 1953, received much attention. He became an authority on the effects of early social experiences in subsequent behaviour patterns. Much of his work was undertaken with motherless children and also later in particular respect to the early experiences of 44 juvenile thieves. His work, although later workers have disagreed with his findings, exerted much influence on the thinking of the day.

Further research was undertaken by a number of workers (the Robertsons and the Clarkes in particular) into the effects of different types of separation. Firstly, those children in whom satisfactory bonding, or attachment, never occurred and secondly, those babies who became attached but who were later separated from their permanent care-giver. The babies who, for whatever reason, did not bond with their mothers in the first few weeks of life appeared to recover from this if the subsequent care given was adequate. (This, of course, has an important bearing on how adopted children form attachments.)

In the second case where separation from the mother, to whom the baby was bonded, occurred for a period of six months or more in children below the age of five years, Bowlby and other workers postulated that this could have long-term effects on personality and emotional health. Examples of this were drawn from the effect seen when a mother had to go into hospital for any length of time. (In the 1950s and 1960s children were rarely able to visit their mothers in hospital and frequently had to be cared for, for long periods of time whilst the father was at work, in nurseries where there was not necessarily a good deal of personal contact.)

Bowlby's views met with a good deal of opposition at the time. It was finally decided that it was the quality of care given to the child during the mother's absence that was of vital importance to the effect that this type of separation had on the child. John Bowlby continued his work by investigating further studies into the development of children who were brought up in institutions. He concluded that separation from the permanent care-giver could have disastrous effects on future healthy emotional development. There are, however, a number of different interpretations that can be put on these studies.

In fact, many of Bowlby's findings were rejected by a number of later workers in this field. Michael Rutter, as part of his important Isle of Wight study (this study was into many aspects of child care and development) considered that arguments and tensions in the home were just as likely to cause developmental delay and delinquency as maternal separation.

In spite of this, Bowlby's views have been influential in changing childcare practice as well as prompting much interest and further work in the subject:

Bowlby's influences
- Hospital accommodation for mothers
- Women encourage to look after their preschool children
- Family allowances
- Keep mother–child bond intact

- In hospital wards, mothers were allowed, and indeed encouraged, to spend as much time as possible with their sick child. Overnight sleeping arrangements were also organized for mothers to stay nearby with their critically ill children.
- Women were encouraged to give up full-time work to look after their preschool age children.
- Social workers were encouraged to keep the mother–child bond intact at all costs.
- Financial help with child care, in the form of family allowances and single parent allowance for example, were also started in the late 1950s and early 1960s.

Whilst many of Bowlby's theories may today be dismissed, it was his influence that inspired much work into the mother–child relationship as well as changing child-care practice.

Taking the idea of attachment further, babies and young children are seen to form attachments to more than one person. There is usually someone to whom the child is most closely attached, but a number of people (often in a hierarchical fashion according to Bowlby) will also belong to the elite of being liked. Evidence of this is seen from the number of attachments formed by children brought up in a kibbutz. Here attachments are made to a number of other people besides the parents.

In the early 1960s Schaffer and Emerson pioneered similar work in Glasgow by the use of naturalistic observations. (This is known as 'ethology', the study of behaviour in natural surroundings.) They concluded that babies, up to the age of around 18 months, can become equally attached to a number of people who interact with them and respond to their general needs. In the days when extended families were the norm (all living close together and taking a share in the care of the young children in the family), this was of importance.

These findings to some extent again contradicted those of Bowlby, namely that the mother–child bond was of paramount importance. Nevertheless, it must always be remembered the enormous influence that Bowlby's work has had on child-care practice, not least because his ideas made other workers think more closely about child–adult relationships.

Situations where attachments may fail

- **Where a child is unplanned and unwanted**. It does not always follow, of course, that an unplanned baby automatically becomes an unwanted baby once he is a reality. Many mothers, even following a difficult, emotionally traumatic pregnancy, dote on their babies and care for them devotedly, but there can also be times when this did not occur and the vital bonding between mother and child never occurs.
- **People who find parenting skills difficult**. The thought of caring, maybe on their own, for the needs of a completely dependent human being can lead to difficulties in attachment. An eminent paediatrician, Dr Hugh Jolly, considered that mothers and babies needed time and the right atmosphere to 'fall in love'. The 'instant love' at birth – so beloved of romantic stories – is by no means invariable. Quality time together for mother and baby, with the help of sympathetic hospital staff and later sympathetic family, is necessary to establish a firm bond.
- **When a baby is born with a physical disability**. The mother may find bonding difficult in the early days. This is especially so when the condition is an obvious one, such as a severe cleft palate and/or hare-lip or a severe skin blemish such as a large port-wine stain. Sympathetic handling and full explanation of how the condition can be managed can do much to help the bonding process. (Photographs of other babies with a similar problem, showing the good results that can be obtained, are also helpful.)

Discussion

Compile a list of the different disabilities with which a baby could be born, e.g. lack of a limb, blindness, cleft lip, heart defect, etc., and the possible effects of each on the bonding process. Write some advisory notes for a nursery nurse on how to help a mother over this difficult time.

- **Early, necessary, separation of mother and baby**. Examples are the premature, or very sick, newborn baby who needs to be nursed – maybe for many weeks – in an incubator. Under these conditions mothers are not able to hold, cuddle, or even care for their babies. It is important that as much contact as is possible is allowed throughout these difficult early days.
- **Postnatal depression** (not just the temporary 'baby-blues' so commonly felt around the third or fourth day after delivery). This condition is thought to affect around 10% of all newly delivered women, and many of these do not get medical help. Close relatives may think that the negative feelings will pass and are just a normal part of child-bearing. Mothers with severe postnatal depression will suffer mood swings ranging from overwhelming love for their baby to totally ignoring her, forgetting to feed her or leaving her alone in the house. Often attempts to help will be spurned. Health visitors can be alerted to signs of depression by signs of general neglect of the baby and the home as well as a general lack of interest in anything. Referral to the woman's general practitioner will be a matter of some urgency where there are severe symptoms. Antidepressant drugs may be necessary, and certainly temporary relief from the full-time care of the baby is vital. Relatives, neighbours and friends can all be enlisted to help with day-to-day care. From the baby's point of view, little harm is done to his emotional health, as long as the substitute care is of good quality.
- **Adverse social factors** (e.g. poor housing, low income, several young children). The new baby is just one more burden for the already overloaded mother. Not all mothers will find bonding difficult in these circumstances and many babies are very much loved and well cared for under the most difficult of conditions.
- **Parents who themselves were abused or deprived in childhood**.

Possible causes of attachment failure
- Unwanted child
- Difficulty with parental skills
- Baby with physical handicap
- Separation of mother and baby
- Postnatal depression
- Adverse social factors
- Parents who were abused or deprived

Situations ('life events') which can affect emotional development

Parental argument and divorce

It would seem unlikely that divorce can occur without children being aware of disharmony between their parents before this event. Ideas as to which situation – disharmony or separation/divorce – is most damaging to children's emotional development have changed through the years. Opinion is now suggesting that continual arguments and disagreements, often involving the children themselves, is more harmful than separation of the parents. Under these circumstances, handling of the children is unlikely to be consistent. So children become confused as to what response is the correct one. Frustration at a continual state of conflict eventually results in behaviour problems, which, of course, will further add to difficulties. These effects can be seen in the playgroup or nursery situation. Aggression, in an attempt to gain sympathetic attention, is a common occurrence. This in turn will alienate the child from his peers and so aggravate his feelings of unwantedness. Yet other children become withdrawn and solitary, complain of tummyaches, headaches or have a return to day-time wetting.

Nannies living with families can have an enormously stabilizing effect on the child in their care whose parents are going through divorce proceedings. Depending on the age of the child concerned, different effects should be looked out for:

- **Under-twos.** Changes in eating, sleeping and toileting patterns are the most common; the child often reverts to an earlier stage of development.
- **2–5-year-old age group**. They are bewildered and afraid that their parents will abandon them; an increasing number of temper tantrums can be the result of this fear; a return to babyish habits such as thumb-sucking or day-time wetting can occur.
- **Early school age (five to seven years)**. Children can become depressed; appetite can be lost and early waking may become a problem; at this age children will be putting into words their feelings of abandonment; self-esteem can be low and the child may feel that the problems of the parents are their fault.

Nannies can best help by being extra attentive to the child's needs, making sure that the child feels loved even in spite of bad behaviour. A secure, well-ordered routine can also do much to help.

The staff in nurseries, too, have an important task to fulfil, firstly in understanding the basic cause for any unusual or antisocial behaviour, then by allowing the child time and space to verbalize his feelings, if he is old enough to do so. Following on from this, care should be taken to handle the child consistently with plenty of opportunity for imaginative play to relieve bottled-up emotions. Stability is the ingredient most needed by the child experiencing problems at home and nursery routine can provide this. Care must also be taken not to excuse unacceptable behaviour just because of the child's situation. Gentle, but firm, control is necessary. Nursery staff must also be sure to keep in close contact with the parents, and report to them any unusual problems that have occurred during the course of the day.

Many children are not permanently affected by the stressful events associated with separation and divorce. When all arguments are over and the main care left in the hands of one parent, children seem to settle readily into the routine of a one-parent family. Some children, however, are permanently emotionally affected by their experiences. It remains to be

Stress signals
- Under 2 years: return to earlier developmental levels
- 2–5 years: thumb-sucking, temper tantrums, bewilderment
- 5–7 years: verbalization, loss of appetite, sleep disturbance

fully seen, when the children themselves become parents, the full effect of parental separation and divorce on the many children so affected these days. Having no role model of happy family life is bound to affect future relationships, bonding and parenting skills. The number of children potentially affected by divorce in their immediate family can be estimated from the known fact that one in three marriages end in divorce in the UK today. Many of these occur within the early years of marriage when there are young children in the home. Remarriage, too, has frequently been found to end in another divorce, with further trauma for the children involved.

Bereavement

Although divorce of parents can seem a type of bereavement to the child involved, death is more usually thought of in bereavement. Although early death is less likely now than a century or so ago, a mother or a father can die or be killed in an accident whilst their children are still young. Also, of course, the death of a much-loved grandparent can be devastating for a young child.

Death is today's taboo subject. Discussion only occurs when it is immediately relevant to a child's experience. Many are the euphemisms associated with the event, such as 'Grandad's gone to heaven'; 'Granny's passed away'. Children, being logical creatures, will want to know 'Where is heaven?' and 'Where has granny passed to?' It is difficult to explain fully to children the exact nature of death, but, over time, they will finally understand that the separation is final. Parents and other family members should not attempt to hide their grief – mourning is an essential part of coming to terms with bereavement. The age at the time of the bereavement will affect the way in which the child accepts the death of a family member. Michael Rutter postulates that, if a parent dies when the child is around three years of age, the effects are greater than if this event occurs when he is older. At this age, role modelling on a parent is important. After about 10 years of age, the normal adult grief reactions – denial, anger, guilt, depression and acceptance – are more in evidence.

The death of a brother or sister can cause much upset to a young child. As well as having to cope with his own loss, the child may feel abandoned by his parents as they themselves grieve for the child they have lost. He may also feel guilt that it was not he that died.

These events can affect behaviour in the nursery situation and staff will need to handle the situation sensitively. Allow the child to grieve, to verbalize his feelings, talk to the bereaved parents about their dead child and the effects on the brother or sister currently attending nursery.

The sudden infant death syndrome (SIDS or 'cot death') is also an event that can affect an older brother or sister. This tragic event is defined as 'the sudden, unexpected death of a previously healthy infant'. For the older brother or sister, the natural feelings of jealousy – probably only just overcome – are replaced by sadness. Again, the grief of the parents may cause the remaining child, or children, to feel lost and bewildered. Help in the nursery, primary school setting or from a live-in nanny is very valuable in consoling children in these circumstances. The Foundation for the Study of Infant Deaths will give advice (see Appendix).

Child abuse

Child abuse has probably always occurred, but the actual size of the problem was highlighted in the 1960s. Professor Kempe first coined the emotive term 'battered baby syndrome' to describe babies that were brought to the Accident and Emergency Departments of hospitals with unexplained – or inadequately explained – bruises, cuts, burns and fractures. It is now known that it is not only babies that are the victims of non-accidental injury; older children, too, suffer from many forms of abuse. Children under five years are most at risk from physical abuse, one reason being their inability to avoid injury.

Erikson, an Austrian psychologist, who had close links in his early days with Freud, majored on the 'whole life' theory of personality development. He postulated that the first year of life was when trust in people and the surrounding environment developed. If this trust was misplaced, as when abuse against the child occurred, for example, serious consequences could be seen in later personality development. So the effects of child abuse early in life can have far-reaching effects – even into the way in which the child's children are handled.

There is no particular class in which child abuse is more common. Children of:

- young mothers/fathers;
- families where pregnancies are close together;
- parents who themselves were abused as children are most at risk from non-accidental injury.

In all these situations there can be seen to be a possible underlying psychological cause for the abuse. (See Chapter 8 for further information on child abuse.)

Development of personality

Defining 'personality' is difficult. The *Shorter Oxford English Dictionary* defines personality as: 'the quality or fact of being a person'. It is a subject that has exercised psychologist's minds for many years, and there are a number of well-known names associated with this particular study. The following section briefly covers the main ideas of some of these psychologists. First, how do children, developmentally, mature into 'personalities'?

Self-concept

This refers to what ideas we have of ourselves; what kind of person we are; what makes us 'tick'. From the age of one year to 18 months babies are largely unaware that they are separate and uniquely different from other people and the other inanimate objects around them. By two years of age they have learnt a good deal about themselves: they are 'a child'; 'a boy' or 'a girl'. In other words they are beginning to categorize themselves. At this age, too, they are beginning to refer to themselves as 'me' and will be well aware of their own name. They will be interested in anything to do with their own bodies and will be able to point to any named part with a fair degree of ease. Slightly later they will be able to recognize themselves in photographs or on video.

Stereotyping and gender

Stereotyping is the way in which we all recognize people. To discuss or study each individual is difficult if one is generalizing, so people with certain common attributes are categorized or stereotyped. For example, a group of women with children could be 'mothers' (even though this may not be true!); a certain race may be stereotyped as 'Americans' or 'the Scots', each group considered to have certain common characteristics; for example: 'All Americans are wealthy' or 'All Scots are careful with money', even though this is patently untrue of many people in each group.

The greatest, and most common, way of stereotyping is by gender: 'men'; 'women'; 'girls'; 'boys'. Sex is determined at conception by the specific sperm which fertilizes an ovum. This is a biological fact and the baby is born with the characteristic anatomy of a male or a female. It is later in childhood that social learning theories of gender exert their influence. Much has changed in recent years regarding the stereotyping of the sexes. Many workers have investigated the way in which social trends determine the way in which boys and girls are brought up. Margaret Mead in the 1930s was one of the earliest workers in this field. She concluded that gender roles were learned rather than being solely the result of genetic inheritance. Later workers considered that peer group pressure, and also the effects of various branches of the media, have great influence on the stereotyping of sex.

Social learning theories consider that children learn gender roles by:
* watching the behaviour of both sexes in their immediate environment;
* imitating members of their own sex;
* being selectively reinforced in their biological gender role by adults.

Kohlberg disagreed with this, and postulated that gender roles were acquired in stages, similar to other cognitive functions. He described three separate stages:
* **Basic gender identity**. Children are aware of their gender from around three years of age.
* **Gender stability**. The child from around five to seven years of age realizes that grown-up life will be the same as that of the same sex parent.
* **Gender consistency**. The child realizes that his/her gender is unchangeable.

In the nursery situation children should be allowed to choose toys and activities which appeal to them personally, rather than stereotyping these activities to gender. For example, boys can play in the domestic corner and girls can ride on trains. (In many cases, however, girls will be seen to prefer stereotyped female activities/toys, and conversely boys prefer stereotyped male activities/toys.)

Nursery staff can actively promote cross-gender play by:

- including both boys and girls in an activity;
- encouraging the children to play with all the toys in the nursery;
- talking to the children about which toys and activities are enjoyed by boys and girls separately and together.

Discussion

From your observations at your place of work experience, make notes on how many of the children play with toys stereotyped to their gender. Bring your findings back to your group and discuss if there should be any change in policy from your observations. Make notes on the discussion adding your own comments and conclusions.

Stereotyping can be long-lasting and fixed. For example, a child who apparently belongs to a 'gang' of children who are behaving badly will automatically be thought of as behaving badly also. Perhaps, in fact, the specific child does not behave in this inappropriate way. This is known as **attribution theory**. Put another way, reasoning persuades us that if a child belongs to that particular group, she must also behave in the same way as the rest of the members. Sometimes this is true and sometimes it is not. A further example applied to one person is if a child is always smiling and friendly, he will be attributed to have a happy personality. The actions and the perception are stereotyped together.

As language skills develop so do skills of comparison. Listen to a group of 3–4-year-olds in conversation. They will be talking about size as 'bigger' or 'smaller', hair colour as 'light' or 'dark'. More subjective traits such as 'kind', 'good', 'naughty' will be being introduced into their speech. The type of words used will depend on the messages passed to them by their parents. Parents who are continually grumbling at their child will find that his speech will be biased towards such words as 'naughty' and 'bad'.

Self-esteem, or lack of it, is also developed at this early age. Again, children whose parents are always telling them that they are 'stupid' or 'wicked' will have a poor self-esteem. In the worst scenario these children will be withdrawn, shy and poor at making social contacts. Children with a high self-esteem (positive self-concept) will be confident, willing to help and participate in activities and so be better able to benefit from early educational activities.

Freud

Sigmund Freud was a Jewish Austrian doctor who lived and worked in the latter part of the nineteenth and early part of the twentieth century. Much of his work concentrated on the unconscious mind. He postulated that two main effects determined personality:

- basic biological make-up;
- childhood experiences.

Freud considered that there were three distinct aspects to personality, all hypothetical but nevertheless describable.

The id

This is the basis of all psychic energy, and seen markedly in very young babies. The id demands immediate attention and satisfaction of needs. In the young baby these are relief of hunger, thirst, cold, pain, etc., all very necessary needs for survival. This is known as the 'oral' **stage**.

Freud considered that if the id did not receive immediate and appropriate satisfaction, frustration and anxiety would supervene and become buried in the unconscious mind. These anxieties could surface in later life and affect personality development.

(As an aside, perhaps the child-rearing suggestions of Truby King in the early part of this century could be said to have an adverse effect on the gratification of the id. Truby King advised that babies were fed on a rigid time-table principle, e.g. four-hourly feeds and not a minute sooner or later, was the ideal for which new mothers should aim.)

The erogenous zone through which the id receives gratification is the mouth – feeding, sucking, etc. This personality stage of development was said to last for the first two years of life.

The ego

This second part of the personality appears at around two years. The child has learned that immediate satisfaction does not always happen in later life – as it did in the very early days. So certain strategies need to be learned to satisfy needs. The erogenous zone at this stage is said to be the anus. This is the time when potty-training is uppermost in skills to be learned. The child realizes that she can control the events in her world, to a certain extent anyway, by expelling or retaining the contents of the bowel. Bladder control, or lack of control, is perceived to have similar results. According to Freud, too strict or too lax a training programme can affect the child's later personality.

The superego

The third part of the personality appears around three years of age. This superego has a sense of right and wrong (albeit limited in the early days) and so is considered to be the basis of morality.

In his earlier writings Freud related the appearance of the superego to basic infantile sexual urges. Children became attracted to the parent of the opposite sex – the Oedipus complex in boys or Electra complex in girls. Freud considered that suppression of these urges could lead to neuroses in later life. He dubbed this stage as the phallic stage.

Freud gained many critics from this sexual aspect of personality development, and he omitted it from his later work. Modern psychology pays little attention to the Oedipus complex.

As can be seen from these three postulated stages of personality devel-

Freud's personality aspects
- Id – from birth
- Ego – around 2 years
- Superego – around 3 years

opment, much emphasis is placed on childhood experiences and the way in which children are cared for in their early years.

After five years of age the various parts of the personality are fused together and the child has usually come to terms with what is required of him from the world in general. From now until puberty has been named the 'latency period'. Outside interests – games, sports, holidays, learning, visits – occupy the child's unlimited energies during this time.

At puberty hormonal influences give rise to wide-ranging changes both physically and mentally. This is known as the 'genital stage' and lasts throughout life. Freud considered that if the earlier stages of personality development had been satisfactorily passed through, the young person would reach sexual maturity with few problems. If, however, development had failed at any one point (e.g. at the oral stage) or there were unresolved problems at any stage, neuroses could result in later life.

Freud's theories gained much credence at the time. Later studies have failed to prove or disprove conclusively the existence of, and the after effects of, his hypothetical stages of personality development. It is possibly:

- the type of people Freud investigated (mainly middle class women in Vienna);
- his way of working (the psychoanalysis of dreams and free association ideas which he based on clinical interviewing techniques);
- the heavy emphasis that he placed on the sexuality of babies

that have led to his theories being viewed with a degree of suspicion.

Jung

Carl Gustav Jung was a doctor working in mental hospitals in Austria. He and Freud were contemporaries, although there was a 20-year difference in age. Initially they had many points of agreement regarding the development of personality. Later Jung disagreed with Freud about the stages of personality development that the latter had postulated. Jung thought of personality as a whole, and gave more credence to the role of the conscious mind in the development of personality.

He described two types of people – 'extroverts' and 'introverts', which could be noticed from an early age. Extroverts were those children who go out to meet the world, and all it may give, with confidence. Introverts tend to look inwards and take more notice of their own thoughts and feelings rather than external events.

In addition to these conscious attributes, Jung postulated that there are two parts to the unconscious mind. He described a 'personal' consciousness which contains forgotten or repressed feelings, and a 'collective' consciousness which represented the vast array of all the experiences of humankind. This latter thinking is in keeping with Jung's religious and mystic background derived from his lonely childhood when he read much on religious and mystical subjects. This is in direct contrast to Freud who had no time for religion or mysticism.

Jung's methods of investigating neuroses in adult life were very similar to those employed by Freud. He considered, however, later personality

Carl Gustav Jung
- Austrian doctor
- Contemporary of Freud (20 years younger)
- Mystic ('collective' consciousness)
- Described 'extroverts' and 'introverts'

problems to be due to an imbalance between conscious and unconscious needs.

Adler

Alfred Adler was also a contemporary – in fact a student – of Freud. He disagreed strongly with Freud about the importance of sexuality in the development of personality in young children.

One of Adler's main contributions to psychology was his description of the 'inferiority complex'. He believed that children, who are initially unable to care for themselves, envy the hold which adults have over them as they care for their physical needs, which they see as 'power'. So they develop a need to gain this power. If this fails, an inferiority complex develops, lasts throughout life and colours all aspects of the personality.

Alfred Adler
- Student of Freud
- Disagreed regarding infant sexuality
- Postulated 'inferiority complex'

Erikson

Erik Erikson was another psychologist who studied under Freud. He did not totally reject Freud's ideas of the stages of development theory. He extended this to encompass further developmental stages occurring throughout life in his 'whole life' theory of development.

Erikson moved to America and there studied groups of both children and adults. Basically he postulated that throughout life a series of goals had to be overcome before the next stage could be reached. It was the failure to attain these goals satisfactorily that could result in neuroses in later life.

Eysenck

H.J. Eysenck, working in London in the middle of the twentieth century, postulated an objective view to personality. He described three basic personality characteristics to be found in everyone. Each person was somewhere along a line between the two extremes. These three characteristics were:
- extroversion — introversion;
- neuroticism — stability;
- psychosis — normality.

There needed to be a balance between the two extremes of each type for a stable personality. Eysenck also considered that there is definite evidence, from physiological as well as psychological studies, for the inheritance of personality characteristics.

Humanistic approach to personality

There has been an upsurge in humanistic psychology since the 1960s. Humanists emphasize the importance of the 'whole being' and not each individual's separate parts. The employed way of study differs from all other streams of psychological thought. Generalizations on group studies are not made. Rather an individual's 'whole life' experience is studied.

Many humanistic ideas are based on the Gestalt school of psychology, whose motto can be summarized as: 'the whole is more than the sum of the parts'. A type of therapy – Gestalt therapy – was developed in America in the 1960s and humanists tend to adhere to these theories. Therapy concentrates on current problems rather than endeavouring to find out what has caused them. Also, individuals are encouraged to discover for themselves what is wrong.

Other therapies, such as Carl Roger's 'client-centred' therapy and existential therapy also have their vogue in humanist circles.

COGNITIVE AND LANGUAGE DEVELOPMENT

OBJECTIVES

1. **Describe theories of cognitive development.**
2. **Identify theories of language and their relationship to thought.**
3. **Understand theories of intelligence and its measurement.**

Cognitive development

Cognition is again a difficult term to understand. The *Oxford English Dictionary* defines cognition as: 'the action, or faculty, of knowing'. The *Penguin Dictionary of Psychology* defines cognition more fully as: 'a broad term which has been traditionally used to describe such activities as thinking, conceiving, reasoning . . . insight, imagery, problem-solving and so forth'. So, from these definitions, it would seem that as soon as babies begin responding to the stimuli around them – human or otherwise – they are in a state of knowing or 'cognition'. The social smile of the 6-week-old baby could thus be described as 'cognitive'.

Piaget

Jean Piaget, a Swiss biologist, became interested in the way in which cognition developed in children. In the early years he based his research largely on the findings from his own three children as he observed them at play ('naturalistic' observation). As they grew older he told them stories, and then later questioned them about the actions of the people in the story to test their emerging reasoning abilities. Piaget was one of the first researchers to suggest that children were not 'mini-adults', but showed quite different powers of cognition to adults. Throughout 50 years of research (until his death in 1980) Piaget used his knowledge of biology to try to correlate cognitive growth with other developmental measurements. In the nature versus nurture debate, he concluded that outside influences acted on maturing biological structures.

Piaget considered that babies are born with minimal basic abilities. They learn – very quickly! – to build up mental ideas on how to deal with the mental stimuli they receive. He termed these mental images 'schemas' ('schemata'). The first schemata are the ones on which survival depends –

the reflex actions of breathing, sucking, crying, etc. Piaget dubbed these as 'action schemata'.

By the age of around two years the child has some command of language and knows the meaning of many words. In other words, symbols are being used – in the form of speech for objects. This was known as the 'symbolic schema' stage.

As the child matures thought becomes more logical and reasoned. By seven years he begins to realize that his environment can be manipulated by his actions. The outcome of an action is known and is predictable. As a simple example, pulling a door handle down will release the mechanism and the door will open. Other more complicated 'cause-and-effect' examples can be given: retribution is certain if he persists in performing some forbidden activity and, conversely, acceptable behaviour is rewarded. In a more concrete way, a child can be taught that pushing down a certain combination of keys on the piano will produce a pleasant sound. Pushing down a different set will not necessarily give such a desired effect. These are the stages of 'operational schemata'.

These stages of cognition and acquisition of schemata are passed through in the same sequence in all children but at varying ages. Childhood 'thinking' changes as the child matures. This in turn is dependent on other developmental processes controlled by both genetic and environmental factors.

Piaget described four stages of cognitive development:

1. Sensory motor stage (0–2 years) in which action schema are in evidence. Direct sensory experience of objects and people are paramount. Activities are solitary. (This correlates to the type of play seen in children in this age group.)
2. Preoperational stage (2–7 years). This age group is developing and learning the symbolic schema. Language is being used with increasingly good effect: at 3–5 years the constant queries of 'why?', 'how?' and 'when?' occur. An enormous amount of learning is taking place without any formal teaching, but positive interaction with adults is of vital importance. Make-believe play is a feature of this stage. The child gives inanimate objects human feelings and motives. Statements such as: 'The naughty door hit me', 'I cross with Teddy' are common. Piaget termed this substage 'preconceptual thought'. A further feature dominates this preoperational stage, that of egocentrism, i.e. everything revolves around the child himself.
3. Concrete operation stage (7–11 years). This coincides with the onset of formal education. Skills of cognition and manipulation of environmental influences are gaining pace. Through manipulation of objects further cognition is developing. For example, by the manipulation of coloured objects children are learning the bases of arithmetic – adding and subtracting. It was this necessary handling of concrete objects that was the basis for terming this the concrete operation stage. As language skills develop further, so do comparative concepts improve; for example, 'smaller' versus 'bigger' is understood.

Piaget
- 'Founding father' of developmental cognitive psychology
- Swiss biologist and psychologist
- Postulated mental 'schemata' – mental strategies used by children
- four stages of cognitive development.

4. Formal operation stage (from 11 years on). The previous necessity for handling concrete objects is no longer required. Adding numbers can be done in the child's head, or at least with only the symbolic representation of written numbers. Thought is no longer about tangible objects and events, but about hypothetical subjects such as what the future will hold both on a personal and wider level, and other aspects of logical and abstract thought. Obviously many years are spent before this stage is complete, if ever. Some people do not progress far along this path.

Piaget stressed that there is a constant dynamic interaction between the emotional and intellectual aspects of cognition. In times of stress and emotional upset children can return to an earlier stage of thinking. Continuing emotional problems or stress situations can stop progression into the next stage of development. In some cases formal logical thought is never attained.

Piaget's theories have influenced educational practice over the years – probably the most succinct way of describing his views on education is 'discovery learning'.

Hughes and Donaldson, psychologists working in the 1970s, both challenged some of Piaget's ideas as to when children reached certain stages of cognition.

Bruner

Jerome Bruner did not reject Piaget's theories. Rather he put greater emphasis on certain aspects of the development of cognition. Whilst Piaget considered that each developmental stage of thought *replaced* the previous stage, Bruner believed that each stage (or 'mode of thought' as he described it) *built on* the previous one. His work focused more on older children and adolescents who were building on their basic concept knowledge.

Language

Language is a peculiarly human attribute. (Several workers have endeavoured to teach chimpanzees – our nearest relative in the primate world – to speak. 'Washoe', an American chimp was the subject of much work by the Gardners. Washoe could communicate by a special sign language, but she never learned to use language as do humans.)

The *Oxford English Dictionary* defines language as: 'words and the method of combining them for the expression of thought'. A further definition is: 'a set of symbols used by humans in order to communicate.'

This latter definition is a wider one and includes the 'sign language' of the profoundly deaf and 'Braille', the means by which blind people communicate the written word. Both these specialized forms of communication are, of course, based on the use of words.

Development of language

This can be divided into specific stages:

1. **Prelinguistic stage** between 0 and 1 year. The baby communicates but has no speech.

2. **Early linguistic stage**, between 1 and 2 years. Single words are being used at the beginning of this stage, but not always with the correct meaning.

3. **Telegraphic speech** between 18 months and $2\frac{1}{2}$ years. Words are strung together, but sentences are not complete or grammatically correct. For example, 'Me run'; 'Daddy car'; 'Teddy gone', and later 'Car in road'; 'Milk all gone'. Even at this early stage children will be heard to be using the basic rules of grammar, that is, the subject of the utterance always comes first. Understanding the meaning of words always precedes the ability to use them. Babies as young as six months can point to certain objects if asked, but as yet are unable to verbalize the name they understand.

Student exercise

From your experience with children build up, over a period of time, a list of examples of 'telegraph speech' and the sentences they represent.

4. From around three years children's language is advancing daily in content, vocabulary and grammatical correctness. About 1000 words are known and pronunciation is generally correct enough to allow strangers to understand.

Theories of language development

There are three major theories of how language develops. These are proposed by B.F. Skinner, Noam Chomsky and our old friend Piaget.

B.F. Skinner was an American psychologist working in the middle of the twentieth century. He based his theory of language development on the 'operant conditioning' approach first proposed by Thorndike, who worked mainly with animals.

An operant condition is defined as: 'a response which can be elicited if the response results in something pleasant occurring'. (This is in distinction from **Ivan Pavlov's** well-known 'classic conditioning' experiments with salivating dogs. Here the response elicited to a stimulus is a reflex one.)

Skinner considered that if sounds made by babies closely resembled speech these can be reinforced by praise from a caring adult. They would then be learned and become part of the child's vocabulary. Sounds which were not reinforced would seldom be repeated. Later, when single words had been learned, combinations of words and finally grammatically correct sentences would also need to be reinforced until learned.

Piaget considered the acquisition of language to be an integral part of the development of cognition. The development of schemata involves also the necessity of learning the right words to describe them. Knowing the appropriate words allows children to communicate better and so develop more sophisticated schema.

Skinner
- American psychologist
- Acquisition of language dependent on operant conditioning
- Introduced ideas of reinforcement
- Also known as a 'behaviourist'

Ivan Pavlov
- Russian physiologist
- Theories of classic conditioning
- Well-known experiments on salivating dogs
- Reflex responses improved by repeated stimuli.

The question of the interaction of language and thought is a difficult one. Is language necessary for thought? Or can babies think before they can speak?

Vygotsky working on this aspect in the 1950s and 1960s considered that language and thought originated separately. These two aspects were only combined later in life when speech became more established.

Piaget and Vygotsky disagreed for some length of time on the purpose of early childhood language. Later they agreed that the egocentric speech of early childhood – 'Me walk dog' – became redundant when such self-given instructions became unnecessary as language became internalized.

Watson in America postulated that thought *was* language, and thought could be defined as manipulating words in the mind.

Whorf, a contemporary of Vygotsky, considered that 'thought is relative to the language in which it is conducted' – the 'linguistic-relativity hypothesis'. This view was later discredited.

Noam Chomsky disagreed strongly with Skinner on the development of language, and considered Piaget's ideas to be too vague. He postulated that human babies were 'programmed' for language development. Anatomical features – in the brain, in the mouth and facial muscles and in the control of breathing – are specific to humans and make speech and language possible. The language centre, situated in a particular part of the left side of the brain is the anatomical structure especially designed to understand language in all its forms – semantics as well as syntax.

A number of tests have been developed to test both the speech and language abilities in children of different ages and to assess the nature and extent of any language difficulty. Differentiation between difficulties in comprehension (understanding) and problems with expression (verbalization) is also assessed. The phonological process (the ability to process sounds in spoken language) can again be tested. All these tests, when used in various combinations, will pin-point specific areas of difficulty.

None of these theories would seem to totally explain how, in the short space of five years, the vast majority of children acquire an enormous vocabulary and use it to express ideas and thoughts in a grammatically correct form.

Intelligence

Discussion

Before reading, or looking up any definition of intelligence, work in small groups and define what you mean by intelligence. Then pool the definitions to establish a commonly agreed definition.

Much is spoken about intelligence in development and learning fields. Difficulties arise from the beginning as intelligence is an almost impossible concept to define. Definitions have ranged from: 'the ability of humans – and animals – to adapt to their environment, and to adapt their environment to their own needs'; 'the ability to profit through experience'; to 'that which intelligence tests measure'! Perhaps the definition proposed by Heim is the most workable one: 'intelligent activity consists of grasping the essentials of a given situation and responding appropriately to them'.

Theories of the development of intelligence involve, once again, the nature/nurture debate. As neither aspect can be measured precisely, intelligence tests have been developed to judge a variety of abilities at different ages. The scores from these tests are not fixed immutably for all time. Many factors are seen to exert an influence on intelligence test scores:

- **Genetic influence.** Whilst it is not possible to tease out all the threads which intermingle to produce an intelligent child, certain studies on twins have shown that our genetic inheritance certainly has something to do with intelligence levels.
- **Physical and sensory abilities.** Children born with physical or sensory problems (for example a child with cerebral palsy who has limited control over the movements of his body, or the child who has a hearing or visual impairment) will have enormous problems in obtaining the same sensory input as a child without these difficulties. Without adequate sensory input learning is harder and intellectual potential can be limited.
- **Different cultures** can also exert an influence on intelligence scores, and yet not on basic intelligence. Different cultures have different methods of solving everyday problems. Spatial perception, too, is thought to differ in people of different ethnic origins. This will influence the way in which they are able to perform certain parts of the standardized western IQ tests. Allowance has to be made for these differences when IQ tests are being scored. Catell tried to devise 'culture fair' IQ tests, but these are not now considered to be helpful.
- **Age.** In general it is considered that mental abilities increase with chronological age up to adolescence – around 14 to 15 years. Some authorities believe that IQ levels stabilize around this time, and after this time there is a slow decline in mental abilities. There are, however, several exceptions to this:
  - continued intellectual education after adolescence can lead to prolonged development;
  - some children's abilities do seem to appear later – and some earlier – than the expected chronological age; such children are termed 'late developers'.
- The **learning environment** in early childhood also has an effect on IQ scores. Children who are deprived of educational toys, books and stimulating visits, for example, may not develop to their full genetic intellectual potential. From the other viewpoint the child who has had much appropriate early interaction with her mother (or regular care-giver), and has had a good deal of interest taken in her will perform better on later IQ testing.

Student exercise

From your experience and observation of children, list the factors you think have the greatest effect on the development of a child's intellectual abilities. Give concrete examples to support the factors chosen.

- **gender**. There is no difference in the IQ scores of boys and girls, but different skills can be seen to develop at different rates in the two sexes. Girls develop language skills earlier than boys and are generally more able in this field throughout life. Early in childhood, up to around six years of age, girls are slightly ahead in arithmetic, but are generally overtaken by boys later. It has been suggested that parental influence *may* play a part; it is thought that boys will be more skilled in the scientific subjects than girls, whilst girls will be more able verbally. So encouragement is given in these two aspects.
- **Family size**. As a generalization only, children from small families are thought to be intellectually more able than those from large families. Maybe they have more day-to-day interaction with adults?

Types of intelligence tests used

Gesell developmental scales

Gesell and his fellow-workers were the first to attempt to standardize children's performance in the 1920s. These were more developmental observations rather than IQ testing. Various groups of abilities – motor skills, language development and social/emotional development – were tested. (In fact these groupings of tests could be said to be the basis of today's developmental tests.) Gesell observed hundreds of children and attempted to establish 'age norms' at which children were able to perform certain tasks.

Binet

Alfred Binet was also an early worker in this field. He worked in Paris around 1905. Initially his work was promoted by the French government. They asked Binet to formulate tests which would identify children of below average ability, and who were thought to be holding other children back. Basically he tried to establish a method of finding out in what particular areas individual children had difficulties. Later on in America at Stanford University, Binet's work was modified and the test known as the Stanford–Binet test became popular and was the norm for measuring children's intelligence. This test measured a child's mental age (MA). This, of course, need not necessarily correlate with the child's chronological age (CA). These tests have been altered and adapted in recent years, and are not now used as frequently.

Stern

Stern, a German psychologist, developed the concept of an 'Intelligence Quotient'. This is arrived at by dividing the mental age by the chronological age and multiplying this by 100, i.e. MA/CA × 100 = Intelligence Quotient. The score thus obtained can be misleading, as it only describes a score from a specific test. The child (or adult) may have great skills in other areas which have not been tested. Again this concept has been largely superseded.

Weschler scales

Devised by David Wechsler in America these scales used to be the most widely used IQ tests in schools. His adult intelligence scale was modified for use with school children between the ages of six and 16 years (Wechsler Intelligence Scales for Children WISC). Two types of skills are scored – verbal ability and non-verbal performance. The results have been found to correlate closely with, and predict future, educational attainment.

A further scale for younger pupils (infants) and preschool children, the Wechsler Preschool and Primary Test of Intelligence (WPPSI), has also been developed. These tests are continually being up-dated, and new versions of both WISC and WPPSI are expected in the near future.

British Ability Scales

These have been used more widely in the UK and standardized on British children, rather than on the American children where WISC was used. ('British Ability Scales 2' started in October 1996.)

Griffiths Mental Development Scales

This test has a large number of subsections and tests which can be used for children in a wide age group – $0-8\frac{1}{2}$ years. This is a very useful test that can be used in a number of different situations with children of all abilities. Strengths and weaknesses are highlighted so that appropriate help can be given in areas of difficulty.

All intelligence scores need, however, to be treated with caution. They are not exact and have a standard error rate of ±6 points. Nevertheless, they do give important information on children's various difficulties so that appropriate help can be given.

Distribution of intelligence

Intelligence can vary widely amongst a large group of children. There will be some very bright children and a few with severe learning difficulties. The vast majority will fall between these two extremes. Binet thought that intelligence amongst the general population followed the 'normal curve of distribution' of many physical and mental attributes. (This is a statistical device which can be used for many variables, for example how many tall and short people there are in a given population.) It has been found that 60% of people have an IQ between 85 and 115 with almost equal numbers above and below this group. (The lower end of the scale is slightly skewed due to the effect of handicapping conditions and accidents.)

When educational provision is being planned for a given population, it can be calculated that most children will fit into the normal school provision. Children with 'general learning difficulties' (GLD) will score between 50 and 70 and some within this group will have 'specific learning difficulties', for example special problems with language. Children with 'severe learning difficulties' (SLD) will score below 50.

So, theoretically, at least, it can be calculated how many places in the educational system will be needed for each group of children. (Practically, of course, this does not always follow for a small area: one part of the country many have a higher, or lower, proportion of children in the SLD group, for example.) In the UK educational policy is for integrated schooling. Pupils with general learning difficulties attend standard schools with extra resources provided to help with their difficulties.

Gifted children are those who have an IQ score of greater than 140. In the UK, no specific provision in the state educational system is available for such children. There are, however, various private groups which cater for the needs of these children. The National Association for Gifted Children (see Appendix) can be contacted for further information. Recently, a group called the International Centre for Inquiring Children (see Appendix) has been looking into ways of helping gifted children to reach their full potential.

Gifted children can have their own problems such as frustration and boredom with repetition of skills and ideas already mastered. Nursery staff will do well to look out for any gifted child in their group who appears to be behaving badly.

PERCEPTION, MEMORY AND LEARNING

OBJECTIVES

1. **Describe the stages in the development of perception.**
2. **Understand theories of memory.**

Perception

Perception can be defined as: 'the process of taking in, and using, information from the environment'. There are many ways in which we perceive things: hearing, vision, touch, olfaction (smell), taste and bodily position in space. In fact all of our special senses are used in this activity. This, however, is only the beginning of perception. Once images have been perceived they will need to be interpreted by the brain in the context of the environment in which they arise. How we decode all the information that is received varies from person to person and depends on how people are actually placed and feeling at the time.

There are two main theories of how this interpretation takes place:

- **Hebb** proposed that, apart from a few basic inborn tendencies to distinguish form and figures, babies and children gradually learn to identify and interpret objects around them. Particular sets of neurones in the brain become associated with particular objects, and so can be recognized again when heard, seen or touched. Later these small images combine into larger groups with more brain cells being involved. Thus Hebb considered perception to be largely an acquired characteristic.
- German psychologists disagreed with this view and considered that perception is an inborn characteristic. They created a school of thinking known as the 'Gestalt school of psychology'. (The word *gestalt* means 'pattern' or 'form') This theory implies that objects are perceived by their total characteristics and not by the sum of their parts. (As mentioned previously, Gestalt theory can be summarized as 'the whole is greater than the sum of the parts'.)

There is a certain degree of evidence for the Gestalt theory. Taking visual perception – one of the easiest aspects of perception to investigate – as an example, look at Figure 6.1 and say which is the longest vertical line: (a) or (b).

Figure 6.1 A visual comparison of two similar line lengths.

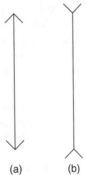

(a)   (b)

They are both actually of the same length, but by perception of the whole (b) appears to be longer.

Perception has practical effects on the way we move. Young children tend to bump into objects more frequently than do older children. They have not yet learned to perceive distance and perspective. From a learning point of view it is important that young children should have plenty of opportunity to explore their environment. Practice with toys of different sizes and shapes in differing situations is also vital.

Before children learn to perceive, however, they will need to acquire 'selective attention'. The surrounding environment is full of sensory images – the sound of the kettle boiling; the sight of the dog walking into the room; the smell of a vase of flowers – as well as a whole host of other smells, tastes and feelings all battling for attention. Children have to learn to filter out some – most! – of these differing stimuli and concentrate on just one particular aspect. In young babies, touching is one of the earliest ways of perception. As vision becomes more competent, visual stimuli take precedence, and hearing, taste and smell all play their part.

Broadbent in the 1950s did much research into selective attention. He proposed a type of physiological filter which regulates the type and amount of information being passed to the brain. He based his theories very much on communication techniques, for example, the sensory stimuli he referred to as 'input channels'. If the input was too great, a bottleneck (or 'limited capacity channel') occurred and only selected stimuli could pass. Other stimuli were stored for a short time in a 'short-term storage system' to be used when and if a channel became free. Broadbent followed this up by postulating that some of the information was passed to a 'long-term storage system' to be used later. He tried to give some explanation of the association between attention, perception and memory.

There are certain stimuli which gain a child's attention to a greater extent than others:
- intense stimuli, e.g. loud noises, bright colours, powerful pressure;
- unusual stimuli gain attention more readily;
- variable stimuli (any mother, or teacher, will tell you how to attract attention by raising, or lowering her voice);
- conditioning (within a very few months babies will 'attend' when their name is mentioned).

As well as the modification of the external stimulus, the internal factors in the child are important as to how attention is gained. For example, a child who is:
- **tired**, will not pay attention so readily as when he is wide awake;
- **ill**, will not be so easily aroused by even a well-known stimulus as when he is well;
- **uninterested** in the particular event or
- **deprived**, will only pay attention to the stimulus if it is an answer to the immediate need. This applies to both physical and social deprivation.

Memory

Memory can be seen to be the logical conclusion to selective attention and perception. Without perception (preceded by selective attention), memory would not exist. With memory an event is stored and, when the event needs to be recalled, retrieval takes place. Information is acquired, or perceived, in a number of different ways, from seeing something (visual memory), hearing something (auditory memory) or even the touch or taste of something. This has an important bearing on how children learn – some children remember everything they see, but have difficulty in remembering anything at all that they hear. It is obvious what problems could arise if this is not understood by teachers.

Storage of information, in whatever way it has been perceived, occurs in two different phases. First of all the information is recognized in the 'short-term memory'. This lasts for an incredibly short time, 20–30 seconds only. Very few perceptions can be stored in the short-term memory at any one time. Further information is then perceived which can alter the situation or action that needs to be taken. Following this either the short-term memory is overwritten or the information is passed to the 'long-term memory'. An everyday example of this is driving a car. Sit in the back seat and watch the driver's eyes in the mirror. Note the visual attention that is being paid to an enormous number of stimuli: the state of the road, the number of pedestrians, the other vehicles on the road. Other sources of information, too, are being received. Auditory ones from the engine and the sound of the surrounding traffic as well as any conversation going on in the confines of the car. Sense of position in the driving seat, the feel of the wheel as inequalities in the road are overcome, all these and many other aspects are passed initially into the short-term memory. The information is being processed, action taken if necessary or short-term memory overwritten. Some pieces of information are being passed and stored in the long-term memory for retrieval should the need arise later in the journey, or on the way back if the route is an unfamiliar one.

Information can be held in the long-term memory for a lifetime. This does not mean to say that memories are necessarily retrievable immediately one needs to remember. This final stage of memory – the **retrieval process** – differs in different people. There are a number of standard ways in which people help themselves to recall facts and events:

- **System of codes** to help the storage process. The mnemonics of student days are an example of coding, each piece of information being coded by a letter, which then makes up a word. (This can have problems if what the letters stand for is forgotten!)
- Using both **auditory** and **visual perceptive methods**. An example of this is saying out loud the telephone number you have just visually looked up. This may save looking up the number again if the last digit is forgotten during the dialling process.
- Organizing the material to be remembered into a **flow chart**.

In spite of all these different aids, everyone forgets at one time or another. A number of reasons have been put forward for this:

- **Lack of adequate perception** in the first place. Lack of attention to the subject matter being presented, or a distraction which meant that part of the information was missed means that this is not a matter of forgetting, rather a matter of never having known in the first place.
- **Interference** in the material stored by similar material being stored at a later date.
- **Repression** of a memory because it brings back painful associations. This was the explanation put forward by Freud and his colleagues and is the basis for the psychoanalytical view of memory.
- **Decay or disease** of the neurones in the brain concerned with memory. Unless constant recall is practised, the information in a certain group of neurones can be lost. This is not probably the entire explanation. How can many elderly people remember how to swim even though they have

not swum for years, whilst they cannot remember the name of the visitor they had yesterday?

There is no doubt that retrieval of information can be improved by practising various techniques. Young people need to practise these techniques in order to further their careers. Older people need also to keep mentally active so that information gained in earlier life is not lost.

For reasons of space, this chapter has only been concerned with basic outlines of psychology/social development in children. For further, more detailed, information, other texts should be consulted.

FURTHER READING

Baddeley, A. (1983), *Your Memory – A User's Guide*, Harmondsworth: Penguin.

Buzan, T. (1982), *Use Your Head*, London: Ariel Books.

Coleman, A. (1988), *What is Psychology?* London: Hutchinson.

Davenport, G. (1994), *An Introduction to Child Development*, London: Harper Collins.

Greene, J. (1987), *Memory, Thinking and Language*, London: Methuen.

Gross, R. (1987), *Psychology*, London: Hodder & Stoughton.

EARLY LEARNING

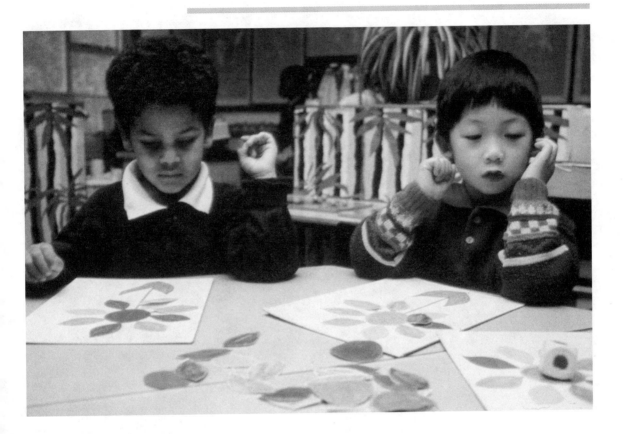

7. EARLY CHILDHOOD LEARNING

OBJECTIVES

1. Understand the nature and purpose of early childhood education from birth to eight years.
2. Acknowledge the work of early educators.
3. Identify different types of play, and be able to provide appropriate resources within a safe environment, bearing in mind the needs of individual children.
4. Understand the structure and function of the National Curriculum.
5. Recognize thematic approaches to play and the curriculum.
6. Knowledge of parenting and educational provision in other countries.

CHILDHOOD EDUCATION

Babies begin to learn from the very day they are born. The instinct for survival is the greatest motivation in these early days, but within a very few weeks the baby will have learned that crying will relieve uncomfortable sensations such as hunger and pain. So, even at a very few weeks of age, communication skills have already begun to be learned.

During the first months of life a baby has to learn to make sense of the world into which she has been born. Her own body and the people and objects immediately around her will occupy her whole attention during this time. As she grows, learns and matures, horizons will be widened to include a wider range of people and situations.

Whilst the learning process – at all ages – must ultimately be a personal one, mothers and carers can do much to help developmental processes. Here a sound knowledge of child development is vital so that toys and activities appropriate to the child's developmental age can be supplied. For example, it is of little use explaining the details of a train set to a 6-month-old baby – but at six years of age he or she will be quite fascinated by this information. Similarly a dangling mobile will be of little interest to a 4-year-old, but will give much pleasure to a baby of four months as well as giving elementary information on movement and distance.

It must be remembered, too, that children should not be forced in any way on to their next developmental stage, whatever their chronological age may be. Carers should be sensitive to the needs of the child at each stage, and share in the enjoyment of the particular activities in which the child is presently engaged.

Student exercise

Watch a 6-month-old baby with a mobile strung across his pram. Note the number of times in 5 minutes that he reaches out to strike it and with which hand, and what else occupies his attention during this time span.

How a child learns

Learning occurs in two different ways, by **direct experience** (learning by trial and error) and by **indirect methods** (learning from other people or inanimate objects such as books, other aspects of the media such as television or from other children).

The baby's initial learning comes from direct experience. The motor skills of movement with head and limbs are the first to be mastered. These progress over the years to the wider skills of running, jumping, riding a bicycle, swimming – the list is endless. Along with these motor skills come the adjacent ones of vision and hearing and eventually language and social skills. Until all these basic practicalities are learned by direct experience, the child will not be able to learn indirectly from others. There are many activities that parents and carers can undertake to help children in learning these tasks. These will be discussed in the section on 'Play'.

By the time the second birthday is reached a secure hold on the world around the child will have been gained. Movements – both large ones and finer ones – will be confident. Much has still to be learned regarding specific tasks, but now is the time that indirect learning plays an increasingly important part. Parents can now **show** their child how to perform many tasks. Much practice – and frustration! – will be needed before the activity can be properly achieved, but the basis of more formal education can now be seen.

Verbally the 2–3-year-old is full of questions such as 'How?', 'Why?' and 'What?'. Explanations need to be given, in simplified form initially, even if they are not understood fully. Talking and querying is very much a learning process at this age, both for gaining understanding of events and activities as well as improving on verbal skills. Solitary play will be accompanied by almost constant chatter with much make-believe content. The child will be telling himself how to perform a certain task and then proceed to do it – or to grumble at himself if it is not done properly! A child will practise all activities – the direct experience again. Carers need to be sensitive to the times when the child needs some help by direct intervention to prevent frustration at being unable to perform some self-imposed task adequately.

Student exercise

Observe a group of 3–4-year-old children for a period of time. Listen to their conversation and watch how they interact with each other. Write down the time and reason for any necessary intervention by an adult, for example when the children started arguing or if they were beginning to get frustrated or when they began tiring of the particular activity.

The child of three years of age will be able to relate past and present events and be able to look forward to not-too-distant future happenings. He is becoming a social being and can be fascinating company as his unfolding personality becomes more obvious. Maybe he is quiet and prefers to play quiet solitary games, or maybe he is active and boisterous, preferring noisy drums to tinkling pianos! Whatever personality is developing the pre-school child will need the security of an adult nearby and a relatively structured timetable of daily events. Whilst she may be 'in charge' of fantasy events – 'Teddy has a tummyache' or 'Teddy is naughty' – real events will need the secure base of a familiar adult.

The preschool years are a time for encouraging children to learn and find out. At this age curiosity is intense. Being sensitive to, and satisfying, this curiosity will sow the seeds for future formal learning.

By the time of school age (five or six years depending on which country the child is living in) indirect learning will be more in evidence than in the earlier years. Books, television, visits and corporate activities will play an important part in the child's life. In the early school years, activities such as play on swings, climbing frames, riding tricycles and bicycles, all play a part in the daily timetable. Agility and control will be improving daily and skills will be being practised in the company of other children in the playground.

Indoor play will have progressed to the enjoyment of board games. Drawing and painting will also show increasingly better results. Story books with pictures are popular. Reading alone, as yet, is not a favourite hobby, as reading skills need to be more secure and this is rarely achieved before the age of around seven years. A bedtime story read by a familiar adult at the end of a busy day is still much enjoyed.

Socially the 5–6-year-old child will be playing happily with many different friends, but more interested in the type of activity than by the people involved. At this age boys and girls play together. Within a brief year or two, however, it is noticeable that friendships of the same sex are made and consolidated which may be lifelong.

Parents and full-time carers will, at this time, no longer have so much control over the child's activities and ideas. Many other sources of information and ideas will be available to the school-age child, but it is important that the child still feels able to confide in, and talk to, parents or a familiar adult within a secure and confidential environment. Worries, frustrations and anxieties all need to be aired and sympathetically treated.

Parents have a definite role to play in early childhood education. From the earliest days they can:
• provide opportunities to learn new skills by the provision of appropriate toys and learning aids;

- give encouragement to try out new skills;
- allow children to find out for themselves through play, but be available to help understand any difficulties encountered;
- let the children in the later preschool and school year help themselves in planning events and activities;
- be available to relieve worries and frustrations;
- set examples of behaviour and teach moral standards.

Obviously those adults in the closer, most frequent, contact with the child will have the greatest influence, but any adult that a child meets can play a part in his early education.

Role of parent in learning
- Provide opportunities
- Encouragement
- Availability
- Set examples

EARLY CHILDHOOD EDUCATORS

Many people over the years have influenced children's education. The nineteenth century was particularly rich in ideas. This ran in parallel with the differing attitudes and knowledge of children's needs and development current around this time. Psychologists such as Piaget, Bruner and Skinner did much work on the basis for knowledge of the way in which children's cognition developed. Workers in other disciplines also began to verbalize their ideas on childhood education. Below is a summary of the work of just some of these people.

Froebel

Friedrich Froebel 1782–1852 was a German teacher who first acknowledged the need of young children to be educated. He began the 'kindergarten' movement for children who hitherto had been considered too young to attend school of any kind. He bought a derelict farm in 1817, and began teaching preschool children. Froebel encouraged children to discover learning for themselves. Trained teachers were available to provide adequate and suitable materials, and gave encouragement and guidance. Graded toys are an important part of Froebel training in providing experience of mathematical and artistic skills.

Pestalozzi

Froebel worked for a time with Johann Pestalozzi (1746–1829), a Swiss educator and reformer. He was much opposed to rote learning and Froebel strongly endorsed this. Pestalozzi set up schools for poor children who were unable to receive any education at all. (All schools at this time were fee-paying and so quite out of the reach of many children.)

Montessori

Maria Montessori (1870–1952) was born in Italy. She eschewed a comfortable social life and, after much difficulty, qualified as a doctor in 1896 – the first woman to do so in Italy. She became interested in paediatrics but later contact with children in the slums of Rome, channelled her considerable energies into teaching these underprivileged children. She believed that, given the opportunity, children were self-motivated to learn and so – in the context of the slum children of Rome – could improve their state. As well as her self-motivation concepts, Maria believed that:

- young children learned by various tactile stimuli – smell, touch, etc.;
- teachers should **encourage** children to learn rather than learn by rote;
- children until the age of around seven years feel more secure in a 'child-sized' environment – small chairs and tables, for example;
- language was learned at a particular stage of development, and a quiet, relaxed environment was necessary for good language development.

Her ideas became popular in Rome and schools began using the Montessori methods of teaching. Maria's son, Mario, continued her work in the UK where a Montessori society was established in 1912. Montessori teaching is still practised – sometimes in a diluted form – in many parts of the world today. Maria Montessori died in 1952 having seen many of her ideas put into practice.

Isaacs

Susan Isaacs (1885–1942), an English woman from Lancashire, was much influenced by Froebel and John Davey (an American educationalist who had very similar ideas to Froebel). Together with her second husband, Nathan Isaacs, she established a school in Cambridge in 1924 for children between the ages of three and seven years. This school allowed children much freedom to express themselves noisily. The Isaacs also started, at the time revolutionary, sex education lessons with reference to animals. The school had to close in 1927 due to local complaints of its permissiveness and lack of discipline. Susan Isaacs also thought that:

- children's ideas should always be listened to, considered and answered;
- children need gentle guidance to make sense of their environment;
- play is vital to good development.

She published a good deal of material on educational projects and shared many ideas with Maria Montessori when the latter was living and working in London.

Early educators
- Froebel
- Pestalozzi
- Montessori
- Isaacs
- Steiner

Steiner

Rudolf Steiner (1861–1925) was an Austrian philosopher, writer and teacher who founded the anthroposophical movement. A number of schools for children with special needs were opened and taught according to Steiner's ideas which related, in some measure, to the occult.

In recent years, an American programme – Highscope – has been adopted in many preschool groups as a forerunner to our National Curriculum. In this programme children have a good deal of choice in their play activities. At the end of each session, the child describes to the group (with the help of an adult if verbalization is difficult) what they have been doing. This is thought to give purpose to their play experience.

Children thus learn to take responsibility for their own actions at an early age. Adults, whilst not playing an actively innovative part in the play, need to be skilful in subtly directing, interacting and channelling the children's activities.

PLAY

Practically all childhood learning is done through play. There are many ways of defining 'play', but perhaps the most useful is 'play is children's work'. In the past, play was seen as merely the way of getting rid of children's surplus energy and passing the time until the child became an adult. It is now realized that play is an essential part of the educative process – basic skills and concepts are learned through this method.

Two main theories of play have been postulated. Firstly, those ideas based on the cognitive developmental thoughts of Piaget and his co-workers. Play is thought of as a series of developmental processes through which the child learns about, and manipulates, the world about him. Play, according to Piaget's concepts, is the practice and perfecting of in-built skills. Other psychologists thought that play also taught the acquisition of new skills. Secondly, the psychoanalytical theories of play postulated by Freud and similar-thinking workers considered play to be the way in which children expressed, and came to terms with, needs and desires. Probably play is a mix of these two differing schools of thought, both of importance in normal development.

Types of play

Two types of play have been described – 'free' play and 'structured' play. The best type of **free play** is in a minimally structured environment where children are given free choice to play with what, where and how they play Time is given to explore and investigate various play materials at the child's own pace. Conversely the worst type of free play is that where the environment is haphazard with minimal learning opportunities.

Covert adult supervision is necessary, of course, for groups of children to play freely. Intervention may be necessary under, for example, any of the following conditions:
- to oversee the safety of the children at play;
- to minimize, and sort out, disputes;
- to encourage shy, diffident children to take part;
- to provide extra suitable equipment to extend the ongoing play session.

Structured play is play under adult guidance with specific aims in any one activity. Here the developmental levels of the children involved must be carefully monitored. Again there is a place for both these aspects of play in early childhood learning

'Hands-on' experience of objects in the environment all teach about shape, colour, texture and size. During active play physical development is enhanced.

Play is children's work

Types of play
- Free play
- Structured play

Student exercise

Watch a group of children at water play and note how increasingly adept they become with utensils involved. From this write a set of guidelines that could be used for assessing a child's ability to improvise, adapt and explore.

Playing with other children develops social skills and the concepts of sharing. Speech is also refined as a means of communication during play. Play also stimulates imagination, the child practising different roles in any number of imaginary scenarios. All these facets of play can be summarized under the general headings:

- discovery play;
- physical play – both gross and fine motor control;
- social play – 'games' play;
- creative play.

Discovery play

This is the play that is begun in the very early days of life. The young infant soon learns the cosy comfort of his mother's arms, the warm milk on his tongue and the softness of clothing. The baby's first toys are likely to be soft woolly animals. Rattles and 'activity gyms' all add the concepts of vision and hearing to the feelings of touch. (The activity gym has hanging objects mounted on a frame under which the baby lies. As she moves her arms and legs the various mobiles move and create sounds. This type of toy is an extension of the stringed beads and other objects across a baby's pram.)

As the baby matures, so will his skills of manipulation. As he starts to sit firmly, the range of toys can be increased. Textures, shapes, sizes can all be discovered by the use of toys in the bath or on the tray of a high chair. Learning to drop objects from a height – for adults to pick up! – is a favourite pastime of the 9–10-month-old baby. This teaches the beginnings of distance and height.

A 1-year-old child will enjoy taking objects out of various containers, but not necessarily returning them again. Simple equipment is eminently suitable for this type of play – a cardboard box or a drawer removed from a chest.

By the time two to three years is reached, many basic materials such as sand, water, dough, plasticine and paints can all be used in discovery play. All these objects will:

- extend **sensory development**: the feel of warm, soapy water as opposed to clear, cold water or the different textures of sand and earth;
- increase knowledge of various **natural materials** and their properties: the ways in which dough and plasticine can be moulded into different shapes with varying degrees of ease or building sand castles

with just the right proportions of sand and water to make a firm structure;
- help understanding of **volume, size and change of state**: for example eggwhites can be whisked to a firmer, and different coloured, texture from the original runny state in a cookery session; water, when frozen, changes its state from a liquid to a solid.

('Messy' play – sand, earth, finger painting – can help children living in an urban environment understand that being 'messy' is not necessarily wrong. Children living in rural areas learn easily that muddy fields are all part of the natural world!)

By four to five years, the child will be extending his play into other discovery channels. Plants, insects and small animals all help in the acquisition of knowledge of the natural world around. These activities will:
- increase understanding of the **life cycles** of animals and plants;
- teach the **continuous care** that is necessary for all living things: for example, a plant that is not watered will quickly wilt and an animal that is not fed will die;
- instil concepts of **basic hygiene**: for example, animals in cages need to be kept clean, hands need washing after digging in a sand-pit or garden;
- give **relief of tension** by vigorous activity such as digging or hammering with special toys, or helping to build a house for the new rabbit or guinea-pig.

Basic resources/equipment for discovery play
The list is endless, and not necessarily expensive:
- For water play:
  - safe containers for water;
  - smaller containers for tipping and filling;
  - sieves – a kitchen colander is ideal;
  - tubing of different sizes – small piece of hose, drinking straws;
  - liquid detergent for making bubbles;
  - sponges.
- For sand play:
  - safe, clean sand pit or tray;
  - containers, plastic cups, buckets, digging instruments;
  - moulds/combs for making patterns;
  - various miniature toy animals/people/plastic flowers for building scenarios.
- For dough, plasticine, clay play:
  - suitably large hard surface;
  - rolling pins;
  - shapes/ biscuit cutters of all kinds.
- For natural world play:
  - small patch of garden, if possible (if not, plastic tubs in which to plant small seeds); damp kitchen paper on which to grow mustard and cress.;
  - various quick growing seeds;
  - possibility of small animals to care for – hamsters, rabbits, guinea pigs;
  - supply of water and seeds (or scraps) for birds during very cold or very hot weather.

- For messy play:
  - cornflour, water, food colourings;
  - finger paints, large sheets of paper.

Student exercise

Write to RSPCA at Causeway, Horsham, West Sussex, RH12 1HG. Ask them to send their 'early years worksheets' on small animals for nursery age children (cost approx. £2.50 inclusive of postage). Use the information on the cards to teach children about the habits, homes, food, etc. required by any animals with which they may have contact, either at home or in the nursery situation.

NB It is vitally important that:
- all equipment is clean and well-maintained;
- all equipment is safe;
- the resources and equipment are appropriate to the age of the children;
- the children should be adequately protected (overalls when playing with water, warmly dressed when outside, suitable footwear out of doors);
- facilities are available for cleaning up afterwards.

These rules, of course, apply to every type of play.

Physical play

This begins in the very early days of life with the large wide-ranging movements of the limbs of small babies. Rattles, activity mats and bath toys all aid physical development.

By the time nine months of age is reached, sitting has been stabilised and so will increase the range of possible physical activities The baby will be starting to crawl and back and limb muscles develop alongside the nervous control of muscles allowing more complex activities. Standing upright will further extend the range and eventually running, jumping, hopping and climbing will all be part of the physical repertoire of the 3–4-year-old child.

Music has many advantages in encouraging active physical movement in even young children. Few people, and children are no exception, are able to resist moving rhythmically to a catchy tune or beat.

Student exercise

Play a number of different types of music tapes to a group of 3-year-old children. Then write down:
- their immediate response;
- the different effects music has,
- the average length of time children will listen.

All these activities relate closely to the developmental profile of each individual child.
- Physical development of the groups of large muscles is encouraged.
- Balance and co-ordination is taught. For example, a 2-year-old child is unable to stand on one leg. By five years of age this is an easy task, and most children of this age will be able to hop – a simple enough movement it would seem, but one which requires much coordination. Catching a ball also requires coordination of muscular action and vision. In addition spatial awareness is becoming a recognizable factor.
- Premathematical concepts of weight, size and momentum are taught. For example, throwing a ball will give information on distance and force needed.
- The need to cooperate with other children and to 'take turns' will be understood. Physical play has a part to play in the learning of social skills also.
- Tension will be relieved. All young animals – and again children are no exception – need to use their abundant energy. If facilities for this are not allowed, frustration and tension build up with possible resultant difficult, or challenging, behaviour.
- From a purely physical viewpoint, physical play encourages adequate circulation of blood and good breathing patterns.

Basic resources/equipment for physical play
Again the list is long, and many simple everyday objects can be valuable for this type of play.
- **Open spaces** are vital for healthy physical play. Ideally at least one physical activity a day, even if only a walk, should be in the open. Weather may preclude this during the winter months. Under these circumstances a large room or hall is a good second choice. All outdoor open spaces must be securely fenced off from contact with traffic, and in rural areas, from dangerous streams and ponds and stray animals. Many areas have purpose-built playgrounds which fulfil all these criteria as well as having safe surfaces under equipment such as bark, rubber or grass, and equipment must be safe and well-maintained. Swings should be of rubber or wood rather than metal and slides should preferably be built into the side of a hill rather than having high steps to the top.
- **Indoor surfaces** must be similarly safe and non-slip and with appropriate matting for running and jumping.

Other equipment should include:
- mobile equipment such as scooters, tricycles and later bicycles;
- balls to throw, ropes to climb and skip with;
- toys to push and pull (to teach concepts of the force necessary to move a given distance as well as developing muscles);
- barrels to crawl through;
- tapes of suitable music for music and movement sessions. (Saint-Saëns'

Physical play
- Encourages physical development
- Teaches balance and coordination
- Teaches premathematical concepts
- Encourages cooperation with peers
- Releases tension

Carnival of the Animals and Prokofiev's *Peter and the Wolf* are all-time favourites to which to listen and move.)

Student exercise

Visit several different playgrounds if possible. Design a table to show the details you notice at each one, e.g. fenced or not, type of surface, number and type of equipment, safety standards, hazards, etc. Write a report on your visits comparing the playgrounds and any suggestions as to how they might be improved.

Social play

From the earliest days, sociability is encouraged by all sorts of games from simple 'peek-a-boo' with a young baby to complicated indoor board games or playground games with rules that need to be kept by the older child. Again, introduction of various types of activity need to run in parallel with the developmental age of the children involved.

Many games played by children have an historical content as well as a cultural one. Marbles, hopscotch and skipping games have been played by generations of children – and fashions in these come and go. Quiet indoor games such as 'Ludo' and 'Snakes and Ladders' have been played over many years.

Pretend play also comes under the category of social play. Here domestic and wider adult activities such as engine-driving or nursing are acted out, often needing cooperation with other children. Dressing-up for various roles is great fun, and also contains a certain social element. Pretend play can also help children come to terms with various worrying, stressful or frightening life events they experience. For example, a hospital visit can be acted out, or the feelings felt by the arrival of a new brother or sister relieved. These aspects of play will encourage and develop:

- cooperation with other children and adults with games in ascending order of difficulty as the child matures;
- communication with others through the medium of play; for example, children who find it difficult to communicate directly, can use a 'pretend' telephone or speak through a finger puppet;
- speech and vocabulary; new situations demand new forms of speech and words if cooperative play is to be achieved;
- imagination; fantasy worlds can be created by adopting the persona of an adult; the difference between fantasy and the real world can also be conceptualized by pretend play.
- 'inner' thought, by the reliving of previous experiences and situations;
- preliteracy skills by 'pretend' writing of shopping list, notes and labels;
- premathematical skills by stacking and grading equipment such as clothes, cutlery or crockery.

Pretend play improves:
- Cooperation
- Communication
- Speech and vocabulary
- Imagination
- 'Inner thinking'
- Preliteracy skills
- Premathematical skills

Student exercise

Write down the number of play situations you can think of that would be provided by:
• six cardboard boxes of different sizes;
• some sticky tape;
• three pots of different coloured paint.
Put your ideas into practice at the eariest opportunity.

Basic resources/equipment for social and pretend play
• **Space**. Ideally, different parts of the nursery should be made ready for differing types of play
• **Home corner** with child-sized equipment of everyday objects and furniture. Thoughtful equipping of such areas can teach much regarding living in different cultures. This can be extended to include items used in shops, hospitals, hairdressers, etc. Packets of everyday groceries can be saved and used for 'shops' as can old Christmas and other cards for stationers. (Much of the potential fear of attending clinic or hospital can be acted out in this type of scenario.)
• **Dressing-up corner**, with a variety of different clothes can be in close proximity to the home corner. This again can teach much about the cultural differences in clothing. Remember to supply a range of different sizes and types of clothing so that imaginations can be stretched. Parents can be helpful in providing items for the dressing-up box.
• **Smaller construction-type toy area**. This should include larger items such as train sets, road lay-outs, etc., as well as Lego and similar construction toys.
• **Sand pits**, preferably outside. Buckets, spades and moulds will also be needed with off-cuts of wood suitably cut and prepared for building houses, cars, boats.
• **Everyday objects**. Cardboard boxes, sticky tape, paints and large sheets of paper make for a variety of imaginative play situations.

Creative play

This type of play comes into its own from around two years onward. The basic skills of running, walking, climbing and fine motor control have been learned and are being continually practised.

Creative play is essentially a quieter occupation than other types of play. Again suitable equipment is endless, but a firm table or other strong surface, of a suitable size with matching sized chairs is a basic requirement.

As well as stimulating creative thinking and imagination, creative play:
• improves hand/eye coordination;
• teaches further size, weight and consistency of materials;
• gives children a sense of achievement when a final product is produced;
• teaches matching of shapes and colours to produce a pleasing end-product;

- teaches further learning of premathematical skills by the weighing and measuring aspects of the creative processes.

Creative play can form the basis for many later adult leisure pursuits, such as painting, sewing, embroidery, collage-making as well as giving basic information on simple cooking procedures.

Adult intervention should be as minimal as possible. Once the basic setting and materials have been provided, children should be allowed a free rein to play with what they wish. Materials need to be replaced when running low or if spoiled and, of course, adults need to be available to advise and sort out creative ideas if a child becomes 'stuck'.

Before starting out on creative activities – which tend to be rather messy at times – children must be adequately protected by overalls. Similarly, adequate washing facilities at the end of the session must be available.

Basic resources/equipment for creative play

- Large and small sheets of paper – plain and coloured – with suitable pens, pencils, paints, brushes and crayons.
- Stiff card, crepe paper, sticky tape, glue.
- Round-ended scissors, rulers, sponges.
- Large needles, thread, material, beads for threading.
- Cooking equipment – bowls, spoons, scales, rolling pins.
- Materials for collage making. This can be all kinds of natural materials such as seeds (take care that seeds used are not of a poisonous variety), nuts (be sure that none of the children has a nut allergy) as well as pieces of material, cotton reels, coloured paper etc.

Finally no play session at the end of the day is complete without a quiet time with a picture or story book, depending on the ages of the children. Old favourites can be read time and time again and interspersed with new characters and situations. These stories help preliteracy skills, introducing concepts of the relationships of symbols, ideas and actions. Rhymes – the old favourite nursery ones as well as more modern, or spontaneously made-up ones – are also valuable, as well as fun.

Cross-cultural stories at this early age help understanding of other children's lives, and parents can be involved in these sessions, to be continued at home if possible. Many nurseries are able to lend appropriate books to parents for this purpose. Younger children will enjoy looking at the pictures as the story is read. In this way, understanding that the printed symbols have meaning is instilled.

Play is an essential part of good child-care practice. Good play opportunities are vital to every child's early learning experience and will lay foundations for later, more formal, education.

ASPECTS OF CURRICULUM

The word 'curriculum' has a wide range of meanings. These range from the more rigid meaning in the school years when the demands of the National Curriculum are paramount, to all experiences and activities in which all ages take part. As has been seen when discussing play, every session, formal or informal, is a learning process for the baby and child, and so can be included in the definition of 'curriculum'.

Early years curriculum

Characteristics of the this curriculum, i.e. that time before formal schooling begins, includes:

- account to be taken of the ways in which children learn at various **developmental levels**: it is vital that activities should be geared to developmental age rather than chronological age;
- recognition that preschool learning is important as a **preparation** for later formal learning and adult life;
- recognition of the importance of the **input of parents**, and other significant influential people in the child's early life; nurseries and day-care centres of all kinds need to be in close touch with parents so that events and activities are common in both parts of the child's life;
- **equal opportunities** for all children independent of race, creed, colour or gender;
- subjects to be presented singly but as part of a **whole range of activities**; for example, one play session could incorporate information and practice on premathematical, prelinguistic and social skills;
- curriculum to be **broad** and **balanced** in outline, encouraging as many learning opportunities as possible at one time.

All play activities, whether in a nursery, day-care centre or a private childminding situation need to bear these characteristics in mind when activities are planned. Later on when the school years begin, the National Curriculum will formalize these aims.

Before discussing more formal schooling, there are certain aspects of child care with which children need to be conversant before starting school. This will make the change – and it is a big one for every child – occur smoothly.

Parents or carers should be sure that their new school-age child is able to:

- dress himself – do up buttons, zips;
- put on shoes – do up buckles or laces;
- go to the toilet without help and wash hands afterwards;
- use a knife and fork;
- know his name and address.

As well as creating independence (and also helping often overstretched teaching staff) children will feel at ease with these self-help skills and so be able to give their full attention to educational activities on offer at school.

National Curriculum

The National Curriculum aims to provide, for children between the ages of five and 16 years, a broad-based education on a definitive range of subjects. In addition, personal and social skills are developed within this context.

There are 10 foundation subjects which are required to be studied at school – mathematics, English, science, history, geography, music, art, physical exercise, technology and (from 11 years on) a foreign language. Maths, English and science are referred to as 'core' subjects. These must be understood, and used, adequately in most of the other subjects.

The curriculum is divided into four 'Key Stages':
- Key Stage 1 – from 5 to 7 years;
- Key Stage 2 – from 7 to 11 years;
- Key Stage 3 – from 11 to 14 years;
- Key Stage 4 – from 14 to 16 years.

Assessment takes place at the end of each key stage. These assessments are known as 'Standard Assessment Tasks' (SATs). The results of these SATs, together with ongoing assessment of each child by the teaching staff, provides teachers with information as to where (if at all) each individual child needs help.

There has been, over the years since the introduction of the National Curriculum, much controversy over the practicalities of the delivery of this, both from the teacher's and the children's point of view. The **planning** for the delivery of the National Curriculum is a specialized and demanding task to which teachers devote much time and thought. As well as planning the best way to **deliver** all the elements contained in the concept of the National Curriculum, **evaluation** of results must be done. Teaching children is a dynamic subject, with differing needs at different times for individual children.

In both early learning and formal schooling **cross-curricula themes** are of great value in a complete educational practice. Basically this means that more than one aspect of the curriculum is being learned in any one activity.

National Curriculum needs:
- Planning
- Delivery
- Evaluation

Thematic play

This can be just as useful in the nursery as can more sophisticated themes for teaching across the curriculum in the early school years. In the nursery the emphasis must be on the development of skills, in keeping with the stage of development reached by the children involved. In the 5–7-year-age group, concepts and facts will be more to the forefront in any planned cross-curricula activity. Whatever is planned, remember that the child should gain as much as possible in all ways from the activity.

An example of cross-curricula activity within a nursery situation could be the use of a child's birthday cake with the appropriate number of candles (perhaps provided by the parent who on this special occasion might manage to be present):
- The texture, taste and colour of the cake (icing?) gives **sensory input** in a number of ways.
- The sharing of the cake, and celebrations, consolidate **social skills**.
- The singing of 'Happy Birthday' teaches **verbal and musical skills**.
- The **scientific principles** of the candles (light, heat, melting wax) could be further explored (perhaps in more detail at a later date?

Student exercise

Make a list of all the activities you can think of with candles as a main theme and extensions to the candle theme that could be used at a later date, for example:
- events in the child's life that could be associated with candles;
- what safety aspects can be taught.

A more sophisticated cross-curricula theme for early school age children could be one on travel. Types of travel could be explored e.g. on foot, on horseback, by car or aeroplane. Children can be asked to find pictures of different forms of travel in magazines, books or newspapers. These could be amalgamated into a 'scrap-book of travel'. Bearing in mind the subjects of the National Curriculum, the following cross-curricula examples could be explored in the context of travel:
- **Maths**: distances travelled, understanding of speeds, focus on money in different countries visited, recording numbers on tickets;
- **English**: widening of vocabulary, looking at different symbols associated with travel, e.g. Highway Code, tape recording a 'pretend' announcement, e.g. 'The train now leaving . . .';
- **Science**: looking at aspects of movement, e.g. horse's hooves, wheels; understanding principles of stopping and starting, and differing speeds of travel;
- **History**: older methods of travel, e.g. pony, penny-farthing bicycle; understanding use of chronological references;
- **Geography**: differing modes of travel in different countries; maps;
- **Art**: drawing different transport systems.

So this one subject of travel gives practice and teaching in many different subjects in an interesting way. This could be extended over several weeks with careful planning.

Student exercise

As a nursery exercise, the older children could be asked to tell you all the different modes of travel that they can think of. Then ask them to draw which they think is:
- the fastest, the slowest;
- used the most, used the least;
- the most modern, the most old-fashioned.

Further aspects of the curriculum are outside the scope of this book and information can be obtained from Her Majesty's Stationary Office (HMSO) who publish leaflets on the curriculum.

Schooling

Schooling in the UK is compulsory from the age of five years. As a legal requirement children have to attend school (or assure education authorities that an acceptable alternative is available) from the beginning of the term after their fifth birthday. This differs from most other European countries where formal schooling begins at six years, but many of these countries have greater nursery provision.

Infant schools provide for children between the ages of five to seven or eight years, depending on which part of the country the child lives in. Then, junior, or middle, schools provide education until 11 or 12 years respectively before secondary school is entered The vast majority of schools are State-run nowadays, LMS (local management of schools) having been taken over by boards of governors. There are also fee-paying schools, or private, infant and junior schools.

The State also run schools for children with specific learning difficulties – although the emphasis today is on integration, if at all possible, into mainstream schools or special units attached to main-stream schools.

A number of parents opt out of State-run and private schooling altogether (for a number of different reasons) and teach their children at home. This is a legal option. The 1944 Education Act made full-time attendance 'either at a school or otherwise' compulsory. An organization 'Education Now' gives advice on alternative forms of education.

CHILD CARE AND EDUCATION IN OTHER COUNTRIES

The child-care practices described relate to those in the UK at present. It is interesting to note the similarities and differences between these and those in other European countries: differing financial arrangements, maternity (and paternity) leave, patterns of parental work as well as educational facilities. Details of half a dozen countries, in alphabetical order, are noted below.

Belgium

Family features
- Maternity leave is 15 weeks.
- Paternity leave is three days.
- Each parent is also entitled to a certain number of days – unpaid leave – to care for a sick child.
- 62% of mothers of children under 10 years work, for an average of 30 hours per week.
- 92% of fathers are also employed.

Belgium is unusual in as much as there are two main communities – French and Flemish – speaking different languages and with welfare and education being the responsibility of each community. This has meant in the past different standards and provision of services.

Education

Around one-third of all under-threes are provided with publicly funded nurseries organized by the welfare services. There are other facilities available in family day-care centres. These centres are available all day, all the year round. Many parents contribute financially. Staffing ratios are one adult to seven children, and three or four children per family day-care workers.

Practically every child has full-time nursery education from three to six years of age provided by the education services. This is free at the point of contact, but all such services are subscribed to by community government legislation. Staffing ratios in nursery schools are one teacher for up to 19 children, and two teachers for up to 38 children.

Denmark

Family features

- Maternity leave is 18 weeks.
- Paternity leave is two weeks.
- There is parental leave (either parent) of 10 weeks with a further three months possible leave for each parent.
- 74% of mothers with children under the age of 10 years are employed for an average of 34 hours per week.
- 85% of fathers are employed.

Denmark is unique in having a well-organized facility for parental leave. There is a high proportion of employed mothers, and fathers are regarded as very much part of the child-care scene. There are strong moves for the provision of workplace child-care facilities.

Education

Unlike many other European Union countries, Denmark has a central ministry – the Ministry of Social Affairs – for both child welfare and education. Nurseries offer accommodation in local authority day-care centres for children from birth to three years of age. Staffing ratios are one adult to three children under three years. There is a maximum of five children for each family day-care worker. Kindergartens, publicly funded, are available for 80% of 3–6-year-olds. Staffing ratio in this age group is one adult to six children. Financially parents contribute to these care facilities through the welfare system, with subsidies being available for low-income families.

France

Family features

- Maternity leave is 16–26 weeks for more than three children.
- No paternity leave.
- Parental leave is shared between parents at three days/parent/year.
- 59% of mothers of children under 10 years are employed for an average of 34 hours per week.

- 90% of fathers are employed.

France has been far ahead of other countries in the provision of nursery schooling for 3–6-year-olds for many years.

Education

There is a range of provision for the under-threes – some nurseries run by local authorities, some by groups of parents coordinating trained nursery staff. Family day-carers also provide a service and are paid by the local authority. Opening hours are all day throughout the year. Staffing ratios are one adult to five children not yet walking and one adult to eight children who are walking. The services are free to parents who contribute through the welfare system.

Full-time nursery schooling for 3–6-year-olds has been available in France for 99% of children for a number of years. Staffing ratio in these schools is usually one teacher to 30 children with the help of classroom assistants.

Germany

Family features

- Maternity leave is 14 weeks.
- No paternity leave.
- Parental leave is shared between parents, up to 25 days per year.
- Mothers work at different rates in east and west Germany, but this is gradually changing. At present these rates are 69% east and 49% west.
- 90% and 93% of fathers are employed respectively.

Germany is the largest EU state, but many federal powers are devolved to 16 states (Lander). Central government provides general guidelines for child care, but this is administered by the 16 states. Since the unification of Germany many changes have been under way and welfare and educational provision are just two of these.

Education

For the under-threes most public provision is in nurseries paid for by the local authorities. Parents contribute to this through the state system. There are also many private unsubsidized family day-carers. Staffing ratios vary in each Lander from one adult to five children to one adult to eight children.

Most 3–6-year-olds attend kindergarten, publicly funded but organized by voluntary organizations. Staffing ratio is one adult to 10–14 children. Numbers are not laid down for family day-care.

Italy

Family features

- Maternity leave is five months.
- No paternity leave.
- Parental leave is six months shared between the parents. This leave is

paid at the rate of 30% of the usual wage, but leave to look after sick children is unpaid.

- 41% of mothers of children under 10 years are employed.
- 93% of fathers are employed.

Again there is a split in welfare and educational services in Italy. There are marked differences in provision between the north and the south of the country. The local authority nurseries, which exist in the north, do not exist in the south. Parents have to rely heavily on family or private arrangements for the care of children. Much work is under way to improve the situation.

Education

Provision for the under-threes is limited to a minimal number of publicly funded nurseries. Staffing ratio is one adult to six children. Relatives or nannies fill this gap. However, 90% of the over-threes are in nursery schools, open during term-time for up to 10 hours per day. These are run by central government, and parents contribute through the welfare system. Other nursery schools are run by private or religious organizations. Staffing ratios are two teachers and one assistant to 25–28 children.

Portugal

Family features
- Maternity leave is between 12 and 22 weeks.
- No paternity leave.
- Parental leave is up to 24 months shared by parents with 30 days leave to care for a sick child; both are unpaid.
- 70% of mothers of children under 10 years are employed, often full-time.
- 95% of fathers are employed.

Portugal has changed over recent years from a dictatorship to a government which has child care very much at heart. Parents, both mothers and fathers, in Portugal tend to work long hours – often at long distances away from home. Services for children are split between welfare and education departments.

Education

Around 12% of under-threes are provided for by publicly funded centres or by non-profit-making organizations. It would seem that many young children are cared for by relatives or private carers. Staffing ratios in the publicly funded centres are one adult to five non-walking children and one adult to 8–10 walking children; four children per family day-carer is the advised ratio. Around half of 3–6-year-olds are catered for by the welfare services, with the other 50% of nursery schools being run by the education department. The welfare-run centres are open full time all through the year. The education run schools are solely concerned with education of the children and are only open from 9 a.m. to 3 p.m. during term-time. Staffing ratio is 1.5 adults to 25 children.

Student exercise

Design and complete a table to show the differences in maternity leave, paternity leave, patterns of parental work and educational facilities between the UK and other European countries. You will need to carry out some research to complete this exercise.

FURTHER READING

Brain, J. and Martin, M.D. (1989), *Child Care and Health*, Cheltenham: Stanley Thornes.
Einon, D. (1985), *Creative Play*, London: Penguin.
Geraghty, P. (1988), *Caring for Children*, London: Baillière Tindall.
Moyles, J.R. (1989), *Just Playing?* Milton Keynes: Open University Press.
O'Hagan, M. and Smith, M. (1993), *Special Issues in Child Care*, London: Baillière Tindall.

8. PROFESSIONAL PRACTICE

OBJECTIVES

1. **Identify and demonstrate the qualities needed for a professional carer.**
2. **Understand working as a member of a caring team, including meeting changing needs and situations.**
3. **Identify, analyse and evaluate own and colleagues' performance as well as that of children.**

QUALITIES NEEDED

Posts available

The possibilities of employment for qualified nursery nurses are both extensive and exciting. Many varied posts are available in which learned skills can be practised and improved. For example:

- in the local authority there are:
  - nursery classes
  - day nurseries
  - infant schools
- in hospitals there are:
  - maternity units
  - children's wards
  - child assessment centres
- in the private sector there are:
  - posts as a nanny
  - posts in workplace crèches
  - childminding needs
  - day nurseries
  - jobs in the holiday industry

to mention just a few.

A brief look at some of the possibilities is of interest. For further detailed information on any one area of work the specific authority should be contacted.

Local authority day nurseries

These are funded by social services and are open for most of the year, only closing for statutory holidays. Availability is from 8.00 a.m. to 5.30 p.m. (or later in some cases) and so are ideal for single parents who need to work full-time. Most children who attend day nurseries are referred there by health visitors, doctors or social service personnel, following breakdown in family dynamics for a wide variety of reasons. The work of the day nursery is often extended into work with the family as a whole and includes parent groups and individual programmes for children in special need or distress.

Staffing levels in these nurseries is high with a usual ratio of one member of staff to every four children. All staff are trained to a high caring standard with special individual training courses where necessary. This type of work requires a good deal of maturity and understanding. Many of the children – and the parents – have long-standing difficulties.

Private day nurseries

These are becoming increasingly in demand to meet the needs of working parents, and many new nurseries are currently being established – often by people with a nursery nursing background. Premises, staffing levels and facilities have to be inspected by social services, fire officers and environmental health officers before being registered. These private nurseries are a valuable provision eking out the meagre state provision in the UK.

Family centres

These centres can be viewed as an extension of the work of the day nurseries in as much as social work with families is undertaken. These centres are funded by a variety of bodies – social services, an education department or voluntary bodies. Each centre will have a different emphasis on various aspects of family care according to local need. For example, mother/toddler groups, day care, resource centres, activity groups are some of the facilities on offer.

Workplace nurseries/crèches

Such nurseries are set up as daily childminding facilities for the workers in a company. Crèches must be registered with social services and checked for facilities, staff and safety. This type of child care facility has not been taken up widely by companies in the UK.

Schools

Schools admitting children of four years of age, and also those for children with special needs, are interesting places for nursery nurses to work, but again work possibilities are restricted due to financial constraints. Special skills for dealing with the needs of children with disabilities are needed for work in special schools or those units attached to existing schools catering for children with less severe difficulties. In some places social services employ peripatetic nursery nurses to give specialized help such as Portage schemes or liaison between home and school for children with special needs.

Hospitals

Some health authorities employ nursery nurses in hospitals (maternity wards and children's wards), to help with general care and play. This work opportunity is gradually reducing due to the increase in high technological medicine and financial cutbacks.

Private nannies

Work as a private nanny is probably one of the most popular choices for a newly qualified nursery nurse. Nannies are employed in a wide variety of situations by professional and business people who are out at work all day. Full daytime charge of the children is the usual rule. Both daily and live-in posts are available and are advertised by agencies who also advertise in such publications as *Nursery World* and *The Lady*. Many posts offer exciting prospects of travel.

It is important that nursery nurses are fully aware of their expected duties (and also other facets of the post such as time off, salary, hours to be worked, sickness arrangements, etc.) at an interview before accepting a post. A contract should be insisted upon to finalize such arrangements.

Working as a nanny can be quite a 'sea-change' from anything previously experienced. Living in close proximity with a family, who may be different in every way from her own and having full charge of the children for a large part of the day, can seem daunting initially. The lack of professional companionship with its sharing of problems as found in college or when working in nursery or hospital settings, can also be worrying at first. But with maturity and a little give and take on either side, both children, wider family and nursery nurse can benefit from the arrangement. Children get the security, stability and stimulation so necessary during the early years, parents can feel happier at leaving their children and the nursery nurse can feel happy at a task well done.

Private nannies need to be aware of:
- Expected duties
- Salary
- Time off
- Hours to be worked
- Sickness arrangements

Holiday industry

The holiday industry is also a source of employment for the adventurous. Hotels, in this country and abroad, which offer facilities for children, employ nursery nurses to care for, and amuse, children whilst parents pursue their own holiday activities.

Childminding

Finally, childminding on a daily basis is a further option, particularly for nursery nurses who have young children of their own at home. This is the most popular child-care arrangement open to working parents. Childminders need to be registered with social services under the Nurseries and Childminders Registration Act (1968). Safety, hygiene, personal health of the childminder, any criminal records of the immediate family all have to be checked out. Recently an organization has been formed, the National Childminding Association (see Appendix). This association gives advice on contracts, insurance and many other aspects of childminding.

This type of work can be very rewarding for a nursery nurse whose circumstances are such that she wishes to be at home with her own children. The atmosphere for the child being minded is homely and relaxed and he/she will have much one-to-one attention as well as having ready-made brothers and sisters to join in play activities.

Holiday/after-school activities
In addition to this broad outline, nursery nurses are an invaluable asset to holiday and after-school care schemes. Respite care schemes, which allow parents of a child with special needs to have a brief rest from full-time care of their child, are also situations where the skills of a nursery nurse are valuable.

Babysitting
Babysitting can also help a nursery nurse on a low income. Parents will always be pleased to employ someone as a babysitter who has had experience and training in the care of children. When babysitting always be sure to know:
- the child's usual routine;
- what to do, and where to contact the parents, in an emergency – this includes knowing the telephone number of the child's doctor;
- where to find refreshments for both child and baby-sitter;
- what time the parents are expected home.

Babysitters need to know:
- Child's usual routine
- Emergency routine
- Where to find food for child and self
- When parents are expected back

Qualities for differing posts
Obviously with such a wide variety of opportunities, emphasis will need to be placed on different aspects of child care depending on the type of work chosen. For example, in a holiday situation, play skills will be important. For a nanny or maternity post a deeper knowledge of the needs of young babies and children will be required.

But all nursery nurses need to have certain basic qualities to care for children from babyhood to the age of eight years:
- The most obvious one is a **love** of children and the ability to give consistent and appropriate care at all times and under all circumstances.
- **Maturity** is needed for the responsibility entailed in looking after other people's children on a long-term basis. Maturity is also vital for the **confidentiality** needed. A live-in nanny will learn much about the private lives of families, and on no account must this implicit trust be betrayed. (Maturity is not necessarily equated with age – an 18-year-old can be more mature than an 80-year-old at times!)
- High standards of **personal integrity** are vital. However hard the going may become, the needs of the children must always come first.
- High standards of **personal behaviour and cleanliness** must be kept. Children learn much by imitation and role models have a duty to show them the highest standards.
- Nursery nurses must also have **good health**. Looking after children is a demanding, physically tiring occupation.
- Nursery nurses must be prepared to undertake work with children who come from a **different culture** than their own. Differences in diet, religious practices, dress, for example, must be understood and adhered to.
- Nursery nurses must be able to work as a **member of a team**. Child care

is a multidisciplinary field which gives much scope for variety and interest. But to fulfil the obligations of the team, **flexibility** must be a quality of the nursery nurse. For example, work in a child assessment centre or hospital situation will involve the sharing of the day-to-day intimate knowledge of the child with other professionals who also have the interest of the child at heart. To do this the nursery nurse must have good **observational skills**, be able to record accurately and take part in discussion. She must also be able to evaluate correctly the differing skills of other professionals and to know when their specific strengths are needed in any particular situation.

Basic qualities for nursery nursing
- Love of children
- Maturity
- Integrity
- Good health
- Ability to work in a team

CHANGING FACE OF THE FAMILY

Both the qualities required for a nursery nurse and the wide variety of work available have, in part, all come about due to the rapidly changing face of the family over the past generation or two.

In Victorian times and at the beginning of the twentieth century families were large, owing both to the fact that many children were conceived from a lack of contraceptive knowledge and the fact that many children did not survive infancy. Fathers were remote figures and mothers played a central part in the rearing of their children having no opportunities to work outside the home. Women had no property, legal or voting rights. Very different life styles were seen in rich and poor families, but at both extremes the wider or extended family were usually available to help with child care. (Wealthy families, of course, were able to afford full-time care from the original prototype Nanny.)

Since this time, many far-reaching changes, both social and economic, have altered the face of the family. These changes are very much interrelated and their effects cannot be separated.

- The **status** of both men and women has altered profoundly since the beginning of the twentieth century and with this the responsibility for the care of the children. Votes for women became law in 1928 as a result of the suffragette movement and the work that had been done in World War I by women. Other legislation, such as the Equal Pay Act and the Sex Discrimination Act as well as the contribution of the activities of women in World War II has markedly changed the picture from that of Victorian and Edwardian days. In many households today, men take a prominent role in the care of young children, quite unheard of in bygone times.

- **Equality of opportunity** in both education and, to a certain extent, in work prospects for both sexes has also affected the care of children.

- **Ease of mobility** from place to place in one country and also from country to country means that no longer do several generations live in one close community: aunts, uncles, cousins and grandparents are no longer necessarily available to help with the care of the children in times of crisis.

- Adequate **contraception** has changed the size of the family. (Improved health of parents and children is also a potent factor in family size.) No longer do couples need to conceive many children in order to have two or three surviving adolescents. The number of children can be chosen, with a fair chance that they will all reach adulthood.
- Divorce has become commonplace, from being a disgrace in Victorian times. This has far-reaching effects on child-rearing practices. Divorce has been a large factor in the number of one-parent families. The struggle to make provision in this situation is hard and help is always needed for child care under these circumstances. Lone parents also arise from children born outside marriage (or long-term cohabitation) as well as the death of a parent. Lone-parent statistics are made up as follows:
  - single mothers 21%;
  - divorced mothers 40%;
  - separated mothers 18%;
  - widowed mothers 12%;
  - lone fathers 9%.
- Life expectancy has increased. No longer are there available house-bound white-haired grannies of 50+ available to care for grandchildren. This age group is fit and is either at work or leading a busy social life.
- **Different cultures** abound in our society today. This means an added dimension and richness to life, but understanding different ways of life – including the upbringing of children – can cause disruption if these differences are not talked through. Nursery nurses may have a number of children from various cultures in their care. They will need to appreciate fully both parental and children's needs.

Partnerships

All these changes contribute to the need for a qualified caring force to cope on a daily basis with children. Nursery nurses fulfil this need. They must be seen as partners in the task of providing a healthy caring environment in which children can grow and develop to their full adult potential. Partnerships must be formed with:

- **Parents**. Nursery/school care must be along the same lines as those pursued by parents at home. Confusion and frustration will be the lot of the child who has to face widely differing standards on a daily basis. Discussion on approaches must start at the outset, when the parent first comes to arrange a child's admission to a nursery, for example, or interviews a nanny for a post. Remember that parents can well be feeling upset and uneasy at leaving their child in someone else's care, whether it be at a nursery or in their own home in the charge of a nanny. They, too, will need understanding and reassurance that their child will be happy and well-cared for in their absence. If at all possible parents should be encouraged to participate in special nursery activities – at various festivals for example. In this way a true partnership can be set up.

Student exercise

List and record the occasions when it might be possible for parents to participate in day nursery activities, and what they might do.

- **Other workers** in the workplace. As mentioned before, many disciplines can be involved in the care of the child in certain work situations. Information about the perceived needs or actions of specific children will need to be shared without hesitation.
- Above all, the nursery nurse must work in partnership with the **child**. It is to the carer that the developing child will look for care, reassurance, comfort and stimulation on a daily basis. He must have full trust in his carer to fulfil all these needs.

From a wider viewpoint, there are a number of specialized situations in which teamwork between professionals and parents is vital. For example, children who have behaviour problems; children who have specific – maybe only temporary – developmental difficulties such as bed-wetting. Of great importance, the nursery nurse must always be aware of the possibility of child abuse in children who appear unusually upset or withdrawn. These special situations will be looked at in more detail later. Nursery nurses should also be aware of the statutory provisions to which parents and children are entitled.

Help available for parents

Social Services
- **Child Benefit** is a weekly cash payment for every child under 16 years (or under 19 years if still in full-time education) This benefit is paid to the person having the full-time care of the child, and is obtainable from Post Offices or can be paid into a bank or building society account.
- **Family Credit** is paid to low-earning families with children under 16 years (or 19 years if still in full-time education). One or other parent must be in work for at least 16 hours per week. The amount paid is dependent on income and savings.
- **Income Support** is paid to those parents whose income is below a certain level and who are not working, or working less than 16 hours per week.
- **One-parent Benefit** can be paid in addition to child benefit to a parent bringing up a child on his or her own.
- **Housing Benefit** can be paid to families who need help with rent and council tax.
- **Maternity Benefits** include:
  - **Statutory Maternity Pay** (SMP) is payable provided various criteria regarding length of work for one employer and the payment of National Insurance

contributions are met. This is paid by the employer, but most can be re-covered from central government.

- **Maternity Allowance** is paid to pregnant women who have paid National Insurance but who do not qualify for SMP because of changed work or being self-employed.
- Provision of day nurseries, fostering and adoption services and some children's homes are offered.
- Social Services also register and inspect, childminders, playgroups and nurseries.

National Health Service
Services offered by the NHS include:
- antenatal clinics and classes;
- family planning and child health clinics;
- school health services.

Student exercise

Visit a local Social Services Department, and obtain as much information in the form of leaflets as you can on statutory benefits associated with children. Prepare a table summarizing these leaflets, e.g. title, reference, date of issue and key words, and any others you can find.

ANALYSING CHILD BEHAVIOUR PROBLEMS

All children misbehave – quite deliberately! – at some time or other. This is all part of the process of growing-up. Learning behaviour that is accept-able for the society in which they find themselves is just one important aspect of this. It is when discipline, and safety, is compromised by certain types of challenging behaviour that definitive action by the team of parents and nursery staff, or nanny, must occur.

Primary school teachers and child-care professionals have been heard to say recently, in many contexts, that 'the problem of discipline is worsen-ing'. Children as young as three or four years old are causing problems. The possible reasons for this are complex. Some workers think that chil-dren today have a poor self-image, and react to this by disobedience and disruptive behaviour. The cause of this poor self-esteem in these children can be caused by stress in the home situation – poor relationship between parents, financial difficulties and general feelings of insecurity, for example.

To counteract this, nursery and school staff need to make the children feel valued, trusted and understood at least whilst they are at school or nursery even if it not possible for staff to alter the home situation. Children need:
- a caring and supportive environment;

- consistent handling with a predictable daily structure;
- someone to listen to them – their worries and fears as well as their joys and excitements.

Parents and nursery staff together should endeavour to give these basics to all children, and especially to those who are low in self-esteem owing to circumstances beyond their control.

Aggression

Probably the most common type of challenging behaviour met with is aggression If allowed to continue, serious bullying can become a problem. To deal with this:

- Try preventative tactics. Remove the child – or object about to be thrown – before the event occurs.
- A firm 'No' in good time can also have the desired effect of quelling a potentially explosive situation.
- Removal of an object – toy or larger piece of equipment, for example – with which the child wants to play can be helpful, i.e. the removal of a 'privilege'.

Role play

As a member of the large and thriving Tiddington Tots & Toddlers (3Ts) Day Nursery you have been asked to join a staff meeting to consider the problem of Robert. He is a 3-year-old who has been at the 3Ts for a few months but is becoming increasingly aggressive both to adults and to the other children. Discuss with your colleagues the possible reasons for this extreme behaviour and make suggestions as to how it may be handled. Make a set of notes summarizing the points considered and the recommendations made.

Verbal aggression

The use of unacceptable swear words can also be part of challenging behaviour. If the child realises that the use of such words produces a reaction in his carers, it will be used all the more frequently as an attention-seeking device. Ways of dealing with this include:

- carers setting an example by never swearing in front of the children themselves;
- not responding to this form of unacceptable verbal abuse from the child; response should only be given when this type of behaviour ceases;
- suggesting a nonsense word – 'sugar', 'bananas', for example – for use in times of stress.

Disruptive aggression

A further aspect of aggression can be general disruptive behaviour, e.g. upsetting other children's activities, calling out in quiet times, running around at inappropriate times, etc. It must be remembered that such behaviour can point to underlying insecurity and emotional disturbance. Staff should liaise with parents to try to unravel any deeper causes for the disruptive behaviour. It can be helpful:

- to allow such children the opportunity to bring their feelings to the surface by either 'acting out' situations causing them pain or by painting/drawing their feelings (clues as to basic anxieties can often be found in these ways);
- to have extra time spent in outdoor activities (this will often relieve pent-up feelings);
- getting specialist help when needed from clinical psychologists in extreme cases.

Student exercise

Prepare a list of the potentially dangerous situations that could arise from disobedience. Note any specific examples, with time date and place, you have come across in your work experience.

Disobedience

Children who persistently refuse to cooperate can cause much disruption to general activities and, unfortunately, this type of behaviour is eminently catching! Helpful ways to overcome this include:

- giving the child a specific responsibility;
- giving positive encouragement when the child responds when asked;
- being firm and deal with disobedience incidents quickly.

Remember that disobedience can lead children into many dangerous situations.

Temper tantrums

These are relatively common between the ages of 18 months and three years. In a tantrum the child will lie on the floor drumming her heels and screaming, shouting or crying. She will not listen to reason and has no intention of stopping until she is ready! There are a number of possible reasons for a temper tantrum:

- frustration at not yet being mature enough, or able, to do what she wants; the inability to verbalize fully thoughts and feelings can also be frustrating;
- 'blackmail' to get her own way; if she learns that throwing a tantrum results in what she wants this will be tried again at a later date.
- emotional needs; frequent temper tantrums can be a cry for more love and attention;
- older children or friends losing their tempers which may be imitated by children.

Trying to unravel the reason for the tantrum is half-way to dealing with it.

Student exercise

Observe a number of children having a temper tantrum in a public place, such as the street or supermarket, and note:
* the probable age of the child;
* gender,
* how the carer, or parents handled the situation;
* whether any physical force or restraint was used and why.
Write what you can learn from these incidences and suggest the most effective way of controlling such situations. Is there is any difference in incidence between boys and girls?

Handling a temper tantrum
* Do not respond to a tantrum by giving in to demands; give lots of love and attention throughout the day.
* Try to understand the difficulties occurring because of lack of communication – and do not lose your own temper!
* Always be positive and praise good points.
* Try to avoid definitive commands; rather, make suggestions and join in with the difficulties the child is experiencing.
* Do not say, for example, 'Why can't you button your coat?'. Say instead something like: 'That's a hard job – let me see if I can help'.

When a temper tantrum has spent itself the child is often exhausted and upset by the strength of her emotions. A quiet cuddle with plenty of reassurance that she is still loved is the best action to take.

Children with positive personalities, plenty of energy and determination are more likely to have temper tantrums than children with a more placid nature. Again, consistent handling by the team of parents and nursery staff is important under such circumstances.

Hyperactivity

Hyperactivity is an emotive word. It is frequently used to describe many aspects of children's behaviour – from the natural 'busyness' of the growing child actively exploring his environment to the truly hyperactive behaviour of the child with a short attention span and constant – often aimless – activity.

It may be that the child just needs more opportunities to release his energy. Outdoor play, with the emphasis on physical action, may be all that is necessary to impose periods of calm when indoors. The onset of hyperactive behaviour after the birth of a brother or sister, or move to a new house, can be a sign that the child is feeling insecure at the change in his life. Discussion with the parents about possible causes and ways of easing tension can ease this hyperactive behaviour.

Student exercise

Observe the activities of a group of children in a nursery and list the behavioural characteristics of any of the children that might be considered to be hyperactive. Note the steps that are taken to control this hyperactivity. Write a 'Guideline' for use within a nursery on ways in which a hyperactive child could be helped by the combined efforts of parent and nursery nurse.

Suggestions over the years have been made that certain food additives may be a contributory cause to hyperactive behaviour. The most common food additive that has been blamed is tartrazine (E number 102). Another additive – 'sunset yellow' (E number 110) – has also been thought to be a factor. Both these additives are used as colouring agents to make food look more attractive. They are to be found in such products as orange squash, cakes, sweets and foods coated with bright yellow breadcrumbs. Cutting out such foods is worth trying, but does not always have any effect.

Some children also may have an allergy to certain foods, for example, eggs, cheese, chocolate, and this can occasionally seem to be connected with hyperactive behaviour. The help of a dietician is valuable if these foods are thought to be a possible factor. Without such skilled help it can be all too easy to miss out some vital factor in the child's diet. Here again the nursery nurse will need to work as a team with doctor, health visitor, dietician as well as the parents.

Habits

Habits are common in early childhood. Most will automatically disappear as the child matures, but sometimes can continue for many years.

Thumb-sucking

This is a more or less universal habit in the young child. It is when the habit persists continually into the early school days that there is the remote possibility that the growth of the front teeth can be impaired. Making sure that the child has plenty to do with his hands during the day is usually all that is required to stop this habit.

When tired or ill, however, the child can often revert to this 'comfort' habit again. Whilst on the subject of 'comfort' habits, many – if not all – children will have a special soft toy or piece of material to cuddle as they drop off to sleep. Much upset occurs if this 'comforter' is mislaid – or even if it is washed! – and it is frequently many years before the toy or material is discarded.

Student exercise

Carry out a survey into one habit common to children in a nursery. Find out how many children have this habit. If it has been stopped, ask the parents when this occurred, and if any steps were taken to cause the habit to stop. Prepare a simple table of your results, e.g. age range, numbers who do, numbers who have stopped, gender, etc.

Nail-biting

Nail-biting is a further common – irritating but harmless – habit. Often the child is quite unaware that he is biting his nails, and often only does it when he is tired, nervous or deep in thought. Many have been the suggested remedies from mustard, or bitter aloes, on the nails to nagging about the habit or some other form of punishment. Usually children grow out of this habit spontaneously by around five years or so. For girls the look of the finger nails is an important factor in the cessation of this particular habit. A few adults, however, do still indulge in this particular habit.

Head-banging/cot-rocking

Head-banging and cot-rocking are both habits which affect younger children of one or two years. Heads are banged on the end of the cot just before sleep and can sound both painful and dangerous. This habit can be just part of the sleep routine. An alternative bedtime routine can often break the habit. Cot-rocking can be part of a similar routine and the same action can be the answer. If either habit persists a look at possible causes of daytime anxieties should be searched for by both nursery staff and parents.

Masturbation

Masturbation (handling the genital organs for pleasure) is another common habit in young children. Discovering their own bodies is all a part of maturation and young children should not be made to feel guilty about this particular habit. Attention should be gently diverted, and older children taught that masturbation is not an acceptable behaviour in public. It is important, however, to be sure that excessive masturbation is not a sign that the child is feeling insecure, worried, bored or frightened. It can also be a sign of sexual abuse (see the section below on Child Abuse).

Enuresis

Enuresis (bed-wetting) can be a big problem for some children. Nannies and those professionals caring for a child full-time will need to practise teamwork with health visitor and/or doctor to help the child with enuresis.

Student exercise

Carry out a media search with reference to bed-wetting and list the references. Write a summary of the advice given to parents. Obtain leaflets on and list the facilities available in your area for advice on enuresis.

The cause of bed-wetting in any one particular child is not fully known, but there does seem to be a familial tendency for bladder control to occur later than usual in the child's life. Too rigid a training schedule has also been blamed, as has too much emphasis on wet beds.

Many children are dry at night by three to four years of age, but around 10% of children still have wet beds at five years, and 1% have similar problems at 10 years of age. Boys are more often affected than are girls. Ways of promoting dry beds are:

- Never grumble at the child who has a wet bed; always praise a dry one.
- Use a star chart to mark up dry nights, perhaps with a special treat after a definite number of dry nights have been achieved.
- Do not cut down on drinks during the day. This will only serve to make the urine more concentrated and so more irritable when in the bladder. It is best, however, to avoid a large – especially fizzy – drink just before bed.
- It can be worthwhile waking the child and taking him to empty his bladder when the parents go to bed. But remember that he must be fully awake when this is done, or it will just seem like a dream. If this waking routine disturbs later sleep, it should not be continued.
- An enuresis clinic, run by the general practitioner's surgery or by the local health authority will be able to provide an alarm system – of which there are several types – which rings whenever the child starts to wet the bed The person running the clinic will also check that there is no infection or other abnormality that is causing the continuation of wet beds.
- Medication used to form part of the treatment for enuresis, but is not now thought to be advisable, and particularly not for children under the age of seven years. Results were only found to be temporary, and a return to bed-wetting occurred when the medication was stopped.

With patience and sympathetic handling most children will learn night-time bladder control, but for some families this can cause much worry and work.

Dealing with enuresis
- Do not grumble
- Praise dry beds
- Use star charts
- Give more fluids during the day, less before bed
- Wake to empty bladder
- Attend enuresis clinics

Student exercise

If possible attend an enuresis clinic. List and classify the different types of alarm available. Draw the main working parts of each system and explain how they work. Write down the advantages and disadvantages of the different types. Suggest an alarm you think would be most acceptable to a 7-year-old boy and give reasons for your choice.

ANALYSING CHILD ABUSE

This can be one of the saddest, and most distressing, aspects of the work of a nursery nurse. It is vitally important, however, that nursery nurses are aware of the possibility of abuse, and are conversant with the signs and symptoms of this possibility.

Child abuse can roughly be divided into four types (there can, of course, be overlap in any one abused child):
• physical abuse, also known as 'non-accidental injury' or NAI;
• emotional abuse;
• sexual abuse;
• neglect.

Physical abuse

Many are the ways in which young vulnerable babies and children can be physically abused.
• Direct physical violence involves punching, beating or deliberately throwing the child on the floor or on furniture. The results of this can be severe bruising or fractures of limb bones. Head injuries, including fracture of the skull, can also occur from direct violence. This latter can in turn cause haemorrhage into the brain, with either fatal results or permanent brain damage.
• Shaking the child violently can cause damage to brain tissue with similar results.
• Deliberate burning of the child's skin with cigarettes or by sitting the child on the top of a hot cooker or fire, or by putting him into a scalding hot bath.
• Biting the child – adult size teeth marks are visible in this type of abuse.
• Damage around the mouth by forcing bottle or spoon into a reluctant, or slow, feeder's mouth.

Physical abuse occurs most frequently in small babies and/or toddlers. Reasons are many and varied (see later), but a persistently crying baby whose parent lives in one room with two other children, for example, can set the scene for loss of control. The baby, being the one least able to defend himself, becomes the outlet for the parent's frustration. Toddlers, too, can be 'punished' excessively for actions which they, as yet, are too immature to alter, for example, the third wet pair of pants in a situation where washing and drying is difficult.

Signs of physical abuse can be difficult to pinpoint, but certain aspects can lead to suspicion:
• The explanation of the injury which does not seem to fit with the obvious physical signs: for example, a round burn on a child's arm said

to be caused by getting too close to an electric fire. In this case the 'roundness' of the burn would fit more with a lighted cigarette end.

- Delay in seeking medical help: for example, a child with a fractured leg who was only brought to the accident and emergency department two days after the injury.
- Injuries in unusual parts of the body: bruising behind the knees is an unlikely place for normal bruising falls. A more likely cause is hitting the child's legs with a hard object. Bruising in the armpits is also unlikely to have occurred due to a normal fall – severe shaking could be the cause.

A word of warning here regarding the interpretation of bruising. Some babies have a bluish discoloration on their buttocks or lower back region known as 'Mongolian blue spot'. This can easily be confused with traumatic bruising if the observer is not aware of this normal finding. Mongolian blue spots occur most frequently in Asian, African or southern European babies. They disappear by school age.

Emotional abuse

This can be one of the most difficult of all types of abuse to detect. It can occur in children who are unwanted and unloved – they are consistently ignored or constantly blamed for anything at all that goes wrong. Emotional abuse can be a cause of failure to grow and develop normally. Obviously physical and other causes for this failure to thrive must all be definitely excluded before emotional abuse is considered.

Student exercise

Draw up an additional list of other ways in which a child could be emotionally abused. Compile a list of actions that would have upset you when a young child.

Threats of inappropriate punishment could include such actions as:
- constant criticism – the child is never any good at anything;
- rejection – the child is being left alone for long periods of time, and never praised or thanked for any action;
- threats to destroy favourite toys or pets.

Sexual abuse

Sexual abuse probably occurs more frequently in girls than in boys. The perpetrator is often a close family relative or friend. Professor Kempe (an American paediatrician who also coined the term 'battered babies' for physically abused children) defined sexual abuse as: 'the involvement of developmentally immature children in sexual activity which they do not truly understand, to which they are unable to give informed consent or that which violates social taboos'.

Sexual abuse can vary greatly in severity – from full sexual intercourse, through fondling, masturbation and 'flashing' to pornographic activities. Children are frightened and confused by these events, and are often black-mailed into silence. The perpetrator will impose secrecy by telling the child of punishments that will occur if she tells anyone of 'our little secret'.

Symptoms that a child may be being sexually abused include:
- fear of a certain adult;
- aggression;
- withdrawal and depression;
- knowledge of sexual matters in advance of years.

Physical signs include:
- recurrent urinary tract infections;
- vaginal infections;
- return to bed-wetting;
- soreness, or irritation, in the vulval area;
- bruising in the genital region;
- nightmares.

All these signs ands symptoms can, of course, be due to other, quite innocent, causes. Great care must be taken to exclude these before sexual abuse is suggested – but again, it is the duty of all child care professionals to protect, in all ways, the children in their care.

Neglect

Neglect occurs when children are not fed adequately or suitably for their age, are not kept warm or clean or are left alone for long periods of time. Again, many are the reasons why this can occur:
- ignorance of normal child care;
- difficult social/financial circumstances;
- lack of love/responsibility for the child.

Suspicions of neglect are aroused by lack of clean clothing, unwashed hair and body, obvious hunger with ultimate loss of weight and failure of growth, lethargy and unwillingness to join in play activities.

Nursery nurses in a nursery situation should report their suspicions – and keep reporting them if no action is forthcoming – to their immediate superior. The manager of the nursery should then sensitively approach the parent and suggest ways in which the child can be helped.

Signs of neglect:
- Not fed adequately
- Not fed suitably
- Not kept warm or clean
- Left alone for long periods

Student exercise

Study a newspaper report of a case of child abuse. Make notes on:
- the people involved;
- the circumstances;
- the end result.

Write a report for workers in this field suggesting how such a situations can be avoided.

Help available for suspected child abuse can be obtained from:

- NSPCC Child Protection Helpline: 0800 800500. This is a freefone number and advice is available 24 hours a day. Children or adults can telephone this number. The address is in the Appendix.
- Childline: 0800 1111. Again this is a freefone number and can be used by any child in danger or who is being abused.
- Local social services department
- Local general practitioner or school health service
- The police in cases where the child is considered to be in immediate danger.

Child abuse is not confined to any one part of the community or to any one social class. A sad, and worrying, fact also is that in around 50% of cases of sexual abuse the offender is well-known to, and trusted by, the child.

A few guidelines exist, but are by no means comprehensive or certain, regarding circumstances and personality types who may be involved in child abuse are:

- youthful parents or those parents who have a childish, dependent personality;
- too frequent pregnancies;
- financial difficulties;
- social loneliness and isolation;
- family history of abuse or neglect.

It must be stressed that it is by no means invariable that any of these factors exist in any one case. Nursery nurses must be aware of the possibility of abuse in any of the children in their charge. As always, teamwork between professionals is a vital part of the protection of the child against abuse. Nursery nurses can be in the forefront of this by virtue of their daily contact with children. Getting to know the local guidelines and people involved with child abuse is important. When every member's special skills are known and recognized, rapid and effective action can be taken if, or when, incidents arise.

COT DEATH OR SUDDEN INFANT DEATH SYNDROME (SIDS)

The death of a child is one of the greatest tragedies that can occur in any family. Nursery nurses can be intimately involved if they are working in a family situation, and it is not unknown for a cot death to occur in a nursery. A cot death is defined as: 'The sudden death of an apparently healthy baby, unexpected by the baby's history, and in which a post-mortem examination fails to demonstrate an adequate cause of death'.

There are a number of facts associated with cot death:

- Most cot deaths (80%) occur in babies between the ages of one and six months, the third month being the most likely time.
- Boys are more likely to be affected than girls.
- Babies born in the winter months are more susceptible.
- Twins, triplets or premature babies appear to be more at risk.

Cot death risks
- 80% in babies between one and six months
- Boys more than girls
- Winter babies more susceptible
- Twins
- Premature babies

Much research has been done – and is continuing – into the possible causes of cot death. Of recent years the incidence has reduced dramatically: 1500 to 2000 babies per year died from cot death in the late 1980s. Between the years 1991 and 1993 this figure was reduced by over 50%, but still 10 babies every week die of cot death in the UK. Latest figures show that there has been no further drop in the figures for this tragedy since 1993.

It is probable that cot death is not due to one single cause, but different causes in individual babies. Possible causes include:

- immaturity of the cardiac and respiratory systems;
- an infection against which the baby's immature immunological system is unable to cope;
- overheating;
- allergic reactions.

Recent advice given by the Department of Health has undoubtedly had a bearing on the reduction in cot deaths in recent years. This advice includes:

- putting the baby to sleep on his back or his side and not lying on his tummy;
- getting medical advice early if the baby appears ill in any way;
- avoiding smoking in rooms where the baby lives (smoking should also be stopped during pregnancy);
- avoiding too many bed coverings in a hot room;
- breast feeding if possible to reduce any possible allergic reactions to cow's milk.

What to do in the event of a cot death

If the baby is found not to be breathing, it is imperative to send for medical aid as soon as possible. Telephone 999 for an ambulance if in a rural situation or, if this is quicker, drive to the accident and emergency department of the nearest hospital. The family's general practitioner can also be phoned, but phoning the ambulance first will save time. But many parents do find their own GP a comforting familiar presence.

Whilst awaiting for help to arrive, clear the baby's nose and airway of any mucus or vomit and attempt mouth-to-mouth or mouth-to-nose resuscitation. The hospital – or GP if this is the first person to see the baby – will continue to try to resuscitate the baby, but if this is unsuccessful will confirm death. If the cause of death is unknown a death certificate cannot be given and the Coroner (Procurator Fiscal in Scotland) has to be informed. This action can be upsetting for parents, but it must be explained that this is necessary to prevent potential harm to babies being done and pass unnoticed.

A post-mortem examination will be necessary to see if there is any possible explanation for the death. Only very occasionally is an inquest also necessary. The Coroner will issue a form so that the death can be registered and arrangements set in train for the funeral. It is important that the parents are allowed the opportunity to see and hold their baby again before the funeral. This can be vital to the grieving process. Feelings of guilt can occur in the parents that they could have done more for their baby or that they should have been present when he died, almost as if this – quite normal – absence at bedtime was some sort of neglect on their part.

Much help and support will be needed, both during the few hours and days after the death and in the succeeding weeks and months. Such everyday problems as to what to do with the baby's clothes and other equipment will need sympathetic handling, for example. Nursery nurses who are closely associated with the family can do much to help – by putting their own feelings of grief and puzzlement temporarily aside. Close liaison with health visitor and general practitioner is also helpful to all concerned. The Foundation of the Study of Infant Death (see Appendix) has a wide and helpful range of literature available. It is also able to provide contact with local supportive groups.

Student exercise

Write to the Foundation for the Study of Infant Death and ask for its literature. Read this, and summarize the points you consider to be particularly helpful.

It must be remembered that other children in the family will also be upset by this event in their young lives. Nannies in particular will need to give comfort and support to these children while their parents cope with their own grief. Sometimes the siblings are sent away to spend time with relatives after a cot death has occurred in the family. This can often add to their confusion and insecurity, and they will need much understanding from the people who are caring for them. Often the brother or sister of a cot death baby can regress, both physically and developmentally for a time. Unexpressed fears that they, too, will die suddenly or that, in some way, they are responsible for their sibling's death, all need to be understood and dealt with sympathetically. Many children, under these circumstances, are afraid to go to sleep, so bedtime must be made a special time of relaxed security and comfort.

In the older child, school performance may well be affected for many months after such an event. This will need to be understood and accounted for by both teachers and nursery nurses if the child is at a nursery.

It is to be hoped that nursery nurses will not be involved in this tragic situation too often during their working lives. When they do, it must be remembered that they have an important part to play in helping the surviving children and their parents.

FOSTERING AND ADOPTION

Fostering
This can be a rewarding undertaking, and anyone with a nursery nursing qualification can be suited to this. Ideally children should remain with, and

be brought up by, their natural parents. The Children Act 1989 states this as the ideal. There are, however, a number of situations in which this is impossible, either in the shorter or the longer term:

- inability of the parents to look after their child, or children, adequately;
- children who have been ill-treated or neglected;
- illness of the parents.

In the first two examples, moving the children will usually be by a Court Order. In the case of illness, or other individual problems, foster care will be worked out in agreement with the parents wishes.

The local authority through the social services will make arrangements for the care of the children. Children's homes used to be the more usual place for the care of such children, but in recent years foster homes have been thought to be preferable. Here children can be involved in a closer, more normal family life. The time that children spend in foster care is very variable, and ranges from a few weeks to many years. Prospective foster parents sign on with a register saying they are willing to foster children. Very detailed investigation of the suitability of potential foster parents has to be undertaken in every case. Payment for food, clothes and any other expenses is given by social services. Many children have, over the years, benefited immensely from the devotion of their foster parents. In fact at times, fostered children have later been adopted by their foster families.

Adoption

Adoption is a legal process whereby the adoptive parents gain complete responsibility for the care of the child. This includes all the legal rights of parents (not so the case with fostered children).

A relative can apply to adopt a child whose parents have died. Similarly on remarriage of the mother and/or father, children of the first marriage can be legally adopted so that the new family becomes more cohesive with a common surname. Other ways of adopting a child are through adoption agencies. Many prospective parents have great difficulty in finding a child to adopt these days. This is due to two main and relatively recent reasons:

- Allowances are now more readily available from the State to help single parents bring up children on their own.
- The wider availability of contraception and abortion means that there are fewer babies born to women who do not wish to raise them.

Much paper work and investigation into the suitability of the prospective parents needs to be done to be sure that the adopted child will have a happy and secure home. A probationary period of 13 weeks before the adoption can be made legal by the County or High Court is necessary A social worker from the adoption agency will visit regularly during this time to make sure that all is going well. After the adoption is made legal the adoptive parents have full legal responsibility for the child, the natural parents having no claim on the child after this event.

When an adopted child reaches the age of 18 years, she is allowed to see her birth certificate if she wishes, and try to regain contact with her natural parents. There are organizations which assist in bringing natural parents and children together.

Student exercise

Obtain, and file, detailed information on fostering and adoption from the British Agencies for Adoption and Fostering (see Appendix).

FURTHER READING

Carson, P. (1987), *Coping Successfully with your Hyperactive Child*, London: Sheldon Press.

Doyle, C. (1994), *Child Sexual Abuse*, London: Chapman & Hall.

O'Hagan, M. and Smith, M. (1993), *Special Issues in Child Care*, London: Baillière Tindall.

SPECIAL ISSUES IN CHILD CARE

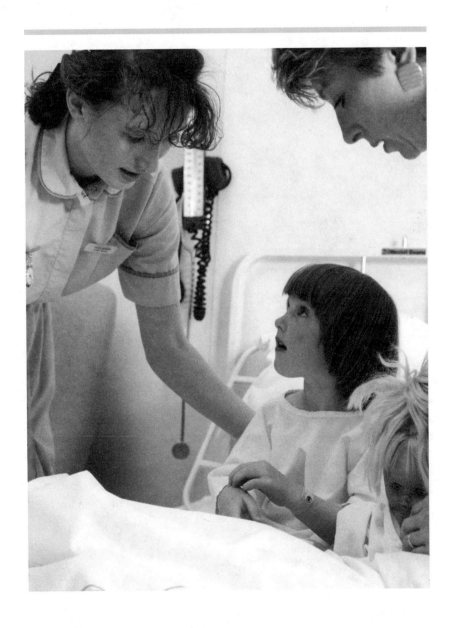

9. CARE OF THE SICK CHILD

OBJECTIVES

1. Appreciate the concepts relating to the different causes of illness.
2. Understand preventative care and hygiene.
3. Recognize signs and symptoms of common illness and the more important uncommon ones.
4. Be aware of, and understand, appropriate special procedures.
5. Develop an understanding of, and feel for, the emotional needs of sick children and their carers.

CAUSES OF ILLNESS

Regretfully illness, at some time in life, is something everyone has to face. Illness in children is different, in many aspects, to that state in adults. There are five main causes of illness.

- **Infection** is probably the most important cause of illness in children owing to their relative lack of resistance.
- **Congenital conditions** have either a genetic basis or other prenatal developmental problems. In other words the baby is born with a specific condition which will cause ill-health. Examples of this type of illness are cystic fibrosis, haemophilia or Down's syndrome, the latter causing developmental problems rather than ill-health (see Chapter 10).
- **New growths, or malignant tumours**, can affect children as well as adults but comparatively rarely. An example of this is a specific tumour of the kidney – known as a Wilm's tumour which can occur in under-fives. Leukaemia, a malignancy of the blood cells, also affects children as well as adults.
- **Degenerative conditions**, which are also relatively rare, include conditions such as Hunter's syndrome and Batten's disease. In these diseases there is a degeneration of nerve tissue in the early years of life with subsequent disability and ill-health.
- **Accident or trauma** account for a relatively high proportion of illness in children. Regretfully **non-accidental injury** (NAI) must also be included in this category.

INFECTION

As this is the most common cause of illness in children, a number of factors need to be looked at in more detail:

- types of infection;
- how infection is passed on from individual to individual;
- protection and treatment;
- prevention;
- specific infections.

Types of infection

Bacterial infection

Bacteria are single-celled micro-organisms which can only be seen under the microscope. Bacteria of all kinds abound in nature, and by no means do all of them cause disease. In fact many of them have useful properties, as, for example, certain bacteria in the lower gut which have an important function in the proper absorption of food.

There are, however, certain groups of bacteria which, if they invade the human body in excess and defence mechanisms are ineffective, cause illness. Each group of bacteria will produce a quite unique set of symptoms.

Bacteria are divided into broad groups according to their shape when visualized under the microscope:

- round-shaped bacteria, named **cocci**. Examples of this type are the streptococcus and the staphylococcus, giving rise to severe sore throats and skin infections respectively.
- rod-shaped bacteria, named **bacilli**. These give rise to such diseases as tuberculosis and tetanus.
- curved bacteria, named **vibrios**, which cause diseases such as cholera.

Bacteria reproduce at a tremendous rate – doubling their number in about 20 minutes given the right conditions! So, unless the body's defences are in good working order and/or appropriate treatment is given, the infection can rapidly become overwhelming. As well as causing direct damage to body tissues, certain bacteria can produce chemical poisons, known as 'toxins', which cause further damage.

Viruses

These are also single-cell micro-organisms, which are even smaller than bacteria. They cannot be visualized under an ordinary microscope, but can be seen with an electron microscope. They act in a somewhat different way to bacteria. It is only when they actually enter a living cell that their effects can be exerted. For this reason infections due to viruses are more difficult to treat than those infections caused by bacteria. More reliance has to be placed on the body's own defence mechanisms. Antibiotics are not active against viruses. Viruses cause many types of disease, examples of which are measles, influenza, rubella as well as common warts.

Bacteria and viruses account for the majority of infectious diseases. There are other organisms, larger and of a more complicated structure than bacteria and viruses, which are also capable of causing symptoms of ill-health.

Fungi
Some fungi widely found in nature cause no harm. Certain types, however, give rise to such conditions as ringworm, athlete's foot and thrush.

Protozoa
These are simple one-celled animals, and certain types can cause disease. An example of this is the amoeba which cause amoebic dysentery.

Parasites
Lice and fleas, threadworms and the mite causing scabies come into this category of infectious disease.

How infections are passed on
Micro-organisms such as bacteria and viruses are able to enter the body in a number of different ways:

- **Inhalation** through the nose and throat. This is the commonest way in which infections are passed on from person to person. Every time we speak we spray out tiny, invisible (usually!) droplets of secretions from our mouths and noses. If there is an infection lurking in the throat or nose this can be passed on to anyone within range. If their defences are poor, or immature as in young babies and children, they, too will soon be suffering from the infection.
- **Ingestion** of organisms which are in food or drink. Food contaminated with pathogenic (those which cause disease) organisms can cause serious illness, such as various types of food poisoning or dysentery.
- **Inoculation**. This occurs when organisms enter the body by cuts or abrasions to the skin. An example of this is when a wound is contaminated by road dirt or soil containing the tetanus bacillus. Injections, whether intentional as with drug-users, or accidental as with a needlestick injury from an infected person, can also transmit infection in this way.
- **Indirect infection** can also occur through:
  - **flies, rats and other animals**. The common house fly feeds on all kinds of rubbish and excrement which can contain pathogenic organisms. If the flies then land on food which is to be eaten, the organisms can be easily transferred to the food. (Flies have an unpleasant habit of regurgitating their stomach contents onto the food before sucking it up again!) Salmonella and typhoid can both be transferred by this means.
  - **hands** which prepare food. If hands are not carefully washed before food preparation or after dealing with a child's cut finger, micro-organisms can again be transferred.
  - **'carriers' of certain diseases**. Some people, having had an infection with a specific organism, can carry the organism for many months after they have completely recovered from their original illness. Examples of this carrier state include the **haemolytic streptococcus bacteria** which can be carried in the throat; whenever the person coughs or sneezes, the bacteria is exhaled in the form of minute droplets. People on the receiving end can then suffer from the severe sore throat caused by this organism. **Diphtheria** can also be passed

on in this way, although cases of diphtheria are extremely rare in the western world today owing to immunization against this bacteria. Another example is **salmonella**, a particularly vicious form of food poisoning, which can persist in the bowel of a one-time sufferer for many months. Unless scrupulous, regular hand-washing is done after a bowel movement, this infection can be passed on to other people in prepared food. Outbreaks of this particular form of food poisoning need careful tracing back to the person who is 'carrying' the organism, so that their carrier state can be treated and so stop the risk of infecting other people.

- **People incubating infection**. This is a somewhat different type of carrier situation, when someone is incubating a specific infection – be it bacterial or viral. The incubation period is that period of time between the original infection and the time when the symptoms appear. This can range from a few hours to – in some unusual infections – many months. The usual incubation period of most infections is measured in days or weeks. During this time the person is 'infectious' and can pass on the disease to other people.

How the body protects against infection

Immunity

This is an enormous, complex subject, detailed knowledge of which forms the basis for all immunization procedures. **Natural immunity** can be defined as: 'the ability of the body to resist infection'. Newborn babies have a certain amount of inborn immunity against infections that has been passed on from their mothers, provided, of course, that the mother herself has had the specific infections. (A certain amount of immunity is also gained from breast milk.) This inborn immunity wanes by around the age of six months. The baby then has to rely on his own immune system to protect against infectious disease.

Active acquired immunity is gained in two main ways:

- If the child has an attack of an infectious disease, e.g. measles or chickenpox, her body will be stimulated to produce 'antibodies'. These antibodies will neutralize the specific infecting agent; then, if at any time during later life, the same infection is encountered again, these antibodies will be ready and able to counteract the infection. (Unfortunately, the viruses responsible for the irritatingly frequent upper respiratory tract infections seen in many children have the nasty habit of changing their structure infinitesimally at regular intervals. So any pre-existing antibodies are not able to neutralize this new form of the virus. A similar pattern is seen with the influenza virus, new 'strains' appearing year after year.)
- A further way of actively protecting against specific diseases is by immunization. Antibodies against the specific disease are produced by the body when a small amount of the weakened – or 'attenuated' – organism is given. Signs and symptoms of the illness do not appear, but the stimulus is sufficient to produce antibodies. These will then be available to fight off later infection with the specific bacteria or virus. Examples of this are many and form the basis of the routine immunization schedules

Spread of infection
- Inhalation
- Ingestion
- Inoculation
- Indirect:
  - animals
  - hands
  - carriers

offered to all babies in the UK. (Details of current immunization schedules are given below.)

Passive acquired immunity is a far less frequently used method of protection against infectious disease. This method involves the giving of serum (the liquid part of the blood) taken from a person who is known to have suffered from the particular disease and so will have antibodies available in his or her blood.

This form of immunization is used to protect weak or ill children from an infection which would have potentially serious consequences for them. For example, a child with leukaemia would be rendered extremely ill if he contracted measles or chickenpox. Passive acquired immunity is not as long-lasting as active acquired immunity, but will protect a sick child adequately.

White cells

White cells or leukocytes in the blood are able to attack and destroy invading micro-organisms. When infection occurs, specially adapted white cells increase in number. They travel, via the blood and lymphatics systems, to the main site of the infection and enter into conflict with the invaders. During the course of this battle the temperature often becomes raised and the child will be feeling hot, lethargic and generally unwell as the body puts all its energies into defence. Lymph glands (congregations of lymphatic tissue in specific parts of the body) can also become swollen and tender. A good example of this is the way in which the cervical lymph glands – situated in the neck under the jaw – become swollen during the course of a throat infection.

Miscellaneous

There are also certain other, more specific, protective mechanisms:
- The **skin** is the biggest natural barrier we have to the many micro-organisms that surround us. It is when a break in the skin occurs that infection can readily enter the underlying tissues.
- The **stomach** contents are high in hydrochloric acid, which will destroy many organisms that are ingested along with food.
- **Tears** have an antiseptic quality which protects the delicate surface of the eye.
- In the **nose**, tiny hairs, called 'cilia', are continually in motion. This has the effect of excreting micro-organisms from the nose along with the nasal secretions which keep the nasal tract lubricated.

Good health

Good general health has a vital part to play in the fight against infection. Good nutrition, along with stimulating physical and mental activities, will provide the best possible state for this purpose. Happy, active children are less likely to succumb to infection than those children who live in difficult, unhappy circumstances. It must be the aim of every parent and child carer

Protection against infection
- Immunity
  - natural
  - active acquired
  - passive acquired
- White cells
- Miscellaneous
  - skin
  - stomach
  - tears
  - nose
- Good health

to ensure that, as well as physical needs, the emotional needs of every child are fully met on a day-to-day basis.

Control of pathogenic organisms

Hygiene

Whilst the body does much to repel and neutralize the effects of invading bacteria and viruses, there is much that needs to be remembered about the ways in which the spread of pathogenic organisms can be controlled on a day-to-day basis. Organisms cannot be eliminated completely from daily contact with children (or adults), but much can be done to ensure that conditions for their reproduction are not ideal.

Micro-organisms need warmth, moisture and food in order to live and reproduce. So denial of these basics is important. There are ways of doing this.

- Milk is pasteurized by excess heat, and fresh food can be frozen or refrigerated when being stored.
- Damp articles, such as towels, tea-towels and sponges should not be allowed to remain in a damp heap, but hung up to dry.
- Places of food preparation and also the hands of food preparers should be kept scrupulously clean.
- Prevention of contamination of food by flies and other animals, such as cats and dogs, is of vital importance.
- Good general hygienic practices in home and nursery are vital in reducing the spread of infection. Children living in dirty, untidy surroundings tend to suffer more from intercurrent infection than those living in clean accommodation.
- All people in charge of children should have the highest personal hygiene. It is also vital that children should be taught good personal hygiene habits by parents and child carers. This is probably one of the most important ways of health promotion – by example and on a one-to-one basis.

Control of the spread of pathogenic organisms from person to person

Whilst this is not, of course, completely possible there are several basic methods of reducing spread to a minimum:

- **Isolation** of the sufferer from the main group of children reduces spread to a certain extent, although many infections are passed on before definite symptoms occur. There is no merit – for nursery staff or children – in carrying on bravely with a streaming cold. It is much better for all concerned to stay at home for a couple of days until the worst of the symptoms have subsided.
- **Disinfection** of clothes, bed-linen and clothes can reduce the risk of reinfection for certain conditions. Washing in hot, soapy water is all that is necessary. Burning of used paper tissues is also important.
- **Quarantine** (the isolation of people who have been in contact with

someone suffering from an infectious condition) was used in the days when treatment for infectious conditions was restricted to nursing care only. With today's powerful drugs (and also the difficulties, with the existing work commitments of many mothers, of keeping a seemingly fit child at home) quarantine is rather an outdated concept. For example, scarlet fever – caused by the haemolytic streptococcus bacteria – used to be a much dreaded disease, and quarantine of contacts was often all that could be done to restrict the spread of the disease. Nowadays, penicillin rapidly cures this infection.

- **Barrier nursing** in hospital may be necessary for some highly infectious diseases, such as infective hepatitis or amoebic dysentery. Gowns and maybe also masks should be worn when attending to a child's needs. Also the child should have his own cutlery, plates, cups, etc., which must also be washed up on their own. Bed linen should be steam-disinfected before coming into contact with any other clothing. (Barrier nursing is also necessary in a different context – that of keeping infection away from a very sick child. For example a child under treatment for leukaemia with powerful cytotoxic drugs is gravely at risk from infection, as are also children in the process of bone marrow transplantation.)

Public health

In the wider sense, public health measures, improved vastly over the past century, have done much to reduce the spread of infectious conditions. The foundations of the modern aspects of public health were laid down in 1848 by the First Public Health Act. Many additions and alterations have occurred over the years, but the basic aims remain the same, namely:

- The community must have a supply of pure water.
- There must be adequate removal and disposal of sewage and rubbish.
- Water and air pollution must be controlled.
- There must a supply of wholesome food available.
- Living accommodation must be healthy.
- Disease must be checked and regulated as far as possible by notification and appropriate measures taken to prevent spread.
- Births and deaths must be registered.
- Provision must be made for the burial of the dead.

(Public health measures are in themselves vast areas of study, and legislation is continually changing. Interested students would do well to spend and hour or two browsing in the appropriate section of a Stationery Office (HMSO) bookshop to appreciate the range of activities undertaken by the Public Health Department of a local authority. Environmental Health Officers administer the regulations on public health.)

Aspects of the public health act

- Pure water
- Disposal of sewage and rubbish
- Water and air pollution control
- Food available
- Healthy living accommodation
- Check on disease
- Register of births and deaths
- Burial of the dead

Immunization

Active immunization against specific infectious illnesses of childhood has greatly reduced the overall incidence of these diseases.

- Some infections such as poliomyelitis and smallpox have been virtually eliminated. Poliomyelitis is still a problem in countries where there is no routine immunization schedule in place.

- Complications of some infectious diseases which can cause permanent disability have been reduced. For example, measles can leave behind deafness and/or brain damage.
- Infections which are particularly dangerous to young babies have been avoided. Whooping cough can be a killer disease in babies under one year of age, whilst meningitis due to the Haemophilus influenzae bacteria is especially common and serious in children under the age of four years.

Immunization has, on several occasions over the years, had a bad press owing to the possible complications from the actual immunization procedure. Parents can, understandably, be very worried about this when it comes to the time for their children to be immunized, particularly so in the case of the whooping cough vaccine. After much research into the subject, as well as intensive testing of vaccines for safety, the conclusion is that the benefits of immunization far outweigh any possible risks.

However, certain precautions must be taken before a baby is given any immunization. The doctor or nurse should be consulted before any vaccine is given, if the child:

- is unwell in any way;
- is receiving any medication;
- has had a severe reaction to previous immunization;
- suffers from any serious immunological defect;
- has had any severe allergic reactions in the past;
- has a history of convulsions or there is a history in the immediate family (brothers, sisters, parents).

The **routine immunization procedures** currently given in the UK are shown in Table 9.1.

Postpone immunization in cases of:

- Illness
- Receiving medication
- Severe reaction to previous immunization
- Severe allergic reactions
- Convulsions in immediate family.

Discussion

Ask several mothers at your place of work experience if their child has received the full course of immunization. Check on the reaction of mothers to immunization in general. Bring the findings back to the group and discuss what is considered to be the general feeling regarding immunization and how best fears could be allayed. Write up your notes on the discussion and summarize in a clear concise manner the points to be remembered when trying to allay a parents fears.

Common infections

Some of these conditions are rare in places where immunization levels are high. Nevertheless it is important that students are aware of the signs and symptoms, complications and natural course of these diseases as they are still encountered on occasions.

Table 9.1 Routine immunization procedures in UK

Age of child	Vaccine
2 months	DPT (triple) + Polio + HiB
3 months	DPT + Polio + HiB
4 months	DPT + Polio + HiB
12–13 months	MMR
4–5 years	Booster DT + Polio
15–16 years	Booster T + Polio

D = Diphtheria; P = Pertussis (whooping cough); T = Tetanus; HiB = *Haemophilus influenzae* (one cause of meningitis, especially in young children); MMR = Measles, Mumps and Rubella.

All infectious diseases follow the same basic pattern:
1. The micro-organism enters the child's body by one or other of the possible routes.
2. There is a period of time (the **incubation period**) when the organism multiplies rapidly. This is the time when the child is most infectious, although there will, as yet, be no specific signs or symptoms of the infection. The child may just be 'off-colour' or irritable.
3. **Manifestation** of the specific disease includes rash, fever, cough or enlarged lymph glands.
4. **Recovery** usually within a specific time scale.
5. Complications may follow.

Table 9.2 lists salient points of the so-called 'childhood infections'. Childhood is not a unique time at which to contract these infections. Adults, too, can suffer from the unpleasant symptoms and complications and can often be more severely affected than children.

Many infections are **notifiable**. This means that doctors have to notify the health authority of each case that they encounter. Important information is thus collected on the prevalence of each specific disease in the community at any given time. This gives valuable help in predicting epidemics of infectious disease and in planning immunization campaigns to control epidemics.

Student exercise

From discussions with parents you come in contact with in your work experience, compile a database of the infections their children have had. Design the database with the most useful headings for future reference rather than analysis, e.g. parts of body affected, mode of spread, effect on child, whether immunization available, etc.

Table 9.2 Common infections

Name	Cause	Notify	Incubation (days)	Immunization availability	Signs & Symptoms	Period of infectivity	Treatment	Complications
Chickenpox (Varicella)	Virus	No	10–21	Not at present	Malaise Mild fever Rash – irritating Small red spots then blisters then scabs, very irritating Usually mild	From 2 days before spots appear until 1 week after rash appears No need to keep off school until all the scabs are off	Light diet Calamine & tepid baths to control irritation	Pneumonia (rarely) Impetigo (from scratching of rash)
Measles	Virus	Yes	10–15	Yes: at 12–14 months in conjunction with mumps & rubella in MMR vaccine	Fever Cough, runny nose Red confluent rash spreading over body Conjuctivitis Koplick spots on inside of cheeks	Onset of cold-like symptoms until 5 days after rash appears	Analgesics (Paracetamol) Light diet Antibiotics (if complications) Tepid sponging (if high fever) Drops to eyes (if necessary) Darkened room (if eyes painful)	Middle ear infection Deafness Encephalitis (may cause permanent damage) Chest infection
Meningitis	Virus and bacteria	Yes	Variable	Yes (Only with HIB infection type)	Severe headache Vomiting Neck stiffness Drowsiness Rash with meningococcol meningitis **URGENT treatment**	Variable	Good nursing care possibly in hospital Antibiotics for meningococcal infection	Deafness Encephalitis (possible permanent damage) Death

Disease	Cause	Incubation period (days)	Vaccine	Symptoms	Infectious period	Treatment	Complications
Mumps	Virus	12–28	Yes: with measles and rubella MMR)	Fever Malaise Swelling on either side of jaw	Until swelling subsides	Analgesics Light diet (liquid through a straw)	Meningitis Orchitis (infection in the testes)
Rubella (German measles)	Virus (unborn baby can be damaged)	10–21	Yes	Mild fever Brief pink rash Swollen glands at back of neck	Onset to end of rash	Rest Light diet (the above only if necessary)	Maybe arthritis in older people
Scarlet fever	Bacteria	2–4	No	Severe sore throat Fever 'Scarlet' rash	Can be up to 2 weeks after onset	Analgesics Penicillin Light diet	Middle ear infection Chest infection Involvement of kidneys (rare nowadays)
Whooping cough	Bacteria	7–12	Yes	Fever Cold-like symptoms Sever cough with 'whoop' and maybe vomiting	From start of cold symptoms up to 3–4 weeks	Rest Support during coughing bouts Re-feed after vomiting, if frequent Young babies may need hospitalization	Pneumonia Encephalitis

Student exercise

Use a spreadsheet to create a list of as many childhood infections, including the more common tropical ones, and their incubation periods, that you can find. Then print:

• the list ordered by name;
• the list ordered by incubation period;
• a bar chart in sequence of incubation period (identify the infection by a three-letter reference on the bar chart).

There are, of course, a multitude of other conditions which make children ill, owing to both infective and other causes. Notes on a few of the commoner conditions are given below.

Coughs, colds:

• common, often as many as four infections a year in early school days;
• usually due to viruses;
• maybe secondary bacterial infection on top of viral infection;
• treat with rest, light diet, paracetamol, decongestants;
• avoid contact with young babies;
• normal part of growing-up and immunity gained.

Ear infections:

• middle ear most commonly affected;
• often in association with a head cold;
• fever;
• earache can be severe;
• possible vomiting;
• if untreated, eardrum can rupture or meningitis can occur;
• treat with antibiotics and pain-killers (analgesics); remember that aspirin must not be given to children under 12 years of age.

Tonsillitis:

• often associated with upper respiratory tract infection;
• tonsils red and swollen;
• neck lymph glands swollen and tender;
• fever;
• sore throat, or maybe only complaint of 'tummyache';
• treat with antibiotics and analgesics;
• mouth washes can be helpful;
• tonsillectomy to be considered if more than four proven attacks yearly.

Bronchitis and pneumonia:

• can occur when upper respiratory tract infection descends to lungs;
• can arise with no preceding cold;

- can arise due to complication of other fevers, e.g. measles;
- fever;
- cough;
- maybe coughing up infected sputum;
- treat with antibiotics.

Croup:
- affects young children up to age four years of age;
- inflammation of larynx (laryngitis in older people);
- hoarse barking cough;
- hoarse voice and cry;
- noisy breathing;
- if occurring suddenly in young baby, contact doctor urgently;
- antibiotic treatment often necessary;
- as emergency treatment, put child in steamy atmosphere, e.g. bathroom.

Bronchiolitis and epiglottitis:
- inflammation of tiny bronchi in lung, or of epiglottis at back of throat;
- seen in young babies and children;
- can be dangerous due to swelling of tiny structures;
- urgent medical help necessary if breathing affected;
- feverish, off food;
- treat with antibiotics;
- hospital admission may be necessary.

Meningitis:
- not common, but urgent treatment necessary;
- a serious infection of the meninges, the covering of the brain;
- due to either bacteria or virus;
- particularly severe and serious if due to meningococcal bacteria;
- severe headache and neck stiffness;
- vomiting;
- fever;
- blotchy rash over body with meningococcal meningitis;
- **immediate action necessary**: call doctor or dial 999;
- if treated in time with antibiotics – full recovery;
- can be rapidly fatal
- the National Meningitis Trust (see Appendix) can offer advice.

Gastroenteritis:
- infection of gastrointestinal tract;
- more common in bottle-fed babies;
- diarrhoea, vomiting, abdominal pain;
- can be rapidly dangerous in young babies due to dehydration;
- check on level of fontanelle: if it is depressed the baby is dehydrated;
- give plenty of bland fluids + 'Dioralyte' (proprietary mix of nutrients);

- if severe, hospital admission maybe necessary;
- give advice on prevention of recurrence.

Role play

In pairs, simulate a worried mother who is difficult because of her concern, asking for advice about her baby, ill with gastroenteritis. Have a leaflet ready to pass on, that you have previously prepared, outlining the ways bottle-fed babies can contract a gastrointestinal infection and how to avoid, as far is possible, a recurrence.

Skin conditions

Eczema

- may, or may not be, allergic in origin;
- often family history of allergy (eczema, hayfever, asthma);
- not contagious (passed on by contact) or infectious;
- red rash, often starting in elbow creases, behind knees or round neck;
- can be dry and scaly or moist;
- very irritating;
- can get secondary infection by child scratching;
- treat by:
  - stopping child scratching/short finger nails/bandage hands;
  - special creams;
  - cotton clothing;
  - bath oils;
  - 'wet bandaging' if very severe;
- often grown out of, but can persist, or recur, into adult life.

Impetigo

- skin rash caused by bacteria;
- often seen round mouth and nose following a cold;
- can spread to other parts of the body;
- highly contagious;
- starts as a red spot leading on to blistering and yellow crusting
- quickly cleared by antibiotic cream;
- be sure flannels and towels are not shared;
- exclude from school/nursery until treated.

'Cradle-cap' or seborrhoeic dermatitis

- can be initially confused with eczema;
- usually only occurs on head, eyebrows and occasionally face;
- brown, or white flaky scales around hair roots;
- not contagious or infectious;
- will disappear on its own within a few months;
- hasten disappearance by applying olive oil overnight and washing off later.

Nettle rash or 'hives'
- lumpy red rash in response to contact with some allergen;
- irritating;
- often disappears quickly;
- treat with antihistamine cream;
- investigate cause if occurs too frequently:
  - allergy to foods, e.g. strawberries;
  - allergy to certain medicines, e.g. penicillin;
  - sensitivity to bites, e.g. from fleas.

Warts
- caused by a virus;
- small, scaly patches;
- non-irritating;
- only very mildly contagious, except for **verrucae** (plantar warts) seen on children's feet:
  - passed on by warm, moist conditions such as in swimming baths;
  - painful due to their position;
  - treat by creams, cautery or by excluding air from foot for three weeks.

Student exercise

Find out, what precautions, if any, are taken at your local swimming baths to prevent the spread of verrucae and record the details and procedures.

Conditions caused by fungi or parasites

Athlete's foot
- caused by a fungus attacking the skin between toes;
- red, sore rash which eventually turns white and peels off;
- treat with antifungal powder or cream;
- clean socks every day;
- often to be seen in children wearing plastic footwear continually.

Ringworm
- similar cause to athlete's foot;
- found anywhere on the body including in the hair;
- can be caught from animals;
- the fungus grows outwards, leaving a red ring;
- treat with special antibiotic.

Scabies
- caused by a parasite – the scabies 'mite';
- female burrows under surface of skin and lays 20–30 eggs;
- eggs are hatched in three to four weeks when cycle is repeated;
- causes severe irritation;

- red, raised linear 'burrows';
- between fingers and around wrists the most usual site;
- very contagious;
- treat with special drug available on prescription;
- treat everyone in the family;
- bed-linen and all clothes must be thoroughly washed.

Student exercise

Write an article for a professional magazine about the more unusual parasitic infections, such as malaria, hookworm, bilharzia, tapeworm. Include a discussion on the situations in which a nursery nurse might come across these parasitic infections.

Lice
- head lice commonest in children;
- high percentage of school-children affected at one time or another;
- passed from child to child by physical contact of heads;
- lice lay eggs ('nits') which stick to hair shafts;
- lice bite scalp to obtain blood – this causes irritation;
- treat with specific shampoo or lotion;
- 'nits' may also need to be removed with a special fine-toothed comb;
- treat all the family;
- frequent hair brushing and combing will reduce likelihood of infection, but remember:
- lice like clean hair – so there is no disgrace.

Threadworms
- again, very common in schoolchildren;
- tiny, white worms about 1 cm long;
- do little harm, but can cause itching around anus especially at night;
- each worm lays around 10 000 eggs which can survive for long periods;
- child is reinfected from finger nails which have been scratching;
- other family members can be infected from bed-linen, clothes, dust;
- treat with specific medication;
- treat all the family;
- prevention:
  - wash hands after using toilet, before meals;
  - clean hands for food preparation;
  - wash raw fruit and salads thoroughly.

Other conditions

Asthma (see also Chapters 10 and 13)
- an allergic condition;
- familial tendency – other members may have hayfever or eczema;

- attacks of wheezing and breathlessness, often occurring initially at night;
- varies in severity;
- attacks can brought on by infection, emotion, exercise, cold weather, animals;
- treat with specific drugs – hospital admission may be necessary for severe attacks;
- physiotherapy and graded exercise useful for severe cases;
- prevent by avoiding known 'triggers';
- can disappear spontaneously as puberty approaches, but can be life-long.

Epilepsy (see also Chapters 10 and 13)
- many different types;
- convulsion (fit) caused by an abnormal electrical discharge in the brain owing to:
  - brain injury;
  - brain tumours;
  - hereditary condition;
  - specific syndromes;
  - unknown;
- treat with specific anticonvulsant drugs;
- investigate any possible underlying cause.

Febrile convulsions
- caused by the reaction of the immature brain to a sudden rise in temperature;
- only seen in children under five years of age;
- twitching of muscles, blue pallor of face;
- may become unconscious briefly;
- treat by cooling:
  - open windows and doors;
  - remove excess clothing;
  - tepid sponging;
  - contact doctor;
- prevent by keeping cool when feverish;
- if occurs frequently rectal Valium can be prescribed.

Student exercise

During your nursery experience, or any other suitable situation, find out how many children have attacks of 'wheezy breathlessness'. Prepare a table showing:
- how many these have been diagnosed as having asthma;
- how many are on regular medication;
- how many have a positive family history of allergy;
- how their condition affect their play.

NURSING A SICK CHILD AT HOME

How to tell if a child is unwell

This may seem at first sight to be obvious, but remember that young children are not sufficiently verbally able to describe how they feel. Also they often complain of something quite different from what could be expected. For example, a child with a severely raw red throat due to tonsillitis will often only complain of a tummyache. So various other clues must be sought to decide if a child is unwell. Parents and carers after some experience of each individual child will recognize these clues, which include:

- unwilling to play as usual;
- irritable and grizzly;
- loss of normal appetite;
- unusual pallor;
- feels hot and looks flushed.

Other signs, such as:

- vomiting;
- diarrhoea;
- a cough; or
- a rash

will make the diagnosis clear.

When to consult a doctor

Throughout childhood, there will be many episodes of sickness, diarrhoea, coughs and colds, all due to relatively trivial causes. A feverish child can become completely well again within a few hours, and conversely a fit child can become seriously ill within a very short time. A few guidelines as to when the services of a doctor or hospital are necessary include the following occasions:

- a severe injury causing excessive bleeding;
- a burn which blisters and covers more than 10% of the body surface;
- a severe bang on the head, e.g. a fall from a bed or a chair;
- severe diarrhoea and/or vomiting, particularly in a small baby where dangerous dehydration is an ever-present worry;
- difficulty in breathing;
- a fit or convulsion;
- swallowing any poisonous substance;
- swallowing any object, for example, button or safety pin;
- a high fever;
- a suspected ear infection;
- a rash accompanied by obvious illness;
- unconsciousness;
- in small babies, any abnormalities in the cry.

Day-to-day care

There are very few conditions which necessitate a child staying in bed all day. He will be far happier playing in a warm, quiet room with normal day-to-day activities going on nearby than being in bed upstairs all on his own. Nevertheless it is important to remember that he is unwell and will not be able to amuse himself in the usual way. Children often regress to an earlier developmental stage when they are ill. They become less self-reliant and are more 'clingy' and prone to tears. A return to bed-wetting, in a child with previous good bladder control, is often one of the first signs of an impending illness.

Routine

All children need the security of routine guidelines for behaviour and activities. This is perhaps even more important when they are unwell. Times at which food is offered – even though it may not be eaten and/or enjoyed as much as when he is well – should be regular. For the younger ones, rest times should be times of quiet, even if it means sitting quietly in someone's arms whilst a book is read or a picture-book examined. In between these 'slots' of time, activities suitable to the child's age and interests will also need to be planned. Attention spans are shortened during bouts of illness and changes of occupation should be frequent, but still with an overall pattern. When children are ill, they can become frightened by the unpleasant feelings they are experiencing. A routine as near as possible to the normal one, given by a familiar person, can help dispel these fears.

Diet

A child who is unwell will not feel like eating. It is important, however, that she has sufficient nourishment to fight off infection and also to continue to provide for growth. Meals should be light and appetizing and presented in small portions with an emphasis on known favourite foods.

Fluids should be readily available throughout the day and the night, and the child should be encouraged to drink as much as possible. This is especially important if much fluid has been lost from the body by diarrhoea and/or vomiting, or if the temperature is high with fluid being lost in perspiration.

Student exercise

Map out a 'care' timetable, e.g. schedule of activity, times of rest, etc., for the guidance of the parents of a child who is over the worst stages of a cold but who still needs to be at home. Also include, for them, a list of suitable activities and foods that might be acceptable at this stage of the illness.

Cleanliness

This is an important part in the control of infection, as well as making the young patient feel more comfortable. A daily bath – or all-over wash if the child is very sick – is necessary. Hair needs to be brushed and it is a good idea to encourage tooth-cleaning, or the use of a mouth-wash, after every meal. This latter will freshen up mouths feeling stale due to the infection.

If the child is in bed for any part of the day, her bed should be made tidy and comfortable at frequent intervals. Clean night-clothes and bed-linen when necessary will also make for comfort and control of infection.

Parents and carers should also be extra vigilant in their own cleanliness. For example, hand-washing before and after attending to the sick child's needs is important in preventing cross-infection to other members of the family. Remember, too, to burn or otherwise carefully dispose of any paper tissues that have been used.

Observing, recording and reporting

This is a vital part in the care of the sick child. Observations on the amount of activity that can be sustained, the amount of food and drink that has been taken, effects of any medication given as well as the normal temperature, pulse and respiration measurements are all necessary in determining if the illness is following the usual course towards recovery, or if any complications are occurring.

Taking a child's temperature

The normal range of body temperature in a child is 36.1–37.2 °C (97–99 °F). Readings are often higher in the evening than in the morning. Readings can also be artificially raised by activity and/or excitement in children, due in part to a child's relatively immature control of temperature.

There are four areas from which a child's temperature can be read:
• in the armpit or the groin;
• in the rectum;
• in the mouth;
• on the brow.

For younger children – under the age of 12 years – it is usual, and safest, to take the temperature in the armpit or groin. Clinical thermometers made of glass can easily be bitten through if the temperature is taken in the mouth. Rectal temperatures can be usefully taken in babies, but this method needs training and experience. With very young children and babies, the fever strip used on the brow is probably the safest method (see below).

When reporting on the level of a child's temperature, always quote where the temperature has been taken. Armpit temperatures are a little lower and rectal temperatures a little higher than those obtained from the mouth.

There are three different types of thermometer in common use:
• The **clinical thermometer** is basically a glass tube with a bulb at one end and containing mercury. This tube is marked with gradations of temperature in degrees Centigrade and Fahrenheit. When the bulb end is put under the child's arm, the mercury will expand and so move up the tube until the temperature of the child's body is reached. (Remember NOT to wash this thermometer after use in boiling water. The mercury will rise and break the glass tube if you do!)

To take the temperature with a clinical thermometer:

1. Be sure the mercury is shaken down so that it is well below the arrow marking a normal temperature. There is a knack in shaking down the mercury: hold the top end of the thermometer firmly and flick downwards rapidly using your wrist. Repeat several times.

2. Place the thermometer in the child's armpit. Sit the child on your knee and hold her arm close to her side for two minutes. Many thermometers state that the temperature can be taken accurately in half a minute, but it is preferable to let the instrument remain for two minutes.

3. Remove the thermometer, and, holding it horizontally and in a good light, read off the temperature measured by the level of the expanded mercury. Record this for reporting later.

4. After use, wash the thermometer in tepid water, and shake the column of mercury down again to the bottom of the markings. Dry carefully and replace in case. (If temperatures need to be taken on a regular basis the thermometer can be kept in an antiseptic solution near the child's bed.)

- The **digital thermometer** is battery-operated. It is easy to read, accurate and safe to put in an older child's mouth. It consists of a narrow probe with a tip sensitive to temperature, a display panel and an on/off switch.

- A **fever strip** will not give an accurate temperature recording, but will tell if the child's temperature is above normal. It consists of an oblong strip of thin plastic containing special crystals which change colour according to whether there is a fever or not. To use, hold it firmly against the child's forehead for about half a minute, when a colour change will be seen. This thermometer is useful for a quick subjective check.

Taking a child's pulse

This measurement gives information on the activity of the heart – its rate of beating and the force of contraction. The pulse can be taken on the thumb side of the wrist in a position where a main artery – the radial artery – passes over one of the bones of the forearm. With gentle compression by two fingers, feel the pulse and record the rate. Be sure you do not attempt to take a pulse with your thumb. The pulse in your thumb, which is near the surface in this part of the body, will fudge the reading of the child's pulse.

Babies and young children have a faster pulse rate than do adults: the pulse rate of a young baby is around 120 beats per minute. As the child matures the pulse rate gradually slows until the adult rate of between 60 and 80 beats per minute is attained.

Count for a full minute – you will need a watch with a second hand – or count for half a minute and multiply by two to get the heart rate per minute.

A child with a fever will have a raised pulse rate due to the excess work the heart is having to do to overcome the infection. Care must always be taken in the interpretation of the pulse rate. Events – exciting or worrying – can also give rise to a raised pulse rate.

Measuring a child's respiratory rate

Respiratory rate is a measurement less often taken routinely, but can give helpful information if the child has a chest infection, for example. Under these conditions the respiratory rate will be higher than the normal rate of between 16 and 20 breaths per minute. By observing the child at rest, a respiratory rate can be counted. This information must be taken into account with the observations on temperature and pulse.

Role play

Practise taking the temperature, pulse and respiratory rate of your colleagues, using different types of thermometers, if possible. Record the results and note any difficulties you experienced, e.g. finding the pulse, and how these were overcome.

Giving medicines

This is a pit for the unwary! It is incredible the number of ways that children can avoid taking necessary medicine if this task is not approached in the right way. Young babies are the easiest age group with which to cope. Medicine for this age must, of course, be in a liquid form. If it is not accepted from a spoon, try trickling the fluid into the baby's mouth with a disposable syringe – without the needle attached, of course!

Liquid forms of medication are also acceptable for children under the age of seven years. Tablets and capsules are difficult to swallow for this age group, but if there is some reason why a liquid form is not available, tablets can be crushed and added to a favourite food or drink. Most liquid medicines for children these days are produced with a pleasant taste and are sugar-free. If the giving is made into a game, with the help of a favourite toy, you will probably succeed. A sweet, a piece of fruit or a drink can be given afterwards.

Medicine must never be forcibly given to a child. There is always the risk of medicine being inhaled into the lungs if the child becomes very upset.

Probably the most usual medicines to be given to a child are antibiotics to treat some infection. It is vital that this is given strictly according to the instructions, and also important that the full course be given, even though the child appears to be vastly improved after a couple of days of treatment. (Also remember that it is dangerous to give anyone medicines prescribed for someone else or to use up any drug, mistakenly left over from a previous occasion).

If you think the medicine is having unwanted side effects (e.g. a

---

Normal rates for children
- Temperature: 36.1–37.2 °C
- Pulse: 60–80 beats per minute (100–120 in babies)
- Respiration: 16–20 breaths per minute

Never force a child to take medicine.

rash) contact your doctor and ask for advice before giving any further dose.

Remember to store all medicines in a cool place well out of reach of children, preferably in a locked cupboard or drawer.

Other medication, such as insulin for diabetic children, has to be given by injection. Parents will be shown how to do this regular treatment when their child is in hospital following the diagnosis of this particular condition. Nursery nurses and other long-term child carers will also need instruction on how to do this for young children with diabetes in their care.

Emotional support

Illness is – thankfully – not an everyday occurrence for most healthy children in the UK. So when some infection, or other health problem, does occur, children can be upset and frightened at the strange feelings that assail them. Parents, too, are concerned and worried about their sick child. Professional child carers can do much to provide emotional support throughout periods of illness. Their advice, calm attitude and knowledge are especially valuable if they are conversant with the natural course of the specific illness, how to treat it and the action to take if any complications should occur. Much confidence can be given by professionals to parents who, because of work commitments, need to leave their sick child in someone else's care throughout a long day.

Convalescence

Most children bounce back relatively quickly to full health after any illness, but it is as well to remember that there may be a day or two following an infection when they are not ready to resume full activities. A couple of days spent with quieter tasks, with definite periods of rest interspersed into the routine will do much to aid the recovery process. An added bonus of this will be that the next infection going the rounds will be shaken off quickly.

Nursery staff should also be aware of the need for a little extra care and attention for a child who has recently been ill.

Admission to hospital

Being admitted to hospital is a shock to anyone at any time. For a child especially this can be an extremely upsetting event. He will:
- be in a strange place with strange people;
- not understand fully the reasons why he is there;
- not have his own familiar bed, toys or bath;
- be eating different food;
- be subjected to a completely different routine, which may be painful.

Paediatric wards, specially designed and staffed with children in mind are very different from the wards to which children were admitted 50 years or so ago. At this time children were usually put into a male or female adult ward with no special facilities or play materials. Sick elderly people must have made very frightening companions for the children of those days.

Today children are admitted into bright, homely wards with play areas, toys, play therapists as well as child-sized beds, cutlery, chairs and tables. Also there are specially trained staff, fully conversant with children's needs, to oversee the medical and nursing care of the child. Parents can visit as often, and for as long as they please. In many hospitals provision is also made for a parent to stay with their very sick child and to cooperate in his care – a very different picture form a few decades ago.

Reasons for admission to hospital

These are many and varied, and can be grouped into four main headings:
- emergency reasons, following an accident or an emergency medical condition such as a severe asthmatic attack;
- an elective surgical procedure such as the repair of a hernia or a tonsillectomy;
- investigations and later treatment of a specific condition such as diabetes or cystic fibrosis;
- specific treatment which is impossible or difficult to carry out at home, or where the home conditions are not suitable for the prescribed treatment.

Reasons for admission to hospital
- Accident
- Emergency medical care
- Elective surgery
- Investigations
- Specific treatments
- Adverse home conditions

Preparing a child for admission to hospital

In all but the first of the reasons for hospital admission there is much that can be done to prepare the child for her stay in hospital.
- Take time to explain fully why she has to go into hospital.
- Be sure to emphasize that she will be coming home again – a worry that can so easily be overlooked.
- If possible, pay a preadmission visit to the ward. (Most paediatric wards are very happy to arrange this.)
- When getting her things together prior to admission be sure to include a favourite toy or 'comforter'.
- Tell (or ideally make a written list for) the nurses of any unusual words or descriptions the child has for everyday bodily functions – such as wanting the toilet.
- If an operation is planned, ask if you can stay with the child until she is under the anaesthetic, and try to be immediately in sight when she wakes up again.
- As you leave her in hospital, do not try and slip quietly away when she is not looking. Say goodbye without fuss, say when you will be back and depart quickly. It can be a good idea to leave a notebook or a scarf for her to 'look after' until you return.

The Action for Sick Children organization (see Appendix) has a number of helpful leaflets for parents. Books for young children explaining what happens in hospitals are also available from bookshops. General practitioners' surgeries also have information available for children about hospitals.

On returning home from hospital children are often unsettled for a short time. Behaviour can deteriorate and skills learned, such as being dry at night, can be temporarily forgotten. Lots of love, sympathy and understanding will reduce this period of time to a minimum and the child will soon be back in the normal daily routine again. Remember, too, that the return to school for a school-age child can be a traumatic experience for the first few days until the familiar routine is once again established.

Support services

After the child has returned home, the community health team will be available for parents to call on for help or to alleviate any worries.

- A telephone call to a local GP, who will have been informed of the child's discharge from hospital, is all that is necessary.
- Health visitors are available to visit and give help and advice to parents of preschool children. In an area with a relatively static population the health visitor will be well-known to the family.
- District nurses will visit after any surgical procedure to be sure wounds are healing well, and to do dressings, as well as to advise on after-care of the young patient.
- In many areas there are school nurses who will be aware of any pupil who has been admitted to hospital. They are available to give help to schoolchildren after a spell in hospital.
- Occupational therapists (either from the hospital or in the community) or physiotherapists are able to help with any equipment a sick child may need at home, e.g. for example, a wheelchair or crutches for a child with a broken leg.
- Nurses with a special expertise in various conditions are available for advice and help in many areas. For example, a nurse with expertise in diabetes will be of immense value to a parent whose child has just been diagnosed as having diabetes.

Preparation for visits to other clinics

However routine a clinic visit is to an adult, to a child it can be a potentially frightening prospect. Children at times may need to visit an audiology or an eye clinic to check on hearing and vision. Explanation beforehand, in rough outline, of what to expect can help allay fears. For example, before a visit to an audiology clinic a description of headphones (if these pieces of equipment are new to the child) is a good idea: let him try on a Walkman if you have one. Eye clinics need to be explained: lights will be shone into the child's eyes as well as pictures shown that he will have to identify.

A further potentially worrying visit is to a child assessment clinic. Such clinics are often housed in, or near, a hospital. Explained that she is not being admitted to hospital, although she may have to spend several days in the assessment clinic. During this time she will see a number of professionals who will assess various aspects of her development. To the child the whole assessment process can seem rather like a day or two at a playgroup, i.e. enjoyable. Nevertheless a little preparation at to what will actually be happening will set the scene for a relaxed few days.

Caring for a sick child at home is bound to come the way of child-care professionals at one time or another, even if only in an advisory capacity. Every illness or accident is different, but as long as basic principles of care

are understood and practised, the correct and most appropriate care can be given in a professional and satisfactory manner.

FURTHER READING

Carson, P. (1987), *Coping Successfully With Your Child's Asthma*, London: Sheldon Press.

Darbyshire, P. (1994), *Living with a Sick Child in Hospital*, London: Chapman & Hall.

Hilton, T. (ed.) (1993), *Great Ormond Street Book of Baby and Child Care*, London: The Bodley Head.

Muller, D.J., Harris, P.J., Wattley, L. and Taylor, J. (1992), *Nursing Children*, London: Chapman & Hall.

Welfare of Children and Young People in Hospital (1991), London: HMSO.

Weller, B. (1980), *Helping Sick Children Play*, London: Baillière Tindall.

10. SPECIAL NEEDS

OBJECTIVES

1. Define the term 'special needs', the various classifications and terminologies.
2. Assess relevant legislation and procedures required to meet special needs.
3. Understand the need for a multidisciplinary approach and partnership with parents as part of assessment procedures.
4. Provide good learning experiences, environment and attitudes for children with special needs.

'Special needs' is the term applied to children having difficulties with learning. There are a multitude of reasons why children have educational difficulties. These range from purely physical ones such as muscular dystrophy, poor vision or hearing to overall developmental delay as a result of either injury, illness or genetic causes. In addition there are those children who have specific speech difficulties which inhibit cooperation with learning activities, and children with dyslexia or the more descriptive term, 'word-blindness'. Again there are children with such conditions as diabetes, epilepsy, cystic fibrosis or haemophilia whose diseases will undoubtedly affect their learning abilities. Finally, there are those children who are particularly gifted – they too have special needs in the educational field.

It is thought that up to 20% of all children can be classified as having 'special needs' at some time or other. The problems experienced need not necessarily be long-term. However, unless these fluctuating difficulties are recognized and appropriate help given, learning abilities will again be restricted. An example of this is the fluctuating deafness that occurs in many children who have frequent head colds and ear infections. At the times when their hearing is poor, because of an infection, much schooling and learning activities that need 100% hearing can be missed. (It is very probable that when the time comes for routine hearing tests to be done that particular child's hearing will be perfect!) In the nursery situation, nursery nurses, with their powers of observation during the daily routine, are in the ideal situation to notice such fluctuating problems.

Other difficulties that can be encountered are the children who have some long-term disease such as cystic fibrosis or diabetes. Whilst these diseases can be managed medically a good deal of time off school is sometimes necessary for treatment or admission to hospital. So, once again, a special needs situation is created when the child returns to school or nursery. Children with cystic fibrosis often need ongoing treatment such as postural drainage and those with diabetes need insulin injections. A number of other conditions will classify children as having 'special needs' for at least some of the time during their early school years.

Student exercise

Write down additional reasons why children may have special needs at some time during their learning years. (Refer to the section later in this chapter for conditions to which this could apply.) Choose just one of these conditions – possibly applying to a child that you know – and keep a diary on how the condition affects the child during nursery/school hours.

In addition to these 20% of children having variable and fluctuating special needs, there are 2% of children who have 'permanent' special needs. These are the children with severe disabilities – often from birth – and who may never be able to lead a completely independent life. Many of these conditions are genetically inherited and are termed 'syndromes' i.e. a collection of physical conditions which make up a definable and repeatable picture. The most well-known syndrome is Down's syndrome where there is a specific chromosomal defect giving rise to the well-known and documented signs and symptoms of Down's syndrome. (Much progress has been made in recent years in the education of Down's syndrome children and many are able to cope in mainstream schooling with extra resources.) The more severe symptoms seen in other syndromes, such as blindness and deafness as well as mental delay, mean that individual care and education usually in a special school setting or unit is needed for these severely disabled children.

Student exercise

In your nursery observe, over a given period of time, one child who has been diagnosed as having learning difficulties. Write down:
• the type of problems they are encountering;
• the help that is being given;
• any other ways in which this particular child could be further helped.

The effect on the parents of having a severely disabled child can be devastating. Reactions on first being told range from complete disbelief to rejection of the child. This latter reaction is rare, but the birth of a disabled child is the cause of some marriage failures. Fortunately today there is much help and support available to these families and the general public are now being better educated to the needs of severely disabled people. (In the past it was the custom to 'hide' disabled people: children were never educated and much sorrow and heartache ensued from these attitudes.)

SUPPORT

Support available to families with a severely disabled child include:

- **Health department**:
  - advice and support from health visitors;
  - multidisciplinary assessment in child development centres (see below);
  - provision of free disposable nappies and incontinence pads for older children with bowel and bladder control problems (e.g. spina bifida);
  - provision of wheelchairs for non-ambulatory children;
  - provision of hearing aids, spectacles and other aids after diagnosis and prescription of appropriate treatment.
- **Social services departments**:
  - support and advice from specialist social worker;
  - help in the home for mothers burdened with the full-time care of a severely disabled child and perhaps several other children;
  - arrangements for 'respite care' so that the rest of the family can have a holiday;
  - attendance allowance – a weekly sum of money for those caring for a severely disabled child over the age of two years;
  - mobility allowance is also available for severely disabled children over five years so that they can be taken out; car tax is also waived under these conditions.
- **Education department**:
  - advice, assessment and support from educational psychologist;
  - suitable education from the age of three years at a residential school if this is thought necessary at any time;
  - free transport to and from nursery or school.
- **Housing departments**:
  - alterations to rented accommodation to assist with the care of the disabled child, e.g. ramps for wheelchairs, downstairs bathroom and toilet facilities;
  - grants available to house owners for similar alterations.
- **Voluntary organizations**:
  - self-help societies of which there are many (listed in the Contact-a-Family (CaF) Directory – see Further reading and Appendix);
  - help from the Family Fund set up by Joseph Rowntree to help the families of disabled children which aims to fill up any gaps in the statutory services.

Family support
- Health Departments
- Social Services Departments
- Education Departments
- Voluntary Organizations

Over recent years much progress has been made in the care and acceptance of children and adults with disabilities. Nowhere is this greater than in the terminology used. Previously 'mental' and 'physical handicap' were the generic terms used. As well as being degrading, they did nothing to explain the different types of disability. Today such terms as 'learning difficulty', 'specific learning difficulty', 'special needs' and 'disability' are in common usage.

HISTORICAL BACKGROUND

Historically, it is interesting to see the enormous changes in thinking and action that have occurred over the past 40 years in the UK.

In the 1950s children with Down's syndrome and other severe disabling conditions were cared for, after the early childhood years at home, in large mental 'subnormality' hospitals. This meant that all facilities for care, bathrooms, toilets, washing machines, etc., were available under one (large!) roof. (It must be remembered that at this time facilities for extra washing, central heating, etc. were not commonly found in most family homes.)

These hospitals were often placed on the outskirts of towns. This meant that families often found great difficulty in visiting their child on a regular basis. Remember, too, the lack of easy personal transport in the 1950s. So after a while disabled children and adults were left to be cared for entirely by the institutions.

Prior to that the **Education Act of 1944** made it legally binding on education authorities to provide education for children with disabilities. A number of categories of disability were defined:
- deaf and partially deaf;
- blind and partially sighted;
- physically disabled;
- delicate;
- diabetic;
- epileptic;
- speech defects;
- educationally sub-normal;
- maladjusted.

(Also children with a measured IQ of below 50 were deemed 'ineducable'.)

The education provided was not always in schools. In fact the children living in the institutions merely had a few hours a day in a schoolroom on-site.

In **1979** a further **Education Act** made commendations to local authorities that the children previously deemed ineducable must receive some educational help. This again was undertaken within the confines of the institution within which the child lived.

Major changes in the education of disabled children were made in 1983 when the **Warnock Report** was published This report laid down specific procedures on education for children with disabilities. The main points in the report were:
- Categories of disability, such as 'mentally defective' and 'delicate' were abolished. This meant that the child had no generic label which could last all their life.
- There was a statutory obligation on local authority education departments to provide suitable educational facilities for children with disabilities categorized as 'mild', 'moderate' or 'severe' disability.

- There must be a positive written statement of the child's needs made as soon after diagnosis as possible. This meant that appropriate care and education would begin early. Assessment procedures must be undertaken with the production of a 'statement' laying out in detail the child's difficulties and specific advice given for further help and education. (See below for details on production of a Statement.)
- Integration with peers was made, if at all possible, so that disabled children could grow up in their own communities.

A further Act, the **Education Reform Act of 1988** made further far-reaching changes in all aspects of education, including those schools supplying facilities for children with special needs. This included:

- more responsibilities for governing bodies;
- new financing methods with the Local Management of Schools (LMS);
- introduction of the National Curriculum which now applied also to children with special needs.

Assessment procedures, resulting in the production of a '**statement**' can be done in the child's home with visiting professionals each doing their specific part, or, more conveniently, in a Child Development Centre where all assessments can be done under one roof. (Assessments can, of course, be done without necessarily a 'statement' being written.)

CHILD DEVELOPMENT CENTRES

There are probably as many ways to organize a Child Development Centre as there are Child Development Centres! Some are attached to District General Hospitals and some are housed on a separate site, but all have adequate room, ideally both indoors and out, for children to play. Toys and other play and assessment materials are available for the whole age range, 18 months to five years.

Children are referred for assessment at a Child Development Centre by paediatricians, general practitioners or health visitors following concerns about either their developmental level (as a result of the routine developmental checks done on all children) or their physical state. Ideally the age at which referral takes place should be as early as possible. This is in order that extra help can be given before formal schooling begins. This means that some children are able to obtain a little extra help in the specific area of development in which there has been found to be a minor problem. (Others, with more severe mental or physical disabilities are offered on-going help at the school that they will be attending at a later date.)

The staffing at a Child Development Centre includes full-time nurses trained in paediatrics, nursery nurses and social workers, together with play-therapists and secretarial back-up. During the time the child is attending the centre various other professionals attend to undertake their particular part of the assessment procedures. These include:

- educational psychologists;

Important Education Acts in Special Needs
- 1944 – education for all children with disabilities
- 1979 – no child is deemed 'ineducable'
- 1983 – Warnock Report
- 1988 – Education Reform Act

Referral to Child Development Centres by:
- Paediatrician
- General Practitioner
- Health Visitor
- School Doctor

- paediatrician;
- speech therapists;
- physiotherapists;
- preschool teachers.

Each will contribute their own special expertise to the assessment.

At the end of the time allocated for an individual child's stay at the Child Development Centre (children usually attend daily, with transport provided) a case conference is held. At this time everyone involved with the child presents their report. Decisions are then made as to future help, and possible recommendations for future schooling, needed by each individual child.

Parents are welcomed and encouraged to take part in the whole assessment process, and also to be present at the case conference. It is vitally important that parents are seen as full partners during this important time when the immediate future of their child is being discussed.

Workers in all child-care fields must always be alert to the needs of parents as well as the needs of their child. Remember that:

- not all parents have good or knowledgeable parenting skills: they need encouragement and information on how best to look after their child;
- different cultures and languages can make it difficult for parents to fully understand what is happening to their child: time must be taken to be sure that they fully understand, and agree with, the implications of assessment;
- parents must be sure of confidentiality when they bring their child for assessment;
- many parents have other stresses in their lives other than that of the individual child being assessed; these cannot be put on one side, even for a short time, and will inevitably colour reactions to the assessment process;
- parents have the right to bring up their child as they wish, within, of course, the bounds of normal care, and if they do not wish assessment their wishes must be taken into account;
- parents are full partners in the assessment process and it will be up to them to ensure that recommendations are followed.

Role play

Make a video recording of a number of simulated interviews of a care worker having to explain the assessment procedure to parents who are not sure that their child needs assessment and have different attitudes, e.g. one couple are almost angry at the suggestion, another disbelieving, another seeing it as an 'entrance test'. The child herself has some speech delay and is always falling over at the age of three. The care worker must also help these parents to understand the benefits of a multidisciplinary assessment for their child. Then, as a group, review the interviews and from the comments write notes on practices to be avoided and useful techniques to be used.

Possible outcomes from assessment

- Admittance to a suitable nursery or playgroup for children below the age of five years, earlier than would normally be possible, is often the ideal solution for children with only a mild delay in one or two areas of development, possibly from understimulation at home or a mild intellectual disability. Nurseries and nursery schools are ideally suited to help such children, having as they do a wide range of activities and play equipment especially designed to stimulate language, motor and perceptual skills. 'Home-start' (an organization which helps families under stress) would be a further option. A 'Portage' scheme or conductive education (see later for details) for severely disabled children below the age of five years would also be a possibility.
- Extra help from one of a variety of therapists – speech, physio or play – will depend on the specific difficulty from which the child is suffering.
- Extra teaching, perhaps on a twice weekly basis, may be available from a preschool teacher, often attached to the Child Development Centre.
- Attendance of parent and child at a family day-care centre can be a life-saver for mothers or fathers with difficulties in parenting skills. Social isolation for both parent and child can be mitigated by this recommendation.
- Help for difficult behaviour problems can be obtained from a family and child guidance clinic.

Every recommendation must be tailored to fit the individual needs of each child with the full understanding, agreement and commitment of the parents.

The above description is just one way of dealing with an assessment procedure. There are many other scenarios, depending on local facilities, but the basic ideas are the same, namely to obtain as much help as possible for each individual child according to their special needs at the time.

Possible outcomes from assessment:
- Nursery or nursery school
- Extra help from appropriate therapist
- Extra teaching from preschool teacher
- Attendance of parent and child at family day centre
- Family and child guidance

Statementing

Following on from a period of assessment a 'statement of the child's educational needs' can be made. This will pinpoint and define the educational needs of the child. Parents must be fully informed at each stage of the process of the local authority's intentions to issue a statement for their child. They have the right to refuse within a specified time limit to agree to the assessment and subsequent statement, but most parents are only too pleased to agree to help being given to their child. Further specific parental agreement is required when the statement has been drafted. If they are in disagreement with any aspect they have the right to appeal.

People involved in the production of a statement are:

- an educational psychologist;
- a medical officer;
- an education officer;
- all therapists and staff involved with the original assessment;
- health visitor and general practitioner connected to the family.

The first three people in the above list must write reports and often act in drawing together the findings of other people concerned.

Nursery nurses have an important role to play in providing information, especially for preschool children. This role includes:

- identification of particular **areas of difficulty** in the child's developmental profile;
- keeping **records of progress**, or otherwise, in these areas, and the ways in which help is being given to the child;
- **keeping parents informed** during assessment procedures.

There are five sections to a 'statement' which must be completed:

- Part 1: an introductory page with relevant details, e.g. name, address, date of birth, etc.
- Part 2: a description of the child's educational needs as identified during the assessment process.
- Part 3: a specification of the educational provision required to meet the child's needs.
- Part 4: the type of placement required, e.g. special nursery, playgroup or school.
- Part 5: details of other needs such as physiotherapy, speech therapy.

On receiving the statement, the local education department will, within the constraints of local facilities, advise on what can be offered to the child. Without the recommendations of a statement, any extra resources necessary for the welfare of the child will not be funded. This is especially important in the case where, for example, a physically disabled child needs to be integrated into mainstream schooling. Lifts, ramps and other aids to mobility will be required to accommodate the child's specific disabilities.

A statement also protects the child's interests. The local authority is bound by this statement to arrange appropriate help to be given; without a statement help may not be forthcoming. An example can be found in speech therapy input to schools. Speech therapists need to attend local schools to give regular therapy to those children who require help. Owing to financial restraints, this – and other – help is being cut back, but a child with a recommendation in her statement for regular speech therapy is legally entitled to this facility and parents can appeal for the service to be reinstated. Without the 'protection' of the statement, this appeal would stand no chance.

Statements have to be reviewed on an annual basis to ensure that the child's needs have not changed, which, of course, they indubitably will over time.

Children below statutory school age can be 'statemented', but local

A statement:
- Advises on extra resources
- Protects child's interest

authorities, with their limited resources, often find difficulty in providing the facilities recommended. For severely disabled children, examples of these recommendations can be:

Portage programme

This was developed in America and consists of specialized teaching programmes in the home. These programmes are organized for each individual child by special Portage teachers. Six main areas of learning skills are identified and matched to the child's disability. These are:

- motor difficulties;
- self help skills;
- language difficulties;
- cognitive difficulties:
- social skills training;
- stimulation.

A structured learning programme is devised for each child breaking down each 'skills' area into small developmentally correct steps. Parents and carers are taught how to continue the work in normal home situations. These schemes have proved very successful as parents feel involved in their child's progress.

Conductive education

This was begun at the Peto Institute in Hungary in the early 1950s and has gained worldwide recognition in helping children who have severe mobility problems, particularly children with cerebral palsy. This type of education needs to be done in special centres by rigorously trained and dedicated staff. Long hours of work with the children on a regular basis on a one-to-one level are necessary. Conductive education has received a certain amount of criticism as to its lasting value. It has been said that the intensiveness of the one-to-one training is in itself what has made the scheme successful. Nevertheless many children have benefited from conductive education

Both of the above programmes are expensive, needing skilled staff and equipment, and local authorities often have difficulty in providing these resources.

A Code of Practice published in 1994 by HMSO is available giving detailed information on statementing procedures. A further document entitled *The Implementation of the Code of Practice for Pupils with Special Educational Needs* was published in 1996.

Student exercise

Try and visit either an institution where conductive education is practised, or arrange to go out with a teacher of Portage. Write a report on your visit, and give reasons why these programmes are of value.

Student exercise

A child with a statement is being admitted to the nursery where you work. Write brief explanatory notes, for the parents, on what the statement means. Identify and list the aspects of nursery life that will be required to provide for a child with special needs in the area of minimal physical disability, mild deafness and speech delay.

Integration

Integration of children with special needs into mainstream schooling is very much part of educational policy today. Previously it was generally accepted that children with specific disabilities should attend an appropriate 'special' school. For example speech and language schools for speech and language problems, schools for the blind for children with visual difficulties and special schools for children with below-average intellectual abilities.

It is still necessary that some children with severely disabling conditions, in all areas of disability (2%) should attend a school where the layout, curriculum and teaching methods are especially geared to their type of disability. But for children with only a minor degree of disability integration into mainstream schooling is preferable.

Role play

In small groups with one taking the role of the parent and the others acting as a counselling team simulate the situation where to everyone's surprise, a parent, whose child has been advised that mainstream schooling will be suitable, is vehement in demanding that her child attend a 'special school'. Do your best, as a team and on an individual basis, to convince her that her child should be integrated into mainstream schooling. The combined groups then produce a 'strategy' or way of handling such problems from which you prepare a set of notes and personal comments for your own record.

Reasons for this can be summarized as:
- **Parental preference**. Previously there seemed to be a stigma attached to the family if a family member attended a special school.
- **Children's preference**. They can attend the same school as their brothers and sisters and local friends.
- **Ease of travel arrangements** if every child in the family attends the same school. Many special schools are, of necessity because of their speciality, at some distance from many children's homes, the 'catchment area' being wide.

- Benefits to the child in **mixing with non-disabled children**. Also, of course, the children with no disabilities will learn of the problems their disabled friends are having to cope with.
- A **wider range of subjects** is on offer as the educational ladder is climbed.

Difficulties have been experienced in making this integration possible due to financial restraints in the provision of appropriate resources in mainstream schools. This is a difficult problem and one which needs to be looked at carefully from each individual child's viewpoint.

Advocacy and empowerment

These are terms which have particular reference to children with special needs. These children are the very ones who are least able to make their wishes known, hence the concept of a responsible person taking this 'advocacy' role on behalf of the child, as well as 'empowerment' to see that the child's wishes are known and followed as far as possible. This concept is specifically recognized in the Children Act of 1989.

FACILITIES IN THE NURSERY SITUATION FOR CHILDREN WITH SPECIAL NEEDS

The first, and most important, facet for helping children with special needs in the nursery is for the nursery nurse to have knowledge and understanding of the difficulties of each child with specific disabilities. Only by understanding the reasons behind problems that the child is having, together with the natural history of the condition, can appropriate and sympathetic help be given.

It must be remembered that many children with special needs will not have had the usual opportunities to mix fully with other children. This may be due directly to their disability, e.g. mobility, visual or hearing loss, or due to parental overprotection or depression regarding their child's disabilities. Integrating the child, slowly and carefully, into the activities of the other children, must be one of the prime initial aims of the nursery nurse.

Play areas must be large enough and free from clutter, for the safety of the disabled child. Play materials, too, may need adapting to the child's needs. Larger toys should be strong and sturdy and made of non-injurious materials for children who have difficulties in controlling their limbs. Play in 'soft areas' is much enjoyed by children with **mobility problems** as also is exercise in water. In this latter environment the water creates buoyancy for wasted, or poorly muscled, limbs and so helps movement.

Young children **unable to walk** need to be provided with play materials on the floor or at a low level. Specially designed equipment can be useful in allowing these children to stand for various play activities. Older children confined to wheelchairs will also need appropriate activities, such as jigsaw puzzles, painting, drawing and modelling.

Student exercise

Design a new play activity for a child confined to a wheelchair, but who has good vision, hearing and fine motor control. Write it up so that it could be used by other nursery nurses.

Children with **visual problems** will need magnifying glasses and a good light. Large print books with clear pictures are also helpful, as are music and stories on tape.

For **deaf children** sign language, or Makaton signing, may be appropriate.

Above all, the worker with disabled children must help the child develop their own self-esteem and a positive attitude to their disabilities. Ways of ensuring that this occurs are:

- Remember to treat the child always as an individual, whatever the disability. (This can be particularly difficult if the child's speech is not easily understood.)
- Make sure that other children do not bully or poke fun at her disabilities. (Children can be cruel if they are not taught positive care of their disabled companions.)
- As a follow-on from the above, make sure that the disabled child mixes with the rest of the nursery children.
- Give praise to even the smallest success.
- Give only tools or play materials with which the child will be able to achieve a sense of success. It can be very depressing never to have your work on display.
- Do not tolerate bad behaviour on the part of the disabled child. He must learn the ground rules of good behaviour as much as the other children.
- Keep closely in touch with the parents on a day-to-day basis regarding the child's progress.

Apart from these general guidelines as to how to help children with special needs, there are other children with difficulties owing to specific conditions. These are described below, in alphabetical order

Care for children with special needs
- Treat child as an individual
- Stop bullying
- Make sure the child mixes with peers
- Give praise
- Give appropriate toys
- Do not tolerate bad behaviour
- Keep in touch with parents

Asthma

Asthma is a condition that is becoming increasingly common. It is thought that there are 1.7 million children in the UK who suffer from asthma at some time during their childhood years. The severity of symptoms varies from child to child, and at least half of these children will grow out of their attacks of asthma by the time they are adult.

Characteristics

- 'Wheezy' breathing occurs with an attack, and certain conditions make this more likely, e.g. when the child has an upper respiratory tract infection, is exercising or when the pollen count is high in the spring and early summer months.

- Symptoms of cough, which can be especially troublesome at night, and breathlessness can also be a problem. These symptoms are produced by:
  - a narrowing of the bronchi by the action of the 'trigger' factor, e.g. pollen or a viral infection in the respiratory tract;
  - swelling of the lining of the bronchi;
  - excess sticky mucus secretions, which further reduce the size of the lumen of the bronchi.

Management

- First-aid treatment for an acute attack of asthma can be found in Chapter 13.
- Avoid the known 'trigger' factors as far as possible. This may mean getting rid of the family pet. In a household where allergic problems occur – and asthma comes into this category – dogs, cats, hamsters and guineapigs can set off symptoms in a susceptible child.
- Give prescribed drugs. These fall into three broad categories:
  - **bronchodilator drugs** which help relax the tiny muscles in the bronchi; these can be given in the form of tablets or as an inhaler or nebulizer;
  - **corticosteroid drugs** which act by reducing swelling and mucus secretion; care needs to be taken with the long-term use of these drugs, as serious side effects can occur;
  - **non-steroidal drugs** which act in a preventative way, and are usually given by an inhaler; it is important that this group of drugs is given on a regular basis, and not just when an attack of asthma occurs; nursery nurses must be sure that children in their charge who should have these drugs actually take them.
- Physical exercise for children with asthma needs to be carefully controlled, as excessive exercise can bring on an attack. Nevertheless it is important that children with asthma do not miss out on sporting activities altogether. Judicious use of preventative drugs and suitable activities will mean that children can join in games with their peers.
- Emotional factors, such as excessive excitement or anxiety need to be avoided as much as possible.
- During the later school years, schooling should be along as normal lines as possible, with, of course, the appropriate medication on hand if needed.

The National Asthma Campaign (see Appendix) has a number of useful leaflets available.

Autism

The main feature of autism is defined as 'a disorder of normal cognitive function and language development'. Children with specific syndromes such as the fragile X syndrome or Asperger's syndrome can show autistic features.

Characteristics

- Interactive play with peers is virtually impossible. Autistic children do not want to socialize or play with other children at all. They are seen by their fellows as cold or eccentric and will eventually be left to play on their own.
- Routine is vital to the autistic child. Alterations to the normal daily routines can be extremely upsetting to the child.
- Speech is often flat and monotonous. Comprehension of language is often behind expressive language, so that it can be difficult to know just what the autistic child does understand.
- Clumsiness with the adoption of odd postures and facial grimaces are a further feature.
- Obsessive behaviour patterns are also frequently apparent, e.g. walking round and round the same piece of pattern on the carpet.

Management

- It is important that all possible help should be given to encourage socialization. Social skills will need to be explained in detail and practised repeatedly before even everyday skills are managed.
- Speech therapy can help pinpoint the areas of specific communication difficulty. If this help is given alongside the teaching of social skills, comprehension will improve.
- Specific behavioural therapy, by a clinical psychologist, can help terminate the obsessive rituals that can be such an intractable problem. Music is often much appreciated by autistic children and can be helpful in difficult behavioural situations. Nursery nurses can help such children by keeping as far as possible to a regular familiar routine throughout the day and by keeping in close touch with therapists.

The National Autistic Society (see Appendix) runs courses and conferences and can provide useful information.

Blindness (rare) or visual impairment

Impaired vision in children with can be due to a wide variety of causes, from direct injury to eyes to various congenital or infective conditions affecting sight. Careful assessment must be carried out to determine the exact amount of visual loss, and this must be a regular on-going task. Visual acuity changes over the years. **Squints** are relatively common in children. Without early and adequate treatment for a squint, vision can be lost in one eye. This is known as **amblyopia**, and is caused by the brain cutting out the double images that can arise from a squinting eye.

Treatment

This includes:
- spectacles to correct any refractive error, long or short sight;
- occlusion (or 'patching') of the non-squinting eye;
- orthoptic exercises;
- surgery.

The exact form of treatment will depend on the type and size of the squint in each individual child.

Nursery staff having the care of a child with a visual impairment will need to be aware of the degree of the child's disability so that:

- safety measures can be taken to reduce accidents due to poor vision to a minimum;
- suitable tasks and activities can be provided with which a visually challenged child can cope;
- spectacles are worn if required, and kept clean!
- a 'patched' eye remains so for the required length of time;
- suitable stimulating material is provided so that developmental delay due to poor vision is reduced to a minimum;
- good light for all tasks is provided (and also possibly magnification);
- the child is helped to come to terms with his disability.

The Royal National Institute for the Blind (see Appendix) will give help and advice.

'Brittle bones' (osteogenesis imperfecta)

This is a rare genetically inherited disorder. Nevertheless it is vitally important that carers, in nurseries and at home, are aware of the condition and handle the affected children appropriately.

Characteristics

- The main effects, as the name implies, are to be seen in the bones. These are especially fragile all over the body, and are prone to fracture even on very minimal injury. Children between the ages of 18 months and four years are particularly liable to sustain fractures. Between these ages, balance is precarious and 'exploration' instincts strong, a good combination for many falls.
- Blood vessels are also fragile. Minimal injury will cause them to rupture, giving rise to bruising.
- In certain types of brittle bone disease, the whites of the eyes are of a blue colour. This is of no significance, and does not affect vision in any way.
- Some children can also have a hearing loss, from problems with the tiny bones in the middle ear.
- Teeth can occasionally also be affected and be particularly liable to break.

Management

- From the carer's point of view, the child with osteogenesis imperfecta must be protected as far as possible from injury of any kind. It can be difficult to strike a balance between overprotection and too lax a regime. Rough games, with possible collision with other children, should be avoided and other, more sedate, activities explored.
- If injury does occur, it is important that the child is taken to the accident and emergency department of the nearest hospital. Broken bones

must be carefully 'set' to ensure that permanent disability does not result.
- Care must be taken in cases of suspected child abuse. With the excessive bruising and possible many fractures seen in this condition, child abuse can be suspected where none exists. Conversely, of course, non-accidental injury can occur and the disease be blamed for the bruising and fractures. Under these difficult circumstances, the safety and care of the child must be paramount.
- The Brittle Bone Society (see Appendix) will give help and advice.

Cerebral palsy

Cerebral palsy can manifest itself in a wide variety of ways, from the severely disabled child to the one who has minimal effects, who is often termed 'clumsy'. Children with severe cerebral palsy will need specialized care, but many children with lesser degrees of disability manage very well in the ordinary nursery and school setting

Characteristics

Basically cerebral palsy is a disorder of movement, and can be divided into three main types, which can overlap in some children:
- **spasticity**: muscles are rigid and stiff and cannot be relaxed;
- **ataxia**: movements are clumsy, owing to poor coordination and balance;
- **athetoid**: the child makes frequent involuntary movements of body and face when attempting to speak or perform any movement.

Intelligence can vary greatly and range from very high to very low. This can often be difficult to assess accurately because of the child's physical inability to respond in an appropriate way, even though he might well know how to respond. So complete multidisciplinary assessment is vital.

Management

This will depend on the severity of the symptoms.
- Physiotherapy to help coordinate movement is valuable; hydrotherapy is especially helpful;
- Various aids to movement may be necessary. It is important that nursery nurses are fully conversant with the proper use of all available aids.
- Conductive education has been most widely used for children with suitable forms of cerebral palsy.
- Activities should be planned in which the effects of the child's disabilities are reduced to a minimum. It is vital that they should be able to succeed in some area of play, and praise is also especially valuable.
- SCOPE (see Appendix) will give help and advice.

Coeliac disease

Coeliac disease is a specific disorder in which the small intestine cannot handle gluten, a protein found in wheat and wheat products.
- The onset of the condition is seen soon after the introduction of mixed feeding, and diagnosis is nearly always made by the time the child is 18

months of age. So, by the time the child starts at nursery, treatment will be well organized.

- Treatment consists of giving a gluten-free diet. Initially this can seem quite a challenge to parents and carers, but with advice from dieticians and the Coeliac Society (see Appendix) the diet can become a routine.
- In the nursery situation, nursery nurses must be aware that children with coeliac disease must not eat, for example, the birthday cake made for one of their contemporaries. A tactful piece of home-made, gluten-free cake should be quietly substituted. (No immediate reaction to a small amount of gluten will happen, but, if gluten is eaten over a length of time, symptoms of abdominal discomfort, diarrhoea and eventually failure to grow, will occur.)

Cystic fibrosis

Cystic fibrosis is an inherited disorder affecting lungs, digestive tract and sweat glands.

Characteristics

- The most severely affected organs are the lungs. There is a build-up of sticky mucus in all the respiratory passages which predisposes the child to frequent bouts of infection. Treatment for this aspect of the disease includes:
  - giving antibiotics early in each bout of infection;
  - giving physiotherapy with postural drainage, to enable the child to cough up some of the sticky mucus that is continually being formed in the lungs. This needs to be done regularly.
- The digestive tract is also involved with deficiency in specific enzymes from the pancreas. This means that food is not digested, or absorbed, adequately. The motions of the child under these conditions will be bulky and offensive from undigested fat. The addition daily of special pancreatic enzymes are needed to alleviate this problem.
- Sweat glands, all over the body, are also affected, with excess salt being excreted. (This fact forms the basis of the confirmatory test for cystic fibrosis.)

Management

- It is the lung problems that cause most concern; much damage can potentially be done to lung tissue by the repeated infections. Postural drainage, three times a day, is a burden that parents and carers, as well as the child involved, have to bear. Nursery nurses involved should, if possible, be taught how to give postural drainage.
- Children lose education because of frequent absences because of infections. This must be remembered when activities are being planned, in case the child with cystic fibrosis has missed a vital piece of information.
- Meals need to be carefully monitored to ensure that the child with cystic fibrosis is getting a nutritious diet, as well as taking the necessary medication.

- Hot weather, or a holiday in a hot climate, can cause problems because of the excessive amount of salt lost from the sweat glands. Adequate salt replacements must always be given in these circumstances.

Student exercise

Obtain all the information you can on cystic fibrosis from the library and the CF Trust. Write a report on the condition for a new member of the nursing staff, highlighting:
- the problems the child might experience;
- any difficulties that could make planning activities awkward;
- the ways of overcoming the effects in the nursery situation.

Deafness

Deafness can be due to a number of causes ranging from a congenital deafness to the fluctuating deafness seen in children with frequent upper respiratory tract infections. Deafness can be categorized into two main types:
- **sensorineural deafness** in which there is damage to the actual nerves of hearing;
- **conductive deafness** in which there is some blockage to the passage of the sound waves to the inner ear (see Chapter 2, the section on 'Organs of special sense').

Most difficulties with hearing are picked up at the routine hearing tests, but fluctuating loss can be harder to pinpoint. Signs that can alert a nursery nurse to the possibility that a child may be deaf include:
- startled reaction to someone unseen approaching;
- disobedience, due to not hearing requests;
- difficult behaviour;
- immature speech patterns.

Management
- Early diagnosis of both the degree and type of deafness is vital.
- Any possible help with hearing aids, medication or surgery should be sought.
- After-effects of any form of treatment or therapy must be closely monitored by those in close daily contact with the child.
- Nursery nurses must be sure that any child in their care who has a hearing loss fully understands what is required of them, at all times.
- Safety aspects must always be remembered and reinforced for deaf children.
- Follow-up examinations and hearing test appointments must be kept.
- The National Deaf Children's Society (see Appendix) will give help and advice.

Student exercise

Record examples of possible unusual behaviour patterns that could lead you to suspect that a child in your care may be having difficulty hearing. List ways of helping a child with a known hearing problem.

Diabetes

Diabetes is a condition that is due to the inability of the pancreas to produce sufficient insulin to keep the level of sugar in the blood stable. Whilst diabetes is not as common in childhood as it is in later life, there are one or two in every 1000 school-age children with diabetes.

Characteristics

- The onset of diabetes in childhood is usually sudden and is a medical emergency.
- Symptoms include:
  - frequent passage of urine, which may first become apparent as a return to bed-wetting in a child who has achieved control;
  - thirst, a very obvious sign – the demand for any type of fluid is constant;
  - rapid loss of weight;
  - general lethargy and tiredness;
  - coma in the most severe cases – treatment is urgent here.

Management

For children with a diagnosed and treated diabetes, there are two arms to the treatment of diabetes:

- **Insulin** is given by injection to restore the levels to normal in order to control the blood sugar levels. Children of quite a young age are remarkably capable of learning to give their own injections.
- **Dietary** carbohydrates must be tailored to the individual child's needs for good control during the growing years in conjunction, of course, with the correct dosage of insulin.

In the nursery or school situation, nursery nurses must:

- be aware of the children in their care who are diabetic;
- be able to identify, and treat, hypoglycaemia (low blood sugar).

Hypoglycaemia is an ever-possible complication for everyone on regular insulin. A number of factors working together can cause a hypoglycaemic attack:

- too little food after an injection of insulin;
- too much exercise combined with too little food.

Signs and symptoms of hypoglycaemia are:

- dizziness and faintness;
- headache;
- nausea, and eventually
- unconsciousness.

Children, unable to verbalize easily how they are feeling, will often just say they 'feel funny'. Parents and carers will soon learn to recognize these symptoms as being those of hypoglycaemia and give a sweet drink or a lump of sugar. Obviously if unconsciousness has occurred a 999 call will be necessary.

- Remember always to inform the parents of a diabetic child if she has had a 'hypo' during the day. It may mean that diet or insulin need adjusting, or that the child is brewing up an infection.
- Monitor the child's diet carefully.
- All activities can be safely pursued by a diabetic child whilst she is under close supervision.
- The Diabetic Association (see Appendix) will give help and advice.

Down's syndrome

Down's syndrome is one of the most widely known of the 'syndromes', and is due to a chromosomal abnormality. A child with Down's syndrome has 47 chromosomes instead of the usual 46.

Characteristics

This syndrome is readily recognizable by certain physical features:
- distinctive facial features, slanting eyes, a short neck and a flat back to the head;
- short limbs with final adult height limited;
- poor muscle tone;
- hands with short fingers and an in-turning little finger and a single palmar crease.

The intellectual abilities of Down's syndrome children can vary, some being severely disabled whilst others function at the low level of 'normal' ability. Young children with Down's syndrome can be integrated happily into a mainstream playgroup, nursery or nursery school situation.

Management

- Down's syndrome children need to be treated in the same way as their contemporaries. It is important, however, to check that the tasks given are not beyond the child's developmental level, whatever the chronological age may be. At they get older, developmental delay will become more obvious, and must be taken into account when schooling is being decided. All Down's syndrome children should have the benefit of a statement.
- Down's syndrome children often suffer excessively from upper respiratory tract infections and can also have a fluctuating deafness.
- Weak muscular tone means that activities requiring balance and coordination can be difficult, so an eye must be kept open for any difficulties experienced.
- Down's syndrome children generally have happy, loving dispositions. Take care that they are not bullied by older, more able, children.

Further information can be obtained from the books listed at the end of the chapter and also from the Down's Syndrome Association (see Appendix).

Epilepsy

Epilepsy is caused by abnormal electrical discharges in the brain. Around four to nine out of every 1000 school-age children suffer from some form of epilepsy. In children under the age of five years **'febrile convulsions'** can occur. This is in response to a sudden rise in body temperature, as seen during the onset of some infection. Children grow out of this type of convulsion by the time they are five years old. Febrile convulsions can happen in a nursery situation. Immediate treatment is to cool the child as quickly as possible: open doors, remove excess clothing and give first-aid treatment when the fit is under way (see Chapter 13). Parents should always be contacted if their child has a fit during a nursery or school day. They may have had experience of a febrile convulsion before and have appropriate medication available. Medical aid should be sought if this is a first fit, and, of course, the underlying infection will need to be treated.

Characteristics

There are two main forms of epilepsy – 'grand mal' seizures and 'petit mal' seizures. (There are also a number of other specialized types of fits.)

- **'Grand mal' fits** occur in about 80% of children with epilepsy and are characterized by:
  - possible – but not invariably so – altered behaviour for an hour or two before the fit occurs; also an 'aura' of unusual sensations can occur;
  - sudden loss of consciousness with rigidity of muscles and temporary cessation of breathing, followed by
  - jerking movements of the limbs;
  - urinary incontinence during a fit;
  - a slow return to consciousness; drowsiness and confusion may be present for a while after a fit.
- **'Petit mal' fits** are also known as **'absences'**. They are not so dramatic as a grand mal fit. In fact they are very easy to miss altogether.
  - There is a short period – a few seconds only – of altered consciousness in which the child will stop what he is doing and stare into space.
  - Immediately afterwards the activity or conversation will be continued as if nothing has interrupted it.
  - These absences can occur many time throughout the day, so affected children will miss many small parts of day-to-day activity and conversation, and so can become confused as to what is expected of them.

Management

- For first aid treatment see Chapter 13.
- Most epilepsies can be successfully managed on a drug regimen tailored to fit each individual child. Nursery nurses should be sure to check that the appropriate drug has been taken daily.
- Activities for children with epilepsy need only be curtailed if there is an associated danger, such as:
  - swimming: only allow this when there is a one-to-one child/adult in the swimming baths;

- climbing to heights, on ropes or equipment should not be allowed;
  - cycling on busy roads when the child gets older should not be allowed.
- Parents must be informed if their child has had a fit during the day.
- Some children, with severe or poorly controlled epilepsy, will need to wear a special helmet to avoid head injury during a fit.
- The British Epilepsy Association (see Appendix) will give help and advice.

Student exercise

Undertake an investigative study into a child with either:
- Down's syndrome;
- epilepsy; *or*
- cystic fibrosis.

Obtain all possible literature on the chosen condition. Contact the parents and discuss any particular problems they may be experiencing (remember confidentiality issues). Write a report which would be of value in the preparation of a statement for a particular child. Include any changes in nursery lay-out or planned activities that would be needed for the daily care of the child.

Haemophilia

Haemophilia is an inherited condition which only affects males. (This is due to the particular mode of inheritance.) Haemophilia is not common and there are varying degrees of severity depending on which particular 'factor' in the blood is deficient. The basic problem in haemophilia is inability of the blood to clot properly. So any bumps, which in other children would be minor, will cause severe bleeding in a boy with haemophilia.

Treatment consists of immediate administration, by injection, of the missing blood factor.

Management
- Take care at all times during any activity when minor trauma could occur. Boys with haemophilia should be encouraged to pursue quieter pursuits. All contact sports must be avoided.
- Nursery nurses should be sure that they are aware of the routine to follow should a haemophiliac boy receive an injury. Parents usually have the appropriate injection available, or the haemophilia centre in charge of the specific child can be contacted.
- Extra support and encouragement need to be given to the boy – it cannot be much fun seeing your friends allowed to kick a ball around.
- The Haemophilia Society (see Appendix) will be helpful in providing advice and leaflets.

Muscular dystrophy

There are a number of different types of muscular dystrophy, but the Duchenne type is the most common. This condition only affects boys and again is due to the particular mode of inheritance.

Characteristics

The signs and symptoms of this condition do not appear until between the ages of 18 months and three years. Nursery staff with good observational skills may well be the first people to notice problems.

- Walking is often late and the gait will be an unusually 'waddling' one. Difficulties with steps and with running will soon become obvious.
- The classical sign – the 'Gower manoeuvre' – occurs when the boy attempts to get up after a fall. He will need to 'walk' up the front of his legs with his hands to do this.
- Muscles in the calves will be enlarged, giving a false appearance of power. This is not due muscle tissue, but to infiltration with fibrous and fatty tissue.

Regretfully, Duchenne muscular dystrophy is a progressive disability and most boys will be wheelchair-bound by the time they are 10 or 12 years old.

Management

- Gentle exercise is important in the early stages of the disease, but too strenuous activity can accelerate the break down of muscular tissue. So, in the nursery, be sure that the child with muscular dystrophy moves around all play areas, but does not join in any competitive sport.
- Suitable play activities should be organized, e.g. emphasis on activities using hands and arms.
- Physiotherapy is important in the early years to keep joints mobile. It is useful if parents and carers can be shown a few simple exercises to follow on a daily basis.
- Support for the boy's family is also important, with close daily contact regarding activities. The progressive nature of the disease can be depressing, especially if one child has already died of the disease.
- The Duchenne Family Support Group (see Appendix) will give help and advice.

Sickle cell anaemia

This is another inherited blood disease. Only certain racial groups are affected: populations around the Mediterranean – Greece, Turkey and Italy – as well as some areas of West Africa and India and black Americans. The incidence of this disease is high in some areas of the UK.

Sickle cell anaemia is a problem affecting the red blood cells these cells: normally of a smooth elliptical shape, they are distorted into a 'sickle' shape. This means that they are more likely to stick together in clumps and block off the blood supply to organs and tissues supplied by the specific vessel. This is known as a 'sickle cell crisis' and is extremely painful. Infections of all kinds and too much strenuous exercise can all precipitate a crisis.

The child with sickle cell anaemia will also be anaemic. This is due to the reduced oxygen-carrying capacity of the deformed red blood cells. It gives rise to tiredness, lethargy, pallor and possibly breathlessness on exertion.

Management
- Any abdominal or chest pain must be immediately reported to parents and/or the child's doctor as it could mean that a crisis is developing.
- Quiet activities and exercise are a necessary part of daily care.
- Any symptoms suggestive of anaemia should be brought to the attention of the parents.
- A nutritionally sound diet is important to keep the child as healthy as possible.
- Close liaison between nursery staff and parents is, once again, a vital part of daily care.

Role play

You are the manager of a nursery. A child of three years with (one of the above conditions) has just been entered into the nursery. Using an OHP with prepared foils/acetates, explain the condition to your staff, reassure them about play activities, suggest suitable types of play and, of course, field their questions. Include in your presentation a typical week's programme for this child, highlighting the areas where changes from the usual routine will need to be made. Then issue the staff with relevant printed copies of the foils/acetates of this information.

THE TERMINALLY ILL AND DYING CHILD

Sadly this is a situation that may have to be faced. Accident and cancer are the two commonest causes of death in young children. Nursery nurses may well encounter children with cancer and as well as coping with the possibility of death, there are side effects of the necessarily aggressive treatments needed to halt the disease which will need handling. Nausea/ vomiting and loss of hair are the commonest of these effects. It is always advisable that the child – however young – should be told of the possibility of these side effects. Parents too will need sympathy and explanations. Often the terminal nature of their child's illness is difficult to come to terms with and all help may be rejected in the initial stages. There are a number of people and organizations that can be of assistance at these times:
- **Hospices** especially for children exist. They not only give full-time care

when required, but are also available for short-term, and emergency, care if the parents wish their child to die at home.

- Nursery nurses working as **play therapists** in children's hospices will be able to do much through play to allay children's fears and misconceptions.
- **Macmillan nurses** visit terminally ill children, as well as adults, and are specially trained to give the best possible support to child and family.
- The **Society of Compassionate Friends** is an organization which also gives support and is able to link people with similar problems together in the same geographical area.
- Specialized **social workers, bereavement counsellors** as well as **religious organizations** are also available to help.

This is a very specialized area of work for nursery nurses to undertake, and one which requires a good deal of maturity and understanding.

FURTHER READING

Contact-a-Family Directory (1994), London: CaF.

Gilbert, M.P. (1995), *A–Z Reference Book of Childhood Conditions*, London: Chapman & Hall.

—— (1996), *A–Z Reference Book of Syndromes and Inherited Disorders*, London: Chapman & Hall.

HMSO (1996), *The Implementation of the Code of Practice for Pupils with Special Educational Needs*, London: HMSO.

McCarthy (ed.) (1992), *Physical Disability in Childhood*, Edinburgh: Churchill Livingstone.

Kerr, S. (1993), *Your Child with Special Needs*, London: Hodder & Stoughton Positive Parenting.

Tossell, D. and Webb, R. (1994), *Inside the Caring Services*, London: Edward Arnold.

TOOLS FOR THE CHILD-CARE PROFESSIONAL

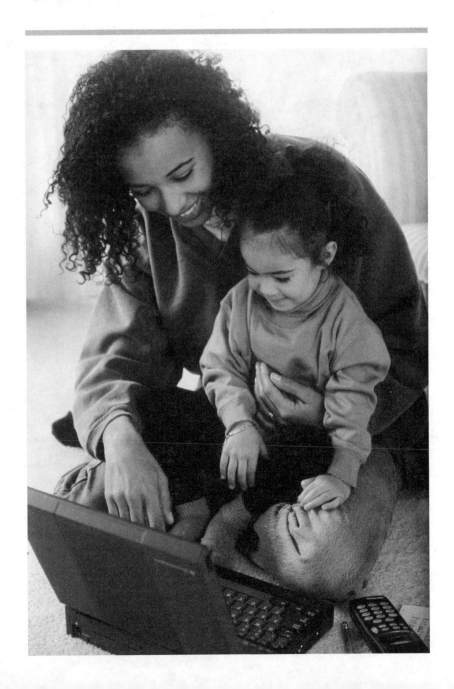

11. DATA INVESTIGATION AND INTERPRETATION

OBJECTIVES

1. Understand and use basic numeral and statistical skills and interpret them to relevant aspects of child care.
2. Recognize the applications of information technology to child care.
3. Gather and present data in an appropriate way to fulfil a community assignment.

All aspects of life demand some knowledge of arithmetical principles. The investigation and interpretation of data, necessary in many everyday aspects of child care, is no exception. Think, for example, of dividing up a box of bricks equally amongst a group of children, or of the effect of breaking six beakers out of 20 when 20 children are demanding a drink! Elementary arithmetic is involved in both these examples, division and subtraction respectively. More complex examples can be thought of, mothers may come to the nursery or school with worries on financial matters concerned with their child's immediate needs. Also, as the management tree is climbed, many arithmetical principles will be needed, for example to determine whether or not an extension to the nursery buildings is financially feasible. Further number procedures, such as percentages and ratios, will also be needed for many operations.

Everyone has a calculator these days, and it does indeed make 'arithmetical' life easier, but it is important to be aware that a calculator calculated answer to a numerical problem can be wrong (such as being 100 times too much) if the wrong information has been keyed in. Without a few skills in basic arithmetical operations much harm can be done, just think of giving a child 100 times the dose of medicine he needs because the decimal place has been keyed in the wrong position.

At the risk of being boring or patronising, we shall discuss a few basic arithmetical rules, from both a mental (or pencil-and-paper) and a calculator viewpoint.

THE FOUR BASIC ARITHMETICAL FUNCTIONS

Addition is the function when two, or any number, of digits are added together. The answer to this particular sum is called the 'sum' of the numbers involved.

Using a calculator to add up a long list of numbers can speed up the process. To do this:

1. Key in the numbers to be added together with the + sign between each.
2. When all the numbers have been entered press the = key. The 'sum' will now appear.

Subtraction is the function when a number, or numbers, of objects are taken away from the whole. The answer is termed the 'difference' between the numbers involved.

Using a calculator for this purpose:

1. Key in the number from which the second number (or group of numbers) is to be taken away with the − sign between each.
2. When all the numbers have been entered, press the = sign and the difference will appear.

Multiplication is the function when two, or more, numbers are multiplied together. The answer is known as the 'product'.

Using a calculator:

1. Key in the numbers to be multiplied together with the × sign between each.
2. When all the numbers have been entered, key in the = sign and the product will appear.

Division is the function when one number is divided by another, the answer being the 'quotient'.

Using a calculator:

1. Key in the number to be divided followed by ÷, then the number to divide the original.
2. Key in the = sign and the quotient will appear.

Sometimes several arithmetical functions need to be done on a group of numbers, for example a multiplication function as well as an adding one. There are certain rules that need to be followed as to the sequence in which these functions need to be done. Brackets, ( ), put round a group of numbers to be added must be worked out before any multiplication is done. When using a calculator remember to key in and calculate the figures inside the brackets first.

Complications also arise when fractions or decimals appear in the calculation.

Fractions (or parts of a whole number) will sometimes need arithmetical functions performed on them.

- **Adding and subtracting**. This cannot be done by simply adding or subtracting the tops and bottoms of the fractions. For example, the sum of $\frac{1}{2}$ and $\frac{2}{5}$ is not $\frac{3}{7}$! Before applying the adding or subtracting function, the fractions must be of the same type, i.e. the bottom figure must be the same in each of the fractions. This figure is known as the 'denominator'. To obtain the denominator in the above example:
  1. Multiply the top and bottom figures of $\frac{1}{2}$ by 5 $= \frac{5}{10}$.
  2. Multiply the top and bottom figures of $\frac{2}{5}$ by 2 $= \frac{4}{10}$. So now both fractions will now have the same denominator, i.e. 10.

3. The top figures are then added (or subtracted), i.e. $\frac{5}{10} + \frac{4}{10} = \frac{9}{10}$.

- **Multiplication** of fractions is easier. The tops and bottoms of the fractions are multiplied together. For example, $\frac{1}{2} \times \frac{2}{5} = \frac{2}{10}$.
- **Division** of fractions is also relatively simple. To divide a fraction by a fraction, turn the second fraction upside-down and multiply. For example, $\frac{1}{2} \div \frac{2}{5} = \frac{1}{2} \times \frac{5}{2} = \frac{5}{4}$.

Unless you have a scientific calculator, manipulating fractions is a complicated procedure. Fortunately today most work is done in **decimals**. Decimals are just another way of writing parts of whole numbers. The **decimal point** divides the whole number from the parts of the whole in the following way:

- the number immediately after the decimal point is the number of tenths;
- the second number after the decimal point is the number of hundredths, and so on.

Using a calculator for decimal functions:

1. Key in the whole number, followed by the button marked . (the decimal point).
2. Key in the parts of the whole number.
3. Then proceed to do ordinary the arithmetical functions required on these numbers.

Accuracy and 'rounding up'. There can be many numbers after the decimal point, making the figure very accurate when a number of decimal places are used. This is important in some calculations, in others this degree of accuracy is unnecessary. Also if counting whole numbers, 'people', for example, it is not possible to have 6.75 people. So, in the above example, the number is 'rounded up' to 7.

PERCENTAGES AND RATIOS

Percentages are specialized forms of fractions; the denominator is always 100. The sign for a percentage is %. Many everyday calculations involve percentage, for example Value Added Tax (VAT) is today $17\frac{1}{2}$%, i.e. for every £100 pounds spent, £17.50 needs to be added on as VAT on many goods.

In an large nursery, it is often necessary to know, for example, how many 3-year-old children there are in the whole nursery, for ordering food, equipment, etc.

Using a calculator for percentages:

1. Key in the number of which you need to know the percentage.
2. Key in a × sign.
3. Key in the percentage number required.
4. Key in the percentage sign (%).

Ratios are used in the comparison of two numbers; in other words, a ratio is the fraction of one number to another. As an example, in a class of 20 mixed-sex children, only five are boys. So the ratio of boys to girls is 5 : 20, or by dividing these numbers down by 5, 1 : 4. (So for every one boy in the class there are four girls.)

STATISTICAL FUNCTIONS

There are a certain number of statistical words that need to be defined and understood when any information on statistics is studied.

The **mean** of a large number of figures is the average of these figures. If, for example, the average length of the hair of a group of children (say 20) is measured and tabulated, the results would probably range from 2 inches to 12 inches, and would look as follows if listed in order:

2, 2, 2.5, 3, 4, 4, 5, 5, 5, 6, 6.5, 7, 7, 9, 9, 9.5, 10, 10, 12, 12 inches.

To find the average, or mean length of hair of this group of children, the numbers should all be added together: 86.5 inches. This figure is then divided by the total number of measurements (20) which equals 6.825 inches. So it can be said that the average, or mean, length of the children's hair is nearly 7 inches.

The **median** is a term that is a specific form of average, but which refers especially to the order in which the numbers appear. For example, if the marks obtained from a SAT are used, the median will be the middle number of the listed marks, i.e. half the marks are greater and half are smaller. Thus:

1. Put the marks in increasing order: 10, 14, 16, 16, 20, 24, 30, 60.
2. Take the two middle numbers: 16 and 20.
3. Half way between them is 18, which is the median.

If just a 'mean' had been calculated, this would have been distorted by the one high ranking figure, the mean of the above example would be 23.7.

The **mode** is yet a third type of average, and is defined as the most commonly occurring number in a set of numbers. In the simple example above, the mode would be 16.

TABLES AND GRAPHS

Any survey, or assignment, will collect a mass of figures which, when looked at just as a series of numbers, is confusing. Also few useful conclusions can be drawn. To interpret the data collected, a number of visual representations will make the task of interpretation easier.

Tables are the simplest form of presenting gathered information. Two variables are selected from what is required and the information on each is put into rows or columns By looking across Table 11.1, with a preconceived idea of what relationships need to be found, you can get an answer.

Various bits of information can be gleaned from this table. For exam-

Table 11.1 Daily attendance at nursery

Age (in years)	0–10 days	10–20 days	20–30 days
2	6	4	2
3	8	3	8
4	2	8	10

ple, the 2-year-olds' attendance was poorer than that of the 3- or 4-year-olds; the 4-year-old children were the most frequent attenders.

Student exercise

Construct a table for finding the most popular toy in a mixed-sex nursery with children aged two, three or four years. (In the age column sex will also need to be a factor, e.g. 2-year-old boys and 2-year-old girls, etc.).

Graphs are an excellent visual way of presenting relationships between certain types of data. Two variables are used, one along the vertical axis and the other along the horizontal axis. A simple example would be to show the relationship of money spent on education in a district over five years (Figure 11.1).

If the figures are plotted and the 'dots' so obtained joined up, the change and increase in expenditure over the five-year period can be seen. (The figures are quite imaginary!)

Figure 11.1 Line graph: educational spend.

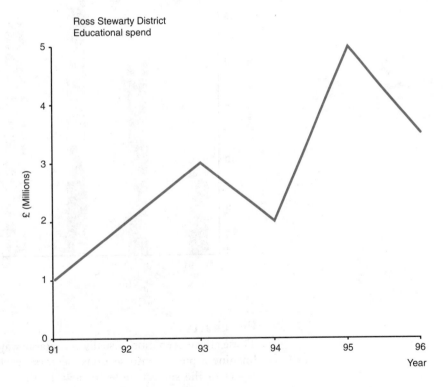

STATISTICAL DIAGRAMS

There are two types of pictorial diagrams used to present statistical information in an easily visualized way.

Bar charts

The numbers found in any survey need to be sorted into groups in order to draw a bar chart. The numbers in each group are then represented by differing lengths of the 'bar'. An example would be to compare, over a five-year period, the number of children of different ages attending a nursery (Figure 11.2).

Again, a number of useful bits of information can be gleaned from this. For example in 1993 the number of boys attending increased dramatically whereas in 1996 the sexes were evenly distributed. Also, a number of indirect inferences could be made from the information, maybe there was an excess of male births in the area in the preceding two to three years to 1993, for example. You must, however, be careful not to extend inferences too far on any one plotted piece of information: there may have been many other factors involved in the case.

Figure 11.2 Bar chart: gender ratios.

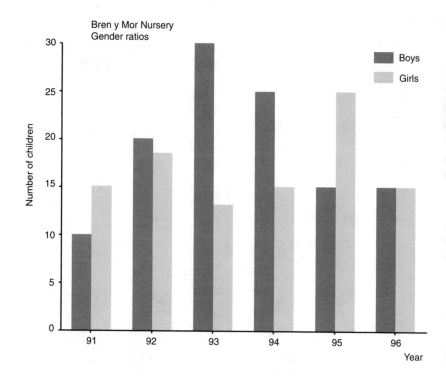

Pie charts

These are an even more visually acceptable way of producing information. Imagine a pie cut into sections (sectors), each section representing one aspect of the subject under review. In this way relative proportions are easily seen. For example, there are many items needing money to be spent in a nursery – equipment, lighting, heating, cleaning, rent, food, to mention just some. The pie chart in Figure 11.3 shows the relative amounts spent, as a proportion of the whole.

Figure 11.3 Pie chart: budget for 1996.

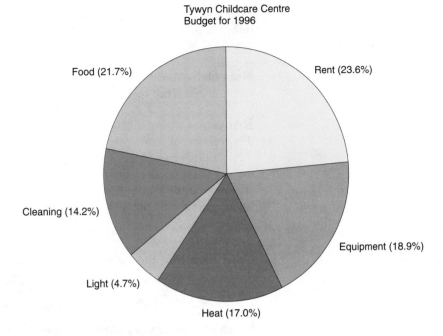

Tywyn Childcare Centre
Budget for 1996

Food (21.7%)

Rent (23.6%)

Cleaning (14.2%)

Equipment (18.9%)

Light (4.7%)

Heat (17.0%)

Student exercise

Using a spreadsheet, draw a pie chart of the number of children using various activities during 'free play' in a nursery over a period of two weeks. Take as your activities:
• large toys;
• home corner;
• construction toys;
• swings;
• water play;
• sand play.
Measure the time of activities over one hour.

POWERS AND ROOTS

There are times, as in statistics, when numbers have to be multiplied by themselves. This is the basis of powers. Reversing the process to get back to the original number is the subject of roots.

Power

This is the value, or 'index', that is used to show the number of identical numbers that are multiplied together. For example :

$$a \times a = a^2 \ (a \text{ squared}), \text{ or}$$
$$a \times a \times a = a^3 \ (a \text{ cubed})$$

where, as can be seen, the power is written as a superscript to the base number. As an example, if

$$a = 4, \text{ then } a^2 = 16 \text{ and } a^3 = 64.$$

Not only is this a convenient shorthand but the indices can in turn be manipulated – but that is for the mathematicians.

Roots

This process of finding the original base number is indicated by the 'root' sign $\sqrt{}$ number or function and, apart from very simple values, this needs the aid of a calculator or spreadsheet to solve it (to avoid a lot of tedious arithmetic!). By convention, if just the $\sqrt{}$ sign is shown it means it is the square root of the number. For example:

$$\sqrt{9} = 3 \ \left(3^2 = 9\right).$$

Other roots have the indices value shown in front of them. For example,
$$\sqrt[3]{27} = 3 \ \left(3^3 = 27\right).$$

STANDARD DEVIATION

Whilst mean, or average values, can be useful guide figures, when used with care, in many situations they do have limitations. An important one is that they do not indicate the spread, or dispersion, of the data elements, i.e. numbers, about the mean value. Thus, comparing the mean of income in different countries can be misleading because in some it clusters close to the mean whilst in others it is very widely spread from very rich to very poor.

Student exercise

Draw a line 10 cm long and put marks on this line at 1, 2, 8 and 9 cm. Treat these as separate lengths, i.e. 1 cm and 2 cm and find their mean. Now place marks at 4.6, 4.8, 5.2 and 5.4 cm and repeat the process. Compare the means and note the disparity in the clustering.

The Standard Deviation is the mathematical 'dodge' used to give a standardized comparison of means and dispersions so they can be more reliably compared and interpreted. In practice one would use:
• a calculator with a STD (Standard Deviation) button for small amounts of data;
• a spreadsheet for middling amounts of data;
• specialized mathematical techniques and programs for very high volumes of data.

However, the general principle behind their calculation is as follows:

1. Rank the numbers in order, smallest to largest (for convenience when calculating).
2. Calculate the mean of these numbers.
3. For each number find the deviation from the mean by subtracting the mean.
4. Square each of the deviation (remember a minus squared is a positive).
5. Find the mean of the deviations.
6. The Standard Deviation is the square root of this mean.

Examples using the figures in the exercise are shown in Table 11.2.

The mean of 1, 2, 8, 9 = 5. The mean of 4.6, 4.8, 5.2, 5.4 = 5. Hence whilst both sets of numbers have the same mean, the Standard Deviation of 3.53 in the first column compared to 0.32 in the second shows how much the first set of numbers is spread, or deviates, from the mean, whereas the second set is much closer.

Table 11.2 Standard deviations

Deviations	Deviations squared	Deviation	Deviation squared
1–5 = –4	16	4.6–5 = –0.4	0.16
2–5 = –3	9	4.8–5 = –0.2	0.04
8–5 = 3	9	5.2–5 = 0.2	0.04
9–5 = 4	16	5.4–5 = 0.4	0.16

Mean of the deviations = 12.5
Square root of mean (or SD) = 3.53

Mean of the deviations = 0.1
Square root of mean (or SD) = 0.32

SAMPLING

When you are conducting surveys, doing epidemiological studies and a host of other types of investigations, practical and/or economic considerations make it is necessary to take only a sample of the total population. Thus great care must be taken in:

- determining the type of sample to ensure that it covers only the variables or factors required.;
- determining the size of the sample to ensure that it is truly representative (there are statistical tables and other techniques which give confidence limits for sample sizes but it is prudent to involve a statistician for any serious and/or professional work);
- randomizing the selection of the items to help establish data that is free from statistical bias or misleading relationships.

INFORMATION TECHNOLOGY

Say IT, or Information Technology, and most people will assume that you are talking about computers. It is true that these play an important role in

Epidemiology
The study of disease in relation to populations of people.
Population (statistical)
All the items with defined parameters.

IT, but with the convergence of technologies many other aspects are now becoming involved e.g. telecommunications.

Any information system, of whatever complexity, can be conveniently considered in one of the four areas of:

- **hardware**, which is all the physical equipment, parts you can see and touch (or stub your toe on!);
- **software**, which is the general term for the programs, or instructions, used by the hardware to process the data;
- **communications**, i.e. moving the data between different parts of the system;
- **systems**, i.e. use of the hardware and software in order to do something useful. It is in this area that most users interact with IT and where most errors occur.

Figure 11.4 The related areas of a system.

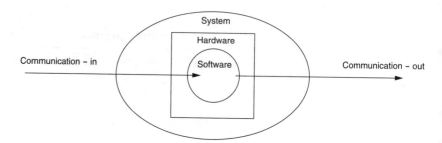

Hardware

A **computer** is in itself a good example of convergent technology arriving via the abacus, Jacquard's weaving loom, Babbage's mechanical computing device, early TV and other technologies, even including the cat's whisker radio; all this has led to the microchip computer of today, be it the mainframe or its desktop equivalent, the PC (personal computer).

A typical computer system consists of:

- the **processor** which does all the calculations and logical decision making under the control of the software;
- the **RAM** (Random Access Memory) which is a limited and temporary store for programs and data making them available very quickly to the processor; switch off and you lose them both – program and data!
- **backing store** which holds programs and files of data, both of which can be of considerable size, and more permanent, i.e. they can be changed but are not lost when you switch off; the programs and data can then be called up by the processor via the RAM as they are required; they are usually known as **hard disks** on PCs and are an integral part of the computer. Other **drives** – devices for reading from, or writing to, a media – are used as an extension to the backing store to accept the exchangeable media of floppy disks and CD-ROM;
- **peripheral devices** found around the computer, hence the term; they are usually near or part of, the computer system but can be located thousands of miles away.

Figure 11.5 The hardware elements of a computer system.

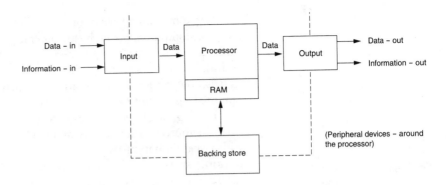

Peripheral devices typically include:

- **input devices**, which convert information or data into a form the computer can use. Common input devices are:
  - the **keyboard** with different clusters of keys – alpha, numeric, control and cursor movement;
  - the **mouse**, used to move the cursor rapidly about the screen, effect control or a drawing device;
  - the **concept keyboard**, a more specialized input device, is made up of a number of pressure pads over which can be laid readily changed templates which in turn can have a wide variety of shapes, sizes and colours printed on to them. As they do not need the precision of an ordinary keyboard and can be programmed for dynamic interaction and feedback, they are particularly suited to teaching those for whom ordinary devices are not suitable;
  - **touch screens** which work in a somewhat similar manner but use a VDU screen (Visual Display Unit) and can be manipulated by touching the screen itself therefore needing a much higher degree of precision; this, combined with their cost, tends to make them more suited to educational applications, such as in museums;
  - **pointers**, special devices usually fitted to the head or other parts of the body for use by severely disabled people;
  - **sensors**, devices for picking up signals which are then input to the IT systems, e.g. specialized monitoring equipment in an intensive care unit;
- **output devices** which convert the processed data into information suitable for the user; these are usually either hard-copy devices, such as printers, which give a permanent printed record or transient devices, such as VDUs, which only provide information on a temporary basis. Common output devices are:
  - the **dot matrix printer**, which is noisy but prints multiple copies at one pass (whilst not suitable for use in a ward, it is acceptable in a lab where several copies of a report may be required); the **ink jet printer**, which is quiet and can print in colour but is relatively slow; and the **laser printer**, which uses photocopier technology to produce very good quality print at a reasonable speed, but in black and white with a wide range of 'grey scales', i.e. shading.
- **VDU** (Visual Display Unit), somewhat like a TV (indeed there is a move back to combine their functions); these are fast and can display text, diagrams, and pictures using either single (mono) or colour screens;

they come in a wide variety of forms from the liquid crystal screen on portable computers through the general purpose ones used on PCs, to those used on specialist equipment such as CAT scanners;

- **sound**, moving away from the 'squeak', 'beep' or other crude alert signals, towards actual voice and music quality with much more spoken output (English not Dalek speak!) likely to be used; this, of course, will give much greater freedom of use when actively doing something, be of value in the educational environment and considerable help to those with visual limitations;

- **backing stores**, mentioned above, an integral part of the computer where the programs and user's data files are stored. However, as a considerable amount of data and programs are stored 'off-line' or transferred using various types of media, they can also be considered a peripheral device. Typical backing store devices with external media are:

  - **floppy disk**, a somewhat dated term as the modern $3\frac{1}{2}$ in. disk is a rigid, reasonably well protected media that is extremely useful for using in conjunction with PCs to store data files and programs; it is cheap and can be both written to and read from or set just to read from for security purposes, but has a somewhat limited capacity;

  - **magnetic tapes**, usually in the form of cartridges, used these days for backing-up the user's programs and data files held on hard disk;

  - **CD-ROM** (Compact Disc–Read Only Memory), becoming very popular for holding very high volumes of data or numerous/large programs; it is cheap for the supplier to copy, cannot be so easily copied as magnetic media and is more robust; an ever-increasing amount of reference information, presented in a dynamic form, with colour and sound, is being produced, therefore becoming very popular in the educational and home market; it does, of course, need a suitable piece of hardware; increasingly computers, even laptops, are being sold with CD-ROM drives.

Off-line
When a peripheral device is not under the active control of the processor even if connected.

Software

(An outstanding mathematician working with Babbage, pioneered and established many of the modern principles of modern programming. Her name was Countess Aida Lovelace, who happened to be married to Lord Byron, the poet. The computer language Aida, in use today, is named after her.)

Software is a general term for the different categories of programs. It is the software that determines what the computer does and how it processes the data. For convenience it can be grouped under four headings:

- **operating systems**, which control and run the computer (analogous to the autonomic nervous system in the human body);

- **user programs** written by or for the user for specialized applications, e.g. calling children for immunization, analysis of signals in a CAT scanner;

- **utilities**, specialized programs used to help sort out problems on other programs or data files;

- **packages**, bought 'off the shelf' complete and ready to 'load and go'.

Typical packages are:

- **word processors**, for editing and manipulating text, e.g. letters, reports, mail-shots;
- **spreadsheets**, in concept rather like a very large piece of squared paper where each cell can be identified and manipulated; reports and graphical output in the form of charts, such as bar and pie charts, can be readily produced; best suited to numeric work which requires tables and analysis, e.g. accounting, statistics;
- **databases**, which can hold large volumes of data, especially text, in a form which can be readily analysed, and produce reports suited to the user's need (it may be necessary to register such data in accordance with the terms of the *Data Protection Act*);
- **DTP** (Desk Top Publishing), somewhat akin to word processors but which are especially suited to produce material combining text, diagrams and pictures, e.g. brochures, newsletters and teaching material;
- **Graphics** and **CAD** (Computer-Aided Design): the former tend to be more suited to freehand or art-like pictures, whereas the latter is for design work involving measurements, e.g. layout of a nursery;
- **accounting**, useful for nurseries, playgroups and the like to gain better control of financial resources, commitments and budgets;
- **teaching**: there is a vast range of these packages, not all of a good standard; they can be used to enhance, not replace, a good teacher;
- **games**, popular with youngsters and when used properly can stimulate, inform and de-stress a child; there is a danger, however, that they become a purpose, rather than a tool, in an educational environment.

COMMUNICATIONS

Apart from the 'computer buff' a computer's internal communications do not normally concern the users. Increasingly, however, users are making, not always consciously, use of communications technology. The only piece of extra hardware often associated with this technology that the user may come across, is the **modem**, plus some software, which **interfaces** the computer with the communications system.

Typical communication systems are:

- **local area networks**: a number of PCs wired together in, for example, an office, schoolroom or building, so that they can share programs, data and exchange messages;
- **wide area or global networks**: private or commercial systems used for sending a wide range of types and volumes of data including that of e-mail;
- **Internet**: this started by linking databases at various American universities but has now gone international and carries a wide range of databases, numerous bulletin boards for special interest groups, a wide variety of services, e-mail and many more facilities; indeed it is becoming so sophisticated that enthusiasts 'surf' the network looking for interesting items; unfortunately the network is also being misused and software is now becoming available to stop children accessing undesirable areas of information.

Interface
A device or procedure to match different system to one another.

E-mail
Electronic mail sent from computer to computer, readily viewed on a VDU.

289

SYSTEMS

This is the area where the user interfaces with the IT system and which needs a lot of care both in design and use. Security is of paramount importance particularly of data files. Hardware and software can be replaced, but corrupted or stolen files could well be irreplaceable. Typical precautions and procedures are:

- **hardware**: locked doors, marking equipment and general anti-theft/vandal techniques;
- **software: virus protection** by very strict control on the loading of new programs:
  - virus detection by the use of programs designed for this work;
  - passwords giving access to programs and parts of programs;
- **communications**: restricted distribution of numbers:
  - **baring**, i.e. electronic control of who can access which numbers;
  - encoding and the use of **cyphers** for very confidential information;
- **systems**: logging of users, use of system:
- **back-up** of files, i.e. copies, on a planned basis;
- **storage** of media in suitable environment, back-ups in different building;
- **data recovery** from back-up files proven, and occasionally practised;
- **controls** to help ensure only valid data and commands used on input;
- access and distribution of output defined and controlled.

Virus
An illicit program designed to impair, or corrupt, other programs and/or data files.

COMMUNITY ASSIGNMENT

All courses in child care include essential practical course work. A community assignment, based on a particular aspect of child care in the community, can be a requirement. The syllabus should be carefully studied before you set out on the assignment, so that the exact requirements are known.

An assignment can take many months to complete, so a good initial definition of the **scope of the assignment** must be the starting point.

- The **time** that is available to be spent on the assignment is important. Do not be caught out by leaving everything, including the actual collecting of information (a time-consuming exercise), until the last few weeks before the assignment is due to be completed.
- Check on the **length of written work** that is required by the particular course.
- Check on the **type of presentation** of your work that will be acceptable. For example, is it going to include:
  - **drawings**, either by yourself or by the children being studied?
  - **graphs, tables**? (Be sure you feel able to present these accurately.)
  - **photographs**? (Be sure they are of good quality, and be sure that you have obtained parental permission for them to be used in your assignment.)
  - **tape-recordings** or **videos** to clarify specific aspects of your study? (Again, be sure permission has been obtained.)
  - **designed items** by you? (For example, mobiles, knitted articles, toys for special purposes, etc., which have particular reference to your study.)

REMEMBER: It is illegal to copy licensed programs, which in practical terms covers most software. Data files holding personal data may well be subject to the Data Protection Act and have to be registered.

- The **age of the child** or children and the **developmental area** you will be investigating are difficult areas for decisions – there always seems to be so many varied and interesting aspects that could be studied.

Remember, too, not to give yourself **too wide a brief**: a smaller aspect of behaviour in a small group of children, or in one child, is easier to control than several aspects of behaviour in a large group. Examples of suitable areas of study would be:

- the **physical growth** and fine motor skills development in one child of a specific age over a period of six months;
- the **free play activities** of a group of children of the same age (e.g. 3–$3\frac{1}{2}$-year-olds) over a total period of time, e.g. 24 hours investigated in 1-hour 'chunks' of time;
- the **resources** you might need, e.g. measuring and weighing equipment, suitable toys to be used in the study, camera, graph paper, access to a computer; any costs entailed must also be considered.

Be sure you keep a check on the **stage** your study has reached, say every month. Check also that you are not wandering off your original brief, and that various aspects of presentation are on schedule, e.g. the child whose photograph that is such a vital part of the finished work is on holiday just before your assignment is due in!

An **action plan**, taking account of the time available, is a good idea, including timings when various stages should have been completed. (This, of course, can be altered at any time during the course of the study if necessary.) Have clear in your mind the type of study you are pursuing: is it a child study? or an investigation into a special aspect of child care that interests you? Do stick to your original decision.

Check that all resources needed at particular times will be available. Much time can be wasted chasing up a resource on the one morning that both you and the study child are free.

Get permission in good time before you start: from parents and your immediate superior at your place of work experience. Finally check with your tutor that the study or investigation you are proposing will be acceptable for the course you are doing.

Collecting the information

There is a wide range of ways in which to do this. If it is a child study you are engaged on, **observation** will be the main way in which you will collect the necessary information Specific times and places must be organized for these observations, and an adequate number must be planned to obtain sufficient material.

Remember not to disturb or distract the observed child in any way, or if this does unexpectedly occur, mention it, and the outcome, in your presentation. Revise the types of observations possible in Chapter 1, e.g. naturalistic, snapshot, etc.

Different types of observations are all valid in an assignment. The type used in any one situation should be recorded.

Different assignments from a child study can be **investigative** in nature, For example, survey the facilities for play for children of two to five years in your immediate locality. This could be restricted to just play-groups or playgrounds, or could be a wider brief with nurseries and nursery schools included (but beware spreading the net too widely).

A further example could be to compare the different milk formulas available for a 6-month-old baby. How do they differ? What are the ones available for special feeding problems? There are a number of different ways to carry out an investigative assignment:

- A **survey**, as in the playground example, is probably one of the simplest to undertake. First choose your aspect of study. Then decide exactly what information you will require to make the survey meaningful. Are the play-grounds suitable and safe? Are they near to children's homes? Make arrangements to visit the places involved in your survey and, finally, record accurately and fully the information you have gained. (If something has been missed or forgotten, don't make it up, it will show! Go back and check again.)

- In a **comparison** such as in the baby milk study, list all the products you are proposing to investigate. If possible obtain a sample of each, so that the contents can be studied carefully. Tables, graphs, bar charts, pie charts and photographs could all be used in this type of study. Further example of a comparative study could be to compare the suitability of different types of disposable nappies. This investigation could include 'hands-on' experimental work in:
  - the ease of putting on the nappy;
  - the ability to keep skin dry;
  - the suitability for boys and girls of different types.

  Good recording for these types of projects are essential. A computer spreadsheet could be a useful adjunct for this.

- Using a preprepared **questionnaire** is also a popular way of doing a survey. This can either be completed by the people asked to contribute to the study, or can be completed during an interview. Examples of questions could be: How much time do children spend watching television? How many babies are up-to-date with their immunization? How many mothers breast feed their babies for longer than three weeks? The sample size is critical in this type of investigation: too few and the results are meaningless, too many and the volume of replies becomes a nightmare to manage. Much initial care is needed in the preparation of a questionnaire, which, in spite of looking easy at first sight, is not an easy option. Also, be sure to set a maximum for the number of questions asked. People are unwilling to fill up long pages of questions.

- **Investigative assignments** could also include a **media search** for relevant information on any manner of subjects connected with child care. The 'media' includes newspapers, magazines, TV documentaries, libraries as well as computer-aided sources of information. If such sources are available, there is much information on the Internet.

When all the appropriate information has been collected the data gained will need to be analysed, the findings evaluated and the final writing-up and presentation of the assignment done.

Analysis of the findings can be made with the help of graphs, tables and spreadsheets to lay out the information in an accessible way. An open mind must be kept when evaluating your findings. Do not start off an assignment with ideas of the result too rigidly conceived – you may be surprised at what you find! If you are surprised, say so on your report and suggest why the results differ from those that you expected initially.

Leave adequate time for writing up your assignment. There is no point in doing a good piece of work if the results are not presented in an attractive, readily accessible, interesting and understandable way. Use photographs, videos, tape recordings or computer-aided design to give body and substance to your work. Remember to state how and where these 'extras' fit into the main part of the assignment.

Community assignments are interesting to do, and give a definite purpose to a work placement, but meticulous planning is necessary for a successful result.

FURTHER READING

Solomon, R. and Winch, C. (1994), *Calculating and Computing for Social Science and Arts Students*, Milton Keynes: Open University Press.

12. LEGAL ASPECTS OF CHILD CARE

OBJECTIVES

1. Understand the basic characteristics and principles of the English legal system, and the influence of European legislation.
2. Identify role of legal personnel and court procedures.
3. Identify main components of the Welfare State.
4. Understand the fundamental principles of the Children Act.
5. Recognize the implications of laws of employment and contract.

THE ENGLISH LEGAL SYSTEM

To understand the principles behind the current English legal system, it helps to consider its historical background. The English legal system, consisting as it does of its courts and tribunals, and the law which they administer, is the end-product of a process which began with the Norman Conquest (1066). The Normans imposed a formal legal structure upon the ancient Anglo–Saxon unwritten laws and customs. From this emerged the beginnings of the 'adversarial' tradition. This means that the parties involved in a case put forward evidence in order to persuade the court where the truth lies. This contrasts with the Roman 'inquisitorial' tradition, found throughout much of Europe and in Scotland. The role of the courts in legal systems of the inquisitorial tradition is to establish the facts and find out the truth for themselves. This points to an important difference between English and Scots law. The succeeding notes refer to the legal system in England and Wales. Much of the law is unwritten. It is divided into two major fields, public law and private law.

   Public law is concerned with:
- the relationship between the State and other states – **international law**;
- the workings of the State – **constitutional law**;
- the relationship between individuals and the State – **criminal law**.
(Criminal law is the means by which the State maintains its basic moral code by outlawing behaviour considered to be harmful or unacceptable to other individuals and by punishing wrongdoers.)

   Private law is concerned with the regulation of the relationships, duties and rights of citizens and is known as **civil law**. (Civil law governs the making and enforcement of contracts [of increasing importance to nursery nurses seeking employment] and the rights and responsibilities concerning land and property.)

From a personal and practical viewpoint, individuals are mainly affected by civil law and criminal law.

The courts

The courts, of which there are a number of subdivisions, dispense civil remedies and administer criminal justice. Some courts, e.g. magistrate's courts, deal with both civil and criminal cases. Below is a brief overview of the type and work of the courts.

The **House of Lords** is at the summit of the court structure, and is the judicial arm of Parliament. It is the court of final appeal, usually as an appeal against a decision given by the 'court of appeal' in civil or criminal matters.

The **Privy Council** also acts as a court of final appeal for some Commonwealth countries.

The **Court of Appeal** is the second most senior of the Courts, the first being the House of Lords. Cases here are decided by judges known as Lord Justices of Appeal, the leader being known as Master of the Rolls. There is both a civil and a criminal division. The cases are mostly appeals from the Crown Court or the High Court.

The **High Court** is a court of 'first instance', i.e. a court in which cases may be heard for the first time. Up to 80 judges are involved in the work of the High Court and it is split into a number of divisions:

- the **Chancery Division** which hears cases involving land and other property disputes, bankruptcy and partnership problems;
- the **Queen's Bench Division** hears contractual disputes and cases involving such civil problems as trespass and personal injury; this is the busiest of the divisions of the High Court;
- the **Family Division** was set up in 1970 specifically to hear disputes within families, particularly those involving marriage, children (adoption, fostering, legitimacy) and matrimonial property; this is an important division with which carers should be conversant, as it is here that the High Court exercises its functions under the Children Act.

The **Crown Court** was created by the Courts Act in 1971, when it took over the work of its predecessors, the Court of Assizes and Quarter Sessions. It has criminal jurisdiction, and is a court of 'first instance' for 'indictable' or 'either-way' offences. Indictable offences are the more serious criminal offences and can only be heard in the Crown Court. Either-way offences can be heard in a magistrate's court or a Crown Court. The Crown Court also hears appeals from the decisions of the magistrate's court.

The **County Courts** hear civil cases only and there is a County Court for each district of England and Wales. These are very busy courts and hear such cases as small claims and disputes over goods and services.

The **Magistrates' Courts** hear both civil and criminal cases, and deal with over 90% of criminal cases in England and Wales. These courts are run by Justices of the Peace (JPs) who are members of the public appointed by the Lord Chancellor to sit in the Magistrates' Courts in their home area. They sit on the 'bench' usually in threes. They have no formal legal training.

Stipendiary magistrates have a legal background and hear the more serious cases. They receive payment for their services, unlike the JPs who give their services free. Magistrates' Courts play an important role in care proceedings and other matters concerning children. For example, they hear applications for 'emergency protection orders' under the Children Act (see below).

Student exercise

If possible get permission to visit a Magistrates' Court. Write a report of the cases heard and the outcome of each.

Tribunals are quicker, less formal courts set up to deal with disputes in a particular field, e.g. industrial tribunals, VAT tribunals, social security tribunals and mental health review tribunals. The members of the tribunal need not necessarily have legal qualifications, but must have professional expertise in the area being dealt with by the tribunal.

General principles of law in England and Wales

The **Rule of Law** means that all functions of the State must be exercised in accordance with the law of the State The law must be observed even by those parties concerned with making laws, such as Government ministries. The High Court can carry out a supervisory role on both central and local government.

The **Rules of Natural Justice** apply to certain administrative and official decisions as well as judicial decisions. There are two main rules:
* the **Rule against Bias**: decision-makers must be impartial and fair, so anyone, e.g. magistrates, must not preside over a case where they have a financial interest or have any family connection;
* the **rule that every party has a right to be heard**: all involved parties must have the opportunity to find out the case against them and be able to put their case in reply.

The **Doctrine of Precedence** assists courts in administering justice in a uniform way. It rests on the ideal that there should be a similar outcome in similar cases.

European legislation and the effect on the English legal system

The United Kingdom, in 1957, became a signatory to the Treaty of Rome when Parliament passed the European Communities Act.

The European Union (as it is now known) has four main institutions:
* the Council of Ministers, which is the law-making organ;
* the Commission, which formulates and enforces policies;
* the Parliament, which has limited budgetary powers;

- the Court of Justice which sits in Luxembourg and is made up of judges from each of the member countries; one of these acts as a presiding judge. The official language of the court is French.

The role of the **Court of Justice** is to make decisions related to legislation made by the European Union. This body has declared that Community law prevails over the national laws of any of the member states. This means that decisions taken in the European Court are binding on member states. Also, if there is a conflict between the European Union legislation and UK legislation, it is the European legislation that must be followed.

There are three main types of European Union legislation:

- **Regulations** are 'directly applicable', meaning that they apply to all member states as they stand.
- **Directives** are of 'direct effect', meaning that each member state is allowed to decide the way in which the directive is to be applied in their own state.
- **Decisions** apply solely to particular cases and are binding only to those to whom they initially applied, states, companies or individuals.

Legal personnel (in England and Wales)

Judges, appointed by the Lord Chancellor, are usually barristers (but must always have a legal qualification) of at least 10 years standing. Initially a judge will start off as an 'assistant recorder', then as a 'circuit judge' sitting in the courts of a given area known as a circuit.

Barristers are the advocates and specialists of the legal profession. They practise as individuals (they are self-employed), but work in a group, known as 'chambers'. Their work comes from solicitors who 'brief' a certain barrister of their choosing on behalf of their client. Solicitors approach barristers (also known as 'counsel') for a researched opinion on legal aspects of their client's case. Once the case comes to court the barrister argues (or advocates) the client's case, usually in the High or Crown Court. Senior barristers are known as **Queen's Counsel** (or 'silks' because they appear in court in silk robes). They are appointed after several years of distinguished work.

Solicitors work in partnerships or 'firms' and are comparable to general practitioners in medicine. Their work involves many different types of legal work, conveyancing, land disputes, divorce, custody of children, tax and insurance problems, personal injuries to mention just a few. In criminal offences, counsel will be briefed if necessary, but solicitors have right of advocacy in Magistrates' and County Courts. They often do much of the work for 'guilty pleas' or 'first appearances'. They also appear frequently in County Courts. Since 1990 under the Courts and Legal Services Act solicitors have been allowed wider rights of advocacy. They now may, after additional training and three years in practice, appear in the Crown Court and the High Court.

Court clerks usually have a legal qualification and their work varies according to the type of court. In a court where there is a judge presiding, the clerk of the court will be responsible for:

- the maintenance of order in court;
- ensuring that the day's work proceeds smoothly and efficiently;
- seeing that the judge, advocates and clients have access to the paperwork of the court.

In a Magistrates' Court or tribunal the court clerk acts as:

- adviser to the lay bench on legal and procedural matters;
- a recorder of all that is said, particularly important in contested hearings;
- the sender of the court's summonses, and other important paperwork.

The **Jury** is a body of lay men and women (12 in number) who are sworn in to give a verdict, or 'truthful answer', to a question posed by the court officials. (In England this practice dates back to the Norman Conquest.) Jurors are selected at random from the electoral register and must be over 18 years and under 70 years. They must also have resided in the UK for at least five years after the age of 13 years. The main role of jurors is in criminal cases in the Crown Court where, under the guidance of the judge, they reach a verdict on the guilt or innocence of the accused person. Changes in the jury system have come about in the twentieth century, and jurors are now used seldom in civil cases. For a number of reasons, further radical reforms have recently been suggested.

THE WELFARE STATE

The UK is a democratic country which means that everyone has a say in how the country is run, through the representatives they elect to Parliament.

- The **House of Commons** which consists of the representatives of over 600 constituencies throughout the country. These parliamentary representatives – or members (MPs) – are elected to their position by the vote of every person over the age of 18 years who is on the electoral roll.
- The **House of Lords** consists of hereditary peers, bishops, law lords and other 'life peers'. Their function is to pass laws proposed, and also passed, by the House of Commons. They also propose amendments to these laws if thought necessary.
- The **Queen** is the constitutional Head of State, but exerts few powers in the actual government of the country. She is kept fully informed, on a weekly basis by the Prime Minister, of current happenings in the country. She gives the Royal Assent before they can become law.

The work of the House of Commons is to govern the country, and this is done by the party who has obtained the largest number of votes in the preceding election. The party who has the next largest number of votes is termed the **Opposition Party**, and acts as a counter-balance to the political party in power, as well as endeavouring to take over power at the next General Election.

New laws are proposed to both Houses of Parliament in the form of **Bills**. After much debate these Bills are voted on and, if passed, by both Houses, become law and **Acts of Parliament** after receiving the Royal Assent.

The **Prime Minister** is the leader of the party currently in power. He or she appoints a **Cabinet** – a group of ministers who take charge of the various departments of government. Each department of the government is staffed by a permanent band of **Civil Servants** whose task it is to implement the Acts of Parliament.

The above brief description is of **Central Government**. Some tasks are passed on to **Local Government** – county, district and city councils. The people making up local government are councillors who are regularly elected to their political positions in local elections.

Local authorities organize local services such as housing, education, social services, highways, and town and country planning. Each local authority, as well as receiving a grant from central government, imposes a charge on local people and businesses in order to fulfil these duties.

Since the end of the Second World War, the Welfare State has been formed by various Acts of Parliament. Before this time, aid to people in need was given by various uncoordinated charities and private people and obviously was very variable from area to area. Education was elementary from the ages of five to 13 years only.

Various acts stand out in importance in the making of the Welfare State:

- the **Education Act 1944**, which provided free education from five to 15 years in three stages – primary, secondary and higher (over 15 years);
- the **Family Allowance Act**, which provided an allowance for each child in the family (initially apart from the first child, which always seemed an enigma!);
- the **National Health Service Act**, which provided free medical care for everyone.

There were, of course, many other Acts passed and amended around this time and subsequently. Further information can be found in various specific books on the subject.

Below is a brief overview of the various provisions available under the umbrella of the Welfare State in the UK today as applied to children. (There are many other aspects of the Welfare State in reference to elderly people, ill people, etc., which is outside the scope of this book.)

Provisions under the Welfare State
- Education
- Social services
- Health
- Dentistry
- Ambulances
- Ophthalmology
- Housing
- Finance
- Environmental health
- Police
- Fire brigade
- Libraries

Education

Education is free and consists of:

- **nursery schools**: compared with other European countries (see Chapter 7) nursery provision is poor in the UK;
- **primary and secondary schools**: for 5–11-year-olds and 11–16-year-olds respectively, all subscribing to the National Curriculum;
- **special schools** or units attached to mainstream schools for children with special needs (see Chapter 10);
- **colleges of further and higher education** for higher diplomas and degrees;
- **universities** for degrees and higher degrees.

(Various changes are made, and are constantly under review, in the two latter groups of education.)

Discussion

Divide into two groups, one in favour of nursery schools and the other against. Debate, after suitable preparation, the advantages and disadvantages of nursery schools. Use for your factual references, information about:

- the Welfare State;
- provision in other countries;
- the role and importance of early childhood education.

Summarize, in writing, the conclusions of the debate, and comment on your own understanding of the role of the nursery school from the debate.

There are also various grants and subsidies for special needs, such as:

- school buses, or fares paid, for children who live over two miles away from their school;
- free transport to and from school for children with special needs;
- free school meals for children from families who are in receipt of income support;
- grants for further and higher education.

As well as these budgetary provisions, money has to be found to pay for:

- teachers, lecturers;
- ancillary helpers in schools and for children with special needs;
- administrative workers at county education level.

With many schools and colleges over the whole country this is a sizeable financial undertaking.

Social services

The existing department of social services arose from the amalgamation, in 1970, of the departments for the elderly, handicapped, mentally ill and children. All local social services departments have a director of social services and a staff of social workers. From the viewpoint of children, social workers:

- work with families who have a wide variety of problems with which to cope;
- assist with various child-care functions under various Acts of Parliament, e.g. Children Act, Nursery and Child-minders Regulations and Adoption Acts;
- supervise the provision for children in nurseries, playgroups and foster homes;
- assist in the investigations for possible child abuse;
- become involved in taking children into care – usually to a foster home

– when parents are unable (for example, through illness) to look after them, or when a Court Order has been made in cases of abuse.

Health

The **National Health Service** has undergone a number of major reorganizations since the original National Health Service Act in 1948. These are complex and largely administrative in nature. Basically as far as the consumer is concerned services are broadly organized as follows:

- The **primary health care team** gives immediate care in case of illness, and undertakes many preventative services. Primary health care teams are situated in doctor's surgeries and consist of:
  - a group, or partnership, of general medical practitioners, from two to 10 doctors in any one practice; there are still a few single-handed practices around, but these are becoming increasingly rare;
  - practice nurses and specialist nurses for different clinics, such as diabetes, hypertension, immunization and family planning;
  - health visitors who are largely concerned with families and young children;
  - midwives who visit mothers who have recently given birth and been discharged from hospital;
  - clerical staff.

Various other optional services are also available at some doctor's surgeries, such as:
- physiotherapy;
- ophthalmology;
- hearing clinics.

(These facilities are also to be found at local hospitals.)

All general practitioners give free medical treatment together with a varied and wide range of preventative medicine facilities. General practitioners must be able to show a prospectus of the services they offer. Also, of recent years, much of the administrative and financial work is being done by the primary health care team in the context of the 'market economy' now occurring in the NHS.

- **Secondary health care** is given by hospitals based in local areas of high density populations. Here, many different specialists in all branches of medicine are present on the same site. Nurses and many therapists are all available to give treatment. Referrals are taken from the primary health care teams in the immediate locality, and from further afield in the case of some specialities. In-patient, out-patient and day surgery are all available on these single sites.
- **Tertiary health care** for special specialized facilities takes place in regional hospitals.

Medicines and drugs prescribed by doctors of the primary health care team or hospitals, are available from pharmacists at a standard charge per item – this is often far below the actual cost of the drug. Prescriptions are free for various groups of people, from the children's viewpoint these cover all children under 16 years, and children under 19 years of age who are still in full-time education.

Dental services are offered by dentists under the National Health Service, although this can be restricted to existing patients in some areas at present. Charges are made for treatment up to a fixed maximum for each type of treatment. Preventative dentistry and oral hygiene is a large part of children's dentistry these days.

Dentistry is free to:
- pregnant women;
- mothers of children under the age of 1 year;
- children under 18 years;
- children up to 19 years who are still in full-time education.

Ophthalmic services are also free to children under 16 years, and up to 19 years for those in full-time education.

Other important aspects of public welfare are also available from the Welfare State. For example, **housing departments** provide:
- council housing for rent;
- accommodation for homeless families;
- rent rebate schemes;
- help with alterations to adapt houses to the needs of handicapped people.

Finance departments, reorganized in 1988 in the new Social Security Act, oversee and administer, from the children's viewpoint, family credits, income support and maternity benefits. (These benefits are itemized in Chapter 8.)

Environmental health services such as clean water, food and air, removal of rubbish and pest control, are all provided by the Welfare State.

There is free **legal aid** for children with guardians *ad litem* (see below) representing children in court who have been abused or neglected.

Finally a number of other services, such as the fire brigade, police, libraries are all provided under the umbrella of the Welfare State.

Money is raised for all these services by the taxation system which is controlled by Parliament and is the subject of several whole books in itself!

CHILDREN ACT 1989

The Children Act came into effect in 1991 and is an enormous and far-reaching piece of legislation relating to child care and law. Not only was existing legislation brought up to date, but reforms regarding child protection and children in need were added, with social services and education departments being given extra responsibilities for children in need.

The Act is complex and covers many different areas of child care. A brief overview of the salient points is given below. It is advisable, however, that nursery nurses and other child-care workers should read at least the HMSO booklet *An Introduction to the Children Act 1989* for further details. Workers in specialized fields, such as day-carers or workers with children with disabilities, can obtain separate volumes (*Guidance and Regulations*) on the specific aspect required from the Department of Health or from bookshops stocking HMSO publications.

The main principles of the Children Act are discussed below.

The **welfare of the child** is of paramount importance in all proceedings involving legal matters – custody, for example. This is an endeavour to protect children against the damaging 'tug-of-love' situations that are, from time to time, reported in the press.

Whenever possible children should be brought up in their own families. This leads into the area of **parental responsibility**, which is defined as: 'all the rights, duties, powers, responsibilities and authority which by law the parent has in relation to the child and his property'. This responsibility cannot be removed until the child is 18 years of age. From a practical viewpoint this means that parents must:

Parental responsibilities
- Physical and moral protection
- Financial responsibility
- Legal responsibility
- Arranging appropriate education
- No harm to or neglect of the child

- give physical and moral protection to their child;
- be financially responsible for their child;
- be legally responsible for his actions;
- arrange appropriate education at the legal age;
- not harm or neglect their child.

Where the parents are married, they both have legal parental responsibility. Otherwise the mother alone has parental responsibility. The father, under these circumstances, can acquire parental responsibility in one of two ways:

- by making a 'parental responsibility' agreement with the mother;
- applying to the court for an order which gives him parental responsibility.

For children who have lost their parents an official **guardian** will be appointed by the courts to take over parental responsibilities. This can be a relative or the social services department.

When dealing with problems relating to children the courts must do this as quickly as possible. This applies both to the actual court proceeding and any action that has been decided. Delays are considered to prejudice the child's welfare and upbringing. Also courts are advised that a Court Order should not be made unless it is considered that to do so would be better than making no order; this adds substance to the view that the child's welfare is paramount.

A **guardian *ad litem*** can be appointed to represent the child in certain court proceedings. New Magistrates' Courts have been set up to hear proceedings under the Children Act. These are known as **Family Proceedings Courts**. The magistrates involved are carefully chosen for their knowledge of children's and family affairs, and have also had special training on the Children Act.

There is a duty put upon local authorities to provide for **children in need**.

- They must identify those who are 'in need', defined as:
  - 'those children who are unlikely to achieve or maintain . . . a reasonable standard of health or development without the provision for him/her of the services of the Local Authority';
  - 'those children whose health/development is likely to be significantly impaired . . . without the provision of such services';
  - 'those children who are disabled'.

Local authorities must take all reasonable steps to identify any such children in their catchment area. They must keep a register of disabled children and ensure that assessments under the relevant Acts are carried out. Local authorities should also publish information regarding their services.

- They must maintain links with the child's family. If possible children in need should be brought up in their own families, and parents should be given all possible help to do this. This includes:
  - advice, guidance and counselling on the child's specific needs;
  - assistance with travel to places of help for the particular disability;
  - help with appropriate activities, including holidays;
  - provision of family centres where the burden of care can be shared.

Children should be **safe**, and protected by adequate intervention if in danger. This is an important part of the Children Act, and has brought together several previous Acts concerned with child care. When a possible case of child abuse or neglect is noted from a case conference that has been called to enquire into the circumstances and possible harm, the following legal actions can be taken:

- The Local Authority or the NSPCC (National Society for the Prevention of Cruelty to Children – see Appendix) can apply to the courts for a **Child Assessment Order**. This ensures that the child's state of health/ development can be assessed. Seven days are allowed for this to be done.
- An **Emergency Protection Order** (EPO) can be applied for, and issued by a court or an individual magistrate, where there is reason to believe that the child could come to a significant degree of harm if not removed from his or her present situation. Once this order has been granted, the person, or authority, applying for it assumes parental responsibilities for a period of up to eight days.
- **Police protection** can be given if it is considered that children will come to significant harm if they remain where they are even for a short length of time.

Following on from this, either a Care Order or a Supervision Order is made by the courts for the further protection of the child.

- A **Care Order** places the child in the care of the local authority or the NSPCC. Parental responsibilities are assumed, and can last until the child is 18 years of age.
- A **Supervision Order** puts the child in the care of the local authority or the Probation Service. No parental rights are altered under these circumstances. The task of the probation officer is to help and assist the child.

This is merely a very brief overview of just some of the complexities of the Children Act. Nursery nurses who are likely to be working is any specialized areas should refer to the appropriate part of the Act.

OTHER SPECIFIC ACTS

There are other Acts which have a bearing on work in the caring services. The **Race Relations Act 1976** is a long Act of Parliament which makes discrimination on grounds of race unlawful in education or employment and in the provision of facilities, services and goods.

From the viewpoint of members of the caring services who deal with children, the sections relating to education and facilities are of relevance. The Act defines 'racial grounds' as differences in colour, nationality or ethnic origin.

An example of discrimination would be if a nursery or playgroup would not admit a child on the grounds that he is black or from a different ethnic origin from the majority of children attending the particular facility.

Similarly, if a care worker, at the request of a parent or group of parents, segregated children to different tasks or different seating arrangements by virtue of colour this would be termed a breach of the Race Relations Act.

The Commission for Racial Equality (CRE) has the authority to investigate possible cases of discrimination. (The Children Act takes antidiscriminatory practices a little further than the Race Relations Act, religion, cultural practices and language being additional aspects of possible discriminatory practices. This has a bearing on such situations as when suitable foster placements, for example, are being decided for a specific child.)

(Detailed information on all aspects of this act can be found in *The Race Relations Act – 1976*.)

The **Sex Discrimination Act 1975** aims to stop anyone being discriminated against on the grounds of sex. As with the Race Relation Act, this will apply to child-care workers in the fields of early education as well as to employment issues. (The **Equal Pay Act 1972** overlaps some of the issues in the Sex Discrimination Act. The Equal Pay Act states that equal pay must be given for equal work regardless of sex. Both these Acts have now been superseded by the **Sex Discrimination Act 1986**, but the basic principles are the same.)

Early on in the childhood years, gender stereotyping in play and learning activities must be avoided. By the age of around three years children are aware of their gender, and care workers must be sure to offer all activities to all children regardless of their gender. There are, of course, physical reasons for 'male' and 'female' roles. Genetically a baby boy will grow into a man with male sexual characteristics, and a baby girl will grow into a woman with female sexual characteristics. This implies a certain amount of physical dissimilarity; for example, only women can bear children and men usually have larger muscles and can exert greater strength. However, whilst these facts must be taken into account, there should be no active encouragement to distinct male and female roles. Children will, of course, learn various dissimilarities in male and female behaviour in their own homes and in the wider world, but in the nursery differences in gender should not be encouraged.

These considerations lead on to **equal opportunities** for both sexes. In the nursery setting both boys and girls should have the same opportunity to play with the whole range of toys.

Equal opportunity will also come within the remit of nursery nurses when work placements are considered. Nursery nursing has, until recent years, been a largely female domain. Today, however, there are not an inconsiderable number of men wishing to find work in the child-care situation.

EMPLOYMENT, CONTRACTS AND UNIONS

Under two Acts of Parliament, the **Employment Protection Act 1978** and the **Employment Acts 1980** and **1982**, all employees who work for longer than 16 hours per week must have a contract stating **terms and conditions of employment**. (Self-employed people and those working in a voluntary capacity are exempt.)

Certain facts are necessary for inclusion in any **contract of employment**:

• name and address of employer and employee;
• job title;
• date of commencement of employment;
• scale of pay;
• number of hours to be worked;
• holiday entitlement;
• sick pay provision;
• length of notice for termination of employment on either side;
• any pension entitlement;
• grievances and disciplinary procedures.

These are all minimum requirements for any contract. All nursery nurses applying for, and obtaining, a full-time post should be sure to be a signatory to a contract. Private nannying is no exception, although there are many times in which this is overlooked.

Student exercise

Design a form of contract for the post of a nanny to look after two children under the age of five years. Make sure all the conditions listed are included.

There is only one **union** specifically for nursery nurses, the **Professional Association of Nursery Nurses** (PANN – see Appendix). This union is not affiliated to the Trades Union Congress (TUC) and so has no power to negotiate at local authority level. It is, however, able to negotiate for members at their place of work.

Other trade unions to which nursery nurses can belong are:

• National Union of Public Employees (NUPE);
• National and Local Government Officers Association (NALGO);
• Confederation of Health Service Employees (COHSE).

By belonging to a union nursery nurses can be involved in furthering their careers and conditions of service. Membership also involves legal protection and support.

Every type of employment has legal requirements and many of these are highly complex and are also liable to changes. For extra, and current, information, the appropriate institution should be contacted.

FURTHER READING

CRE (1996), *From Cradle to School: A Practical Guide to Race Equality and Child Care*, Commission for Racial Equality.

Hendrick, J. (1993), *Child Care Law for Health Professionals*, Oxford: Radcliffe Medical Press.

NCB, *Working with the Children Act*, London: National Children's Bureau.

Thane, P. (1982), *Foundations of the Welfare State*, London: Longman.

HMSO (London) publishes all the Acts mentioned in this chapter.

13. FIRST AID AND SAFETY

A knowledge of first aid needs to go hand-in-hand with safety measures to avoid, as far as possible, the need for first aid.

People in charge of children, of any age, have a vital responsibility to ensure their safety at all times and in all situations. This includes adequate protection from weather, animals, insects and other natural hazards as well as the provision of safe areas in which to play and live. This latter includes safety in the home, nursery, playground and school. Home is the place where the majority of accidents occur, and especially where there are young children and/or frail elderly people. Regulations exist to protect our health and safety at work, in schools, public places, restaurants and on the roads, but it is up to each one of us personally to make sure our homes, and other places where children spend their time, are as safe as possible. This, of course, is very important to professionals having the care of children on a continuing long-term basis.

However careful child-care professionals are, the adage 'accidents will happen' is true. An accident can be defined as 'an event without an apparent cause' or 'an unforeseen course of events'. These events make up an important factor in the continuing health of children. Many young lives have been permanently blighted as the result of an accident. A few facts show the size of the problem:

- On average, three children are killed every day as the result of an accident.
- Accidents are the commonest cause of death amongst both toddlers and older children.
- Every year, one child in five attends a hospital accident and emergency department.
- One in every four of all patients in an accident and emergency department is a child.
- One in every six children in hospital is there because of an accident.

The causes of the 'unexpected events' are many – two, three or more factors all coming together at a particular point in time and resulting in an accident. It is thought that 80% of these events are due in some way to human behaviour and 15% due to environmental factors, the remaining 5% being utterly unexpected and unpredictable.

Discussion

Outline to your colleagues an accident you have experienced, together with the events and situations leading up to the incident. Then as a group consider how each specific accident could have been avoided. Write up a summary of 'Safety Attitudes' for both management and users, e.g. a provision for safety equipment should be in the budget, everyone must be 'safety aware', etc.

Many aspects of human behaviour can have an input into the occurrence of an accident. Children and elderly people are more prone to accidents than any other **age group** – children due to their inexperience of danger and elderly people due to frailty. The type of likely accident is very much determined by the developmental level of the child. For example, a baby of six months is not able to turn on a hot water tap, but a 3-year-old is quite capable of getting scalded by this action. Similarly, sharp objects such as knives kept in a drawer are of little danger to a 1-year-old, but a 2-year-old will be able to open the drawer and play with a sharp knife with a potentially serious outcome. The lesson to be learned is that dangers of potential accidents must always be related to the developmental level of the child.

Physiological factors such as illness, even a simple head cold can impair judgement, and this applies also, of course, to professional child carers. Dangers to children – so obvious when completely well – can easily be missed when suffering from the miseries of a severe head cold. (Remember, too, that more accidents occur during the immediate premenstrual phase than at any other time during the menstrual cycle. So special care should be taken by women at this time.)

Psychological factors such as anger, grief and worry can lead to less than perfect safety precautions.

Education in all aspects of safety is important. Safety precautions have to be recognized and learned – they are not necessarily known by instinct.

There is a **gender difference**. Boys are known to suffer a greater number of accidents than girls by a ratio of 3 to 2. This may be because boys by nature tend to be more adventurous than girls, or is it possibly because carers allow boys to take more risks than girls?

Other aspects of human behaviour resulting in accidents include **recreational and sporting activities**, together with **exploration** of the child's environment. These are all very necessary and excellent aspects of growing-up, but nevertheless can result in accident.

Environmental factors leading to possible accidents include:
• **Physical surroundings**. This includes layout of homes, schools, nurseries and their potential for the avoidance, or otherwise, of accidents.

Roads, the countryside and industrial areas all have their own specific problems. Much care needs to be taken, by authorities responsible for design and layout of public places, to reduce accident potential to a minimum.

- **Equipment**. As with the physical surroundings where people congregate the design of various pieces of equipment requires much thought and attention. Into this category, with particular reference to children, comes the design of toys and playground equipment. There is much legislation concerned with the safety of such products in daily use, and this applies especially to products used solely by children.
- **Weather**. Unusual weather can cause accidents. Heavy rain, for example, makes for poor visibility on roads; high winds can bring down branches from trees and even excessive heat can cause carelessness in many situations.

So it can be seen that it is virtually impossible to avoid accidents altogether. Every effort must be made, both individually and nationally, to reduce the number of tragedies due to accidents. Everyone having the care of children will need to have a basic knowledge of first aid to cope with these, sadly inevitable, events.

The Red Cross and St John Ambulance provide **first-aid courses**, at varying levels, in many centres across the country. All people in charge of children should be able to administer first aid in an accident situation to these standards. (Addresses of the headquarters of these organizations can be found in the Appendix. Local addresses are to be found in the appropriate local telephone directory.) You will gain much confidence by acquiring knowledge of first aid, so that when an accident does occur, immediate appropriate action can be taken.

Discussion

Arrange a seminar for, say, half a day in pleasant and comfortable surroundings, including the provision of coffee/tea, for both your group and other invited people interested in 'First Aid in the Nursery'. Either individually or in pairs give a 10-minute presentation and allow 5 minutes for questions on a related topic, e.g. risk-taking by children at play, nursery layout, staff hazards. (Remember too that staff can be at risk from both the children themselves as well as hazards in the nursery.)

AIMS OF FIRST AID: THE THREE PS

1. *Preserve life*. This is, of course, the most obvious aim. It is the person first on the scene of an accident who will be able to give help to the victim, and in the case of serious accidents to determine whether or not the casualty lives. An example is the rapid control of massive bleeding.

Unless the loss of blood is staunched within minutes, there will be insufficient blood volume left to support life. It has been estimated that 30% of people suffering from a heart attack lose their lives because of inadequate first-aid attention within the first few minutes after the event.

2. **Promote recovery**. Once the initial life-saving actions have been taken, the first-aider can do much to aid the full recovery of the accident victim. It can take anything up to 20 minutes for skilled paramedical help to arrive at an out-of-the-way location. During this time the first-aider can make sure that the child – or adult – is as comfortable as possible, is warm and is reassured. Confidence in first-aid abilities will do much to reassure the sufferer.

3. **Prevent further injury**. It is important that neither the accident victim nor any bystanders take any action that will worsen the original injury. Remember:
   - continue immobilization of the head if there has been a neck injury, as in a whiplash injury;
   - continue firm pressure on a wound to ensure that bleeding remains under control.

Aims of first aid
- Preserve life
- Promote recovery
- Prevent further injury

PRIORITIES AT AN ACCIDENT

The vast majority of accidents are relatively minor and are quickly and easily treated by someone with a knowledge of basic first aid. Occasionally, however, first-aiders will be called upon to deal with major life-threatening incident, either in their place of work or in the immediate environs, e.g. in a nearby roadway. Under these circumstances, a knowledge of the routine to be followed is vital. As an example, take the following scenario:

> The early-leavers from the nursery are waiting to go home. Coats are on, favourite toys are ready. A nursery nurse is standing with the children by the door. Her attention is briefly distracted by a shout from one of the children behind her in the nursery. At that critical moment 4-year-old Elspeth sees her mother coming round the corner. She dashes out to meet her, steps momentarily onto the road to avoid a hurrying pedestrian and is knocked over by a passing cyclist.

The routine to be followed by a first-aider under these circumstances would be:

1. Keep calm; assess and take control of the situation.
2. Make sure the other children in the nursery are safe with someone in charge who will immediately organize an activity for them.
3. Ask a passer-by (the 'hurrying pedestrian'?) to control any traffic that may be around. Even a relatively minor accident can become a major one if other traffic becomes involved.
4. Quickly assess the child's injuries. Is there excessive bleeding? Has the child been unconscious?

5. If there are serious injuries, deal appropriately with these.
6. Summon help – ask a colleague to dial 999 if you think the child has been seriously injured. As many details as possible about the accident should be given: how many people involved; their approximate age; whether the injuries are serious. In the given scenario, it is important that the ambulance service should be aware that it is a child that has been involved.
7. Keep the casualty warm with blankets or coats, and do not move unless absolutely necessary.
8. Reassure the mother.

Each and every accident is quite unique. The detailed action taken will depend on what is found when the situation is assessed. For example, in the above scenario, the child could have received a severe laceration from the passing bicycle. Under these conditions, first aid to stop the bleeding would be a priority. Again, if the child were unconscious, action to check the Airway, Breathing and Circulation would be necessary – the ABC of dealing with unconscious casualties. (See below under 'Unconsciousness'.)

Ongoing throughout the treatment of the casualty, as much information should be obtained about the accident:

- **history**: asking the casualty and/or bystanders what actually happened;
- **symptoms**: subjective sensations felt and verbalized by the casualty;
- **signs**: objective and noted by the first-aider by sight, hearing, touch and smell;
- **external aids**: 'medicalert' bracelet/necklace or card found in the pocket of the casualty. These will alert the first-aider to any long-standing condition such as diabetes or epilepsy that may have had a bearing on the accident or may affect treatment.

ASPHYXIA AND RESUSCITATION

Asphyxia occurs when there is insufficient oxygen available for use by the tissues of the body. Without a continuous supply of oxygen all tissues deteriorate rapidly. Vital nerve cells in the brain will die if they are starved of oxygen for longer than four minutes. Causes include:

- **Obstructed airway**, due to:
  - the tongue falling back into the throat of an unconscious person;
  - food stuck in the back of the throat;
  - swelling in the throat region due to, for example, stings in the mouth;
- **Suffocation** when air is prevented from reaching the lungs (soft pillows, plastic bag over a child's head, for example);
- **Severe injuries to the chest**;
- **Poisoning**;
- **Electrocution**. These two latter causes affect the nerves controlling respiration;
- Air which contains **insufficient oxygen**, e.g. in cases of fire where thick smoke is a problem.

Signs and symptoms of asphyxia

- Difficulty in breathing. Initially breathing is increased in both depth and rate in an attempt to obtain sufficient oxygen. Later gurgling sounds will be heard.
- The face and lips will become blue.
- The casualty will become confused.
- The casualty will fall unconscious.

Treatment

The cause of the asphyxia must be determined and treated. For example, remove a plastic bag from a child's head (never allowed one near a young child in the first place!); take quick action to release an obstructing particle of food (see below under 'choking'). In all cases of asphyxia leading to unconsciousness (and also, of course, in all cases of unconsciousness for whatever cause) the ABC rule must be followed.

- The **A**irway must be opened.
- **B**reathing must be checked.
- **C**irculation must be checked.

The **airway** (i.e. the passage from the exterior through the mouth, down the trachea to the lungs) must be opened. This is done quickly by lifting the chin upwards and forwards. This action will bring the tongue forwards so that there is no risk of this thick, heavy organ blocking the throat. To maintain an open airway, the casualty's chin must be held in this position, or the unconscious person put into the 'recovery position' (see below) with the head in the well-back position.

To check **breathing**:

1. Place your cheek close to the person's nose and mouth. If breathing is present, you will feel the air on your cheek as they breathe out.
2. Whilst performing this action, look down along the line of the casualty's chest. If they are breathing the chest will rise and fall regularly.

To check **circulation**:

1. Place the first two fingers of your hand on one of the carotid pulses. These pulses are to be found on either side of the windpipe just below the chin. With each beat of the heart, blood is pumped through the arteries and this 'beat' can be felt. Other pulses can be felt in the wrist, the upper arm and the groin.
2. Look at the casualty's colour.

If the casualty is not breathing but has a heart beat, **mouth-to-mouth** (or expired air) **resuscitation** (Figure 13.1) must be given:

1. Ensure that there is nothing in the mouth that is obstructing breathing.
2. Lift chin up and tilt head back, to open the airway.
3. Pinch nostrils tightly between thumb and forefinger: this will ensure that the breath you are going to breath into the casualty does not escape down the nose.
4. Take a deep breath in.
5. Make a seal around the casualty's mouth with your mouth and blow.
6. Watch to be sure that the casualty's chest rises as the air enters.

Figure 13.1 Mouth-to-mouth resuscitation.

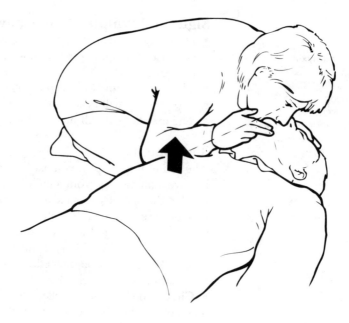

Artificial resuscitation for a small child, or baby, will require some modification:
- Both the child's mouth and nose can be covered by an adult's mouth.
- The force of the expired air will need to be much less than that necessary for an adult.

Cardiac compression for a small child or baby – finger tip pressure only is necessary. The rate should also be increased to around 100 to 120 per minute.

7. Remove your mouth and take another deep breath in.
8. Repeat this process at approximately 10 times a minute – each sequence to be done to a slow count of 6.
9. This will need to be continued until either help arrives or the casualty starts to breathe again

The above procedure will ensure that oxygen is again available to the casualty as long as the heart is still beating to move the oxygenated blood around the body. If the heart has stopped beating (cardiac arrest), **cardiac compression**, or 'chest thrusts', will be necessary (Figure 13.2):

1. The casualty will need to be lying on his back.
2. Kneel beside him.
3. Find the lower end of the sternum (breastbone), and move two finger-breadths upwards.
4. In this position, in the middle of the chest and using the heel of your hand with fingers interlocked, press down rhythmically 4–5 cm ($1\frac{1}{2}$–2 in.).
5. Repeat this 60 to 80 times a minute.

Artificial respiration will need to be continued at the same time as the chest thrusts: two breaths followed by 15 compressions is the rhythm to aim for. This is an extremely tiring procedure to continue for any length of time, so ideally there should be one or more other first-aiders available to take over.

If the casualty starts to breath spontaneously again and the heart is beating, he must be put into the **recovery position** (Figure 13.3). This is

Figure 13.2 Cardiac compression.

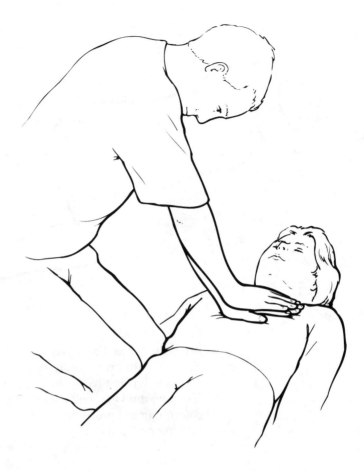

the position in which an unconscious casualty should be placed if there are no other life-threatening injuries. An unconscious person lying on his back is in danger of choking owing to:

- the tongue falling limply into the back of the throat and so obstructing the passage of air into the lungs.
- vomiting; being unconscious, he will be unable to cough or gag to prevent the vomit entering his lungs; if this does happen a life-threatening pneumonia can result.

With the chin lifted, the tongue will be pulled forward and the airway opened. After this, turning the casualty onto his side will allow any vomit or other secretions to drain out of the mouth.

To turn a casualty into the recovery position (Figure 13.3):

1. Loosen any tight clothing and remove spectacles if worn.
2. Kneel beside casualty.
3. Place nearest arm in the raised 'stop' position on the floor.

Figure 13.3 Recovery position.

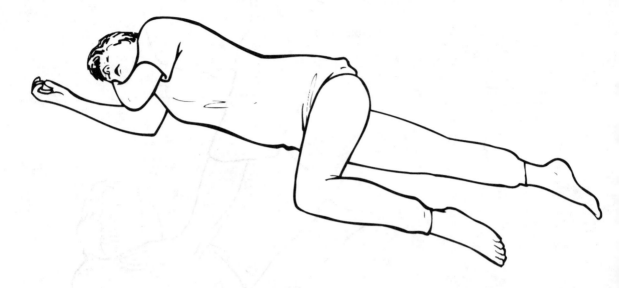

4. Bring the furthest arm over the casualty's chest and cradle the back of his hand onto his cheek nearest to you.
5. Bend the furthest leg at the knee with the foot flat on the ground.
6. Grasping this knee, pull the casualty over towards you onto your knees, controlling and protecting the head with your other hand. He will now be lying on his side.
7. To stabilize the position, bring the top knee up to form a right angle with his body.
8. Make sure his head is tilted well back to maintain an open airway.

(It is very much easier to be shown how to place a person in the recovery position than to explain it! Students should spend time practising putting each other into the recovery position.)

BLEEDING

Bleeding occurs when either an artery or a vein is ruptured due to an injury. Bleeding from veins is the most usual type of injury, as these blood-vessels are nearest the surface of the body. Blood from veins is dark red in colour and tends to ooze relatively slowly from the wound. Arterial blood, when an artery is damaged, is bright red in colour and will spurt out with each beat of the heart.

Bruising occurs when blood vessels are damaged but the overlying skin is not broken. The bleeding under these circumstances is self-limiting because of the tautness of the overlying skin. (It is nevertheless still a painful event!)

Medical help should be obtained if the bruising is severe or if there are associated injuries. Otherwise treat with a cold compress – a handkerchief or piece of towelling wrung out in cold water and left on the wound for 10 minutes. Repeat this treatment again if necessary. (A pack of frozen peas from the freezer can make an excellent ice-pack.)

Bruising from a bang on the head happens quite often in children. The size and speed of the swelling can be quite alarming. Most bumps on the head can be treated as for bruising on any other part of the body. The child should, however, be watched carefully for 24 hours following a bump on the head. If she becomes drowsy, complains of a headache, double vision or vomiting, seek urgent medical advice to check on possible damage to the underlying brain tissue.

OLD WIVES' TALE

Steak on a black eye will reduce the swelling.

Not true! If the steak is cold, the lowering of the temperature of the wound will have an effect. But even the most expensive steak has no magical properties.

Minor cuts

Most minor cuts bleed relatively little. (The bleeding itself serves the purpose of carrying away dirt and bacteria from the wound.) These small wounds need to be cleaned with a swab of cottonwool soaked in an antiseptic solution. Be sure to read carefully the instructions on each bottle of antiseptic solution before use, regarding any necessary dilution. Too strong a solution can damage tissues further. If there is no antiseptic solution available, plain water is quite satisfactory.

A small sticky dressing is usually all that is necessary for a minor cut. This can be removed after 24 hours once healing has begun. Leaving the wound open to the air will allow healing to proceed more quickly.

A **graze** is when a relatively large area of skin is removed, often as the result of a sliding injury. This type of skidding injury is very frequently seen on children's knees. Grazes are often more painful than deeper cuts as it is the outer layer of skin that contains the pain-sensitive nerves. Grazes are often contaminated with dirt or grit. This should be gently removed with a piece of dampened cottonwool as far as possible – swabbing from the centre of the wound outwards. Finally, cover the area with dry gauze until a scab starts to form.

Puncture wounds sustained by treading on a drawing-pin or nail, for example, can be more serious than they originally seem. There can be very little bleeding so that the dirt carried in at the time of the wound is not removed by the flow of blood. Any bleeding that does occur should be encouraged. If the object trodden on is dirty, a visit to the Accident and Emergency Department of the local hospital should be the course of action. An antitetanus and/or antibiotic injection may be necessary.

Major cuts, particularly if the bleeding is thought to be from a severed artery, will need hospital treatment. As a first-aid measure, apply firm pressure over the wound and raise the affected limb above the level of the heart. Take the casualty to the Accident and Emergency Department of the nearest hospital, or dial 999 if the wound is severe and transport is not readily available. Stitching will most likely be with 'butterfly' stitches of the adhesive type. An antitetanus and/or antibiotic injection will also probably be necessary.

OLD WIVES' TALE

Tie a tourniquet tightly above the wound.

This must never be done. Serious and permanent damage, with possible loss of the limb, can result from this mistaken treatment.

Bleeding can occur from particular areas.

Scalp
Wounds to the head bleed freely due to the good blood supply to this area of the body. Children and elderly people are the most common sufferers from this type of wound. The usual treatment for bleeding, i.e. firm direct pressure, must be carried out with care in these cases. There is always a danger that the bony scalp may have been fractured. So any pressure will push the fractured bone into the delicate brain tissue beneath. If there is any doubt as to the possibility of a fracture, pressure should be applied around the edges of the wound in an attempt to stem the bleeding. This can done by building up a dressing around the wound before covering with another dressing. All head wounds – except for the most slight – should receive medical attention.

Ears
Bleeding from the ear can arise from two causes:
• A severe **head injury** can result in fracture of the base of the skull. Urgent medical treatment is necessary under these circumstances.
• Rupture of the eardrum can occur following a middle ear infection. The child will have been complaining of earache previously and will probably also be feverish. Again medical attention is necessary. A clean dry dressing should be placed gently over the affected ear.

Nose
This is a relatively common occurrence. A blow on the nose or the aftermath of a cold can be the cause or there may be no apparent reason at all; 8–10-year-old boys seem especially liable to nose-bleeds for no obvious reason. Treatment is to lean the patient forwards over a bowl or sink and pinch the nose firmly just below the bony part. This should be kept up

for 10 minutes, by which time most nose-bleeds have stopped. If the bleeding has not ceased after 20 minutes, medical help should be obtained. Do not allow him to blow his nose for several hours following a nose-bleed, as this will dislodge the scab and start the whole process all over again.

OLD WIVES' TALE

Lie the person with a nose-bleed down.

No! This will ensure that the blood passes down the back of the throat and is swallowed; this blood will be vomited later. Choking can also occur with this dangerous treatment.

Gums

Bleeding from gums is most common after a tooth extraction. If this is excessive get the child to bite hard on a cottonwool roll, and revisit the dentist if the bleeding continues. Tongue and cheeks can also bleed excessively. Again lean the child forward so that the blood is not swallowed, and take to the Accident and Emergency Department if it is severe.

Palm of the hand

A wound to this part of the body must be treated with care. Vital tendons and blood vessels are near the surface and long-term disability can result from these injuries. To control bleeding, raise the casualty's arm and get him to hold tightly onto a roll of gauze or other clean material. Bandage this into place, put into an elevation sling and take to hospital.

Students must be conversant with the use of manufactured wound dressings. They should also be able to improvise dressings from any material readily available at the scene of the accident. Arm and elevation slings should be demonstrated and practised.

Student exercise

List and discuss the suitability of materials normally found in a nursery – or at home – which could be used to control bleeding.

Internal bleeding

This is a serious form of bleeding which occurs following an injury involving one of the internal organs of the body, or some major internal catastrophe following an accident. Although there is no external signs of bleeding, blood is still being lost from the main circulation into the tissues. So the effects will be the same as in those with a massive external bleed.

Signs of internal bleeding include:

- possible history of a severe injury, or some previous existing condition, such as a gastric ulcer;
- pain and tenderness around the injured part of the body;
- signs and symptoms of shock.

Removal to hospital is urgent under these circumstances. Meanwhile, lay the casualty down, loosen tight clothing, keep warm and reassure. Breathing and pulse rate should be checked regularly and noted down to give to the ambulance personnel when they arrive.

SHOCK

This is a specific clinical condition, and has nothing at all to do with the feelings of 'shock' when we are surprised by people or events! Medical shock is the term used to describe the collection of symptoms occurring when organs of the body – and this includes the brain – are deprived of oxygen for any reason.

Causes of shock

- severe bleeding – external or internal;
- severe abdominal emergencies, such as a ruptured appendix;
- a severe heart attack; here the heart is so damaged as to be unable to pump the blood round the circulation adequately;
- severe burns or scalds: large amounts of body fluid can lost to the circulation under these circumstances;
- severe diarrhoea and/or vomiting; again, large amounts of fluid can be lost.

Signs and symptoms of shock include:

- cold clammy skin;
- shivery feelings;
- rapid, shallow breathing;
- feeble, rapid pulse;
- faintness, giddiness;
- nausea, vomiting;
- confused, anxious;
- thirsty.

The underlying cause for the shock must be found and first aid given as far as is possible, e.g. the control of excessive bleeding. Any person in true medical shock will need hospital treatment. Whilst you are awaiting the arrival of the ambulance the following actions need to be taken:

1. Lie the casualty down with her feet raised, turning her head to the side in case vomiting occurs.
2. Loosen tight clothing.
3. Keep warm, with blankets underneath as well as on top. Do not use hot water bottles as there is always a danger of burns.
4. If she becomes unconscious, turn her into the recovery position.

OLD WIVES' TALE

Give a tot of brandy to someone in shock.

This must not be done. Alcohol will dilate the small blood vessels in the skin. This in turn will further remove blood from the vital internal organs.

FAINTING

Initially the signs and symptoms of fainting may seem very similar to those associated with a person in shock. However, a faint is cause by a temporary lack of blood to the brain and not due to any of the serious conditions that can be associated with shock.

Causes of fainting include:
- standing for long periods of time;
- excessive heat or cold;
- emotional upset;
- a painful injury.

Consciousness can be lost for a short period of time if the person has not been able to sit down.

To **treat** a faint:
1. Lie the person down, or sit her down and bend her forwards.
2. Loosen tight clothing.
3. Get adequate fresh air.

Most faints are over within a few minutes and the casualty returns to full consciousness. The cause of the faint should be found, and similar circumstance avoided in future if at all possible.

Some children who are undergoing a particularly rapid spurt of growth can feel faint if they are required to stand still for any length of time in a hot, stuffy atmosphere.

BURNS AND SCALDS

A burn is caused by dry heat; a scald is caused by wet heat, but the effects on the skin are the same in both cases. Not only is the skin damaged (in all but the most superficial of burns), but the tiny blood vessels just below the skin are also involved. This will cause plasma – a colourless fluid – to leak into the surrounding tissues. As the skin frequently stays intact over the site of a burn, a blister will be formed. If the burn is a large one (covering more than 10% of the body surface, e.g. an arm, a leg or the chest), a good deal of plasma will be lost from the circulation. Under these conditions the casualty will be in a state of **shock**. So treatment for shock will be necessary as well as the first-aid treatment of the burn itself.

The other potent danger with burns is **infection**. To avoid this it is vitally important that the blisters produced by a severe burn or scald are NOT broken. The skin acts as the best possible barrier to infection and must be kept intact.

The burned part should be held under running cold water, or fully immersed in cold water, for at least 10 minutes. This will effectively remove as much heat as possible from the burn. Following this dry the burn carefully and cover with a sterile dry dressing.

Any burn covering an area more than $7\,cm^2$ ($3\,in.^2$) must receive medical attention, as much plasma will have been lost into this area of burning. Also any burns on the face or hands, however small, should receive attention to avoid as far as possible the formation of scar tissue in these vulnerable places.

OLD WIVES' TALE

Put butter on a burn.

This should NEVER be done. The fat will keep the heat in, and so cause further damage. It will also have to be removed later, so causing further problems.

FRACTURES AND SPRAINS

The bones of the body can be broken by:
• a direct blow
• an indirect 'jarring' accident, e.g. a collar-bone can be fractured by a fall on outstretched hands, or the spine can be fractured by sitting down suddenly and unexpectedly.

There are three types of fracture:
• an 'open' fracture in which the broken bone is protruding through the skin;
• a 'closed' fracture when the skin is not broken;
• a 'greenstick' fracture seen in the pliable bones of young children in which the bone bends rather than breaks.

Signs and symptoms of a fracture include:
• severe pain at the site of the injury; any attempt at movement will intensify this pain;
• swelling round the region of the break;
• deformity if the break results in an angulation of the bone;
• shock, when the injury is so severe as to break a bone.

It can be difficult to tell whether or not a bone is broken or if the injury has just resulted in a severe sprain. Only an X-ray examination will be able to differentiate between the two conditions.

The aim for **treatment** of a fracture is to immobilize the broken part so as to avoid any further damage to the surrounding tissues. Medical attention should be obtained as soon as possible. Meanwhile make the casualty as comfortable as possible without movement of the fractured part. A broken **arm** will feel more comfortable if an arm sling is provided to support the weight of the arm; similarly a fractured **collar-bone** will be better immobilized in an elevation sling. (Students should be shown how to apply arm and elevation slings, and should gain adequate practise.)

A broken **leg** can be immobilized safely and securely by binding it to the uninjured leg with whatever may be at hand – scarves, bandages, ties, etc. Adequate soft padding between the legs will make the casualty more comfortable and further reduce unwanted movement in the broken limb.

Fracture of the **neck** or **spine** is a serious condition and it is vital that no movement in the fracture should take place. Damage to the enclosed spinal cord with resultant paralysis can occur if the damaged bones impinge on this vital structure. A conscious patient with a fractured neck or spine may complain of severe pain at the site of the injury, or may have some loss of control of the limbs below the site of the injury. Sometimes these signs are not immediately apparent. So in any accident which may involve a fractured neck, e.g. a whiplash injury in a shunting accident, the casualty must be treated for a fracture until proved otherwise. The prime aim of the first-aider is to KEEP the casualty STILL. Send for help, keep the casualty warm and reassure him.

It is important in all cases of fractures not to give the casualty anything to eat or drink An anaesthetic may be necessary to reduce the fracture and this may have to be delayed if food or drink has been taken.

STRAINS AND SPRAINS

Both have a similar origin, i.e. overstretching or overuse of a specific part of the body: a **strain** is said to apply to damage to muscular tissue, whilst a **sprain** occurs when the tissues around a joint are overstretched. Both types of injuries are common in children.

Muscular strains occur after excessive use of a certain group of muscles. There can be a sharp initial pain following by generalized aching. More usually only the aching pain is paramount. Rest and a hot bath is all that is usually required for a complete cure.

Joint sprains occur when the tough ligaments protecting the joint are overstretched, e.g. when an ankle is 'turned over'. Occasionally the ligament may be actually torn. This is a far more serious injury than a muscular strain. It can be difficult, or impossible, to differentiate this injury from a fracture without the help of an X-ray. Treatment is by rest, a cold compress on the injured part and a crepe bandage for support. If this treatment has not produced a marked improvement within 24 hours, attendance at the Accident and Emergency Department for an X-ray is necessary.

Dislocations at joints – especially shoulders, fingers and knee – can also closely mimic a fracture, although the amount of deformity is often greater. Keep the injured site immobilized and the casualty as comfortable as possible until transport to hospital can be arranged.

POISONING

It is usually children who are in need of first aid following accidental poisoning. They are unaware of the dangers of swallowing some tempting looking 'fruit' from the hedgerows or taking a drink from a bottle that looks vaguely familiar but is in reality some corrosive substance. It is in this particular area of child safety that parents and child carers can do much to avoid such dangers.

Some poisons may cause abdominal pain and vomiting. If the **vomiting** occurs immediately after the substance has been swallowed it is likely that most of the poison will have been eliminated from the body. Nevertheless, medical attention should always be sought under these circumstances.

If vomiting has not occurred the poison will be absorbed into the blood stream and so exert its effects in many widespread parts of the body. Depending on the type of poison taken, respiratory, cardiac or nervous systems can be involved. First-aid care under these conditions will be:

1. Telephone immediately for an ambulance.
2. Reassure the child who has eaten or drunk the poisonous substance. Remember she will be frightened at the reaction produced by – to her – an innocent act.
3. Do NOT attempt to make her sick. This is especially important if the substance that has been swallowed is a corrosive poison such as bleach, paint thinner, or ammonia (all substances often kept in the cupboard under the sink in the kitchen.) If the child is sick the substance will burn the lining of the oesophagus as much on the way up as it did on the way down.
4. If it is a corrosive substance that has been taken, give a drink of tepid water or milk. This will help to dilute the poison.
5. Carefully wipe away traces of the poison from the child's lips.
6. Keep a sample of the substance/pills/garden berries that have been swallowed for the ambulance staff when they arrive. This is important so that a specific antidote to the poison can be given.
7. If the child has vomited, also keep a sample.
8. Keep a careful check on the casualty's level of consciousness, heart rate and breathing.

Common household poisonous substances
- Bleach
- Lavatory cleaner
- Oven cleaner
- Metal polish
- Paint thinner
- Paraffin
- Detergents
- Polish
- Slug pellets (from the garden shed) looking very like sweets.

UNCONSCIOUSNESS

Probably one of the most worrying incidents to occur to anyone in charge of children is when a child becomes unconscious. There are many reasons for this which include:
- head injuries;
- poisoning;
- epilepsy;
- hypoglycaemia (in a diabetic child);

- fainting;
- shock (for a wide number of reasons).

The first action (as with all first-aid procedures) is to assess the situation and make sure that everyone in the vicinity, including the first-aider (you are no use as a first-aider if you are also injured!), is safe from further danger, as in the case of a road accident, for example.

The probable cause of unconsciousness must then be ascertained, and appropriate treatment given. Help, if this is thought to be necessary, and indeed almost always is when a child becomes unconscious, must be summoned. If the child remains unconscious, she should be put into the recovery position, kept warm and her vital signs (respiration, pulse and level of consciousness) monitored regularly.

It is important to try and make an assessment of the level of consciousness initially and again at regular intervals. Recording this will give valuable information. There are three main ways in which the level of consciousness can be monitored:

- the movements of the casualty;
- his speech;
- reaction of his eyes.

Movements: ask yourself the following questions:
- Does the casualty respond at all to commands, however slowly?
- If he does move, is it obviously with pain?
- Does he make no response at all?

Speech: ask yourself the following questions:
- Does the casualty answer questions at all?
- Is the response sensible or is it confused or inappropriate?
- Is there no speech at all?

Eyes: note:
- whether the eyes are open;
- if they open when asked;
- if there is a visual response to pain.

Changes in the level of consciousness over time gives helpful clues as to what is happening in the brain, particularly in the case of head injuries, and is of immense use to those people subsequently treating the person in hospital.

Role play

Ask, nicely, two smallish students to represent two children. Set the scene with an ironing board with the iron plugged in, a cooker with the saucepan handles visible over the side and a quantity of toys scattered about the floor. One small child sits crying and nursing a burnt hand from the hot iron. The other child – slightly older – has rushed to stop the saucepan boiling over. In doing so she falls over the strewn toys and is sitting quietly sobbing and nursing a bleeding leg. Each member of the group in turn is the 'first-aider' who enters into this scene and acts, within a limited time period such as five minutes, all of which is videoed. The group then assesses the video for the actions taken: whether in correct sequence; with regard to further safety and aid given to casualties, etc.

MISCELLANEOUS CONDITIONS

The following are all conditions which are frequently encountered by child carers on a daily basis. Some of the conditions are trivial, but nevertheless will need some commonsense first-aid measures. Others are potentially more serious and may need specialized help, but which still need knowledgeable handling initially. (The conditions are arranged alphabetically, and not in order of seriousness or frequency.)

Asthma

During an asthma attack, the tiny muscles surrounding the air passages go into spasm. This effectively restricts the size of the bronchi and so causes breathing difficulties, especially on breathing out. Children who are known to have asthma usually have medication available to control an attack.

During an attack, the child will :
- have difficulty in breathing;
- have breathing that is 'wheezy';
- become blue in the face owing to lack of oxygen;
- be distressed and anxious.

To treat an attack:
1. Sit the child down: leaning forwards onto a table is often the most comfortable position.
2. Reassure him: remember anxiety levels will be high and this can worsen an attack.
3. Open nearby windows to ensure an adequate supply of fresh air.
4. Give any available medication. Nurseries and schools should be informed if any of their charges suffer from asthma, know what medication is available, where it is to be found and how to give it in the case of an attack.
5. If the attack is a first one, if it is prolonged or if it does not respond to medication – dial 999.
6. After the attack has stopped, be sure that the child's parent knows what has happened during the course of the day.

Choking

Choking on objects put into the mouth or on food is a common occurrence in childhood. Children under three years of age are most at risk, and choking is the largest cause of accidental death in children under one year of age.

If the child is under one year of age:

1. Lay her down on your thigh with her face down and head low.
2. Give up to five firm slaps between the shoulder-blades.
3. If this does not work, lie her on her back again with the head low and give up to five firm chest thrusts.

If the child is over one year of age:

1. Bend the child forwards and give up to five firm back slaps.
2. If this does not work, lie child down and give up to five chest thrusts.
3. If still no result, give up to five abdominal thrusts upwards, in the region just below the lower end of the sternum.

If the child has stopped breathing start mouth-to-mouth resuscitation. (If the obstruction is only partial, it may be possible to get sufficient air into her lungs until the emergency services arrive.) Choking is an emergency and a 999 call is vital if simple first aid measures do not succeed.

Convulsions

This term covers a wide range of conditions ranging from true epilepsy through petit mal to febrile convulsions; the latter are not unusual in the under-fives. (For further information see Chapter 10.)

A **febrile convulsion** is a fit (or convulsion) which occurs in children under five in response to a sudden rise in body temperature. The aim of treatment is to cool the child as quickly as possible. This can be done by:
- opening doors and windows to reduce the heat in the room;
- removing excess clothes from the child;
- sponging him down with tepid (not cold) water.

Other measures are to:
- reassure him (a fit is a frightening event to the sufferer as well as the onlooker!);
- obtain medical help and/or advice;
- try to put the child into the recovery position in case a further fit should occur;
- never leave the child alone.

Epilepsy

Uncoordinated electrical discharges in the brain cause fits to occur. Emergency treatment includes:

1. If the child is seen to fall down at the onset of the fit, try to ensure that he does not injure himself as he falls.
2. Move any nearby furniture, toys or other objects on which injury could occur.
3. Do NOT try to restrain the child whilst the convulsive movements are occurring. This will only result in further injury.
4. When the convulsions cease, reassure the child – he will probably be confused and drowsy – and lie him in the recovery position.
5. If a further fit occurs, dial 999
6. If this is a first fit, contact a doctor. If the child is a known sufferer from epilepsy, check with his doctor that his medication is still satisfactory.

Put something between a convulsing person's teeth to prevent them biting their tongue.

This must NOT be done. Further injury can easily be caused by this action. Also the tongue is rarely bitten during a fit.

Foreign bodies

Eyes

Dust, insects and grit are but a few of the substances that can blow into a child's eyes. The natural reaction of tears and rapid blinking may be all that is necessary to remove the foreign body. If this does not happen:

- Examine the eye in a good light.
- If the object, a small fly for example, can be seen on the white part of the eye, try gently removing this with a dampened wisp of cottonwool or tissue. (The white part of the eye – the sclera – is a relatively tough part of the eye. The cornea, the part of the eye immediately over the iris and the pupil, is very delicate.)
- If the object is on the cornea, attempt to wash it out with PLENTY of water. If this is not successful, visit the Accident and Emergency Department of the nearest hospital. (Rough attempts to remove objects from the cornea can result in scratching of this delicate membrane with subsequent scarring.)
- Remember to try to stop the child from rubbing the eye, as this can also damage the cornea.

Accidental splashing of chemicals into the eye, such as various household cleansing products, can cause damage rapidly. It is vital that quick action is taken to wash the eye with plenty of water is taken.

Ears

Small children are likely to put objects – usually small and round and often sticky – in their ears at any time! Both types are difficult to remove successfully. Damage to the eardrum can easily be done by attempts to do this. It is worth trying to float the object out on a drop of warm olive-oil placed gently into the ear. Pull backwards on the ear lobe as you insert this – this will straighten the ear canal. If this does not remove the foreign body, obtain medical help.

Nose

Any object up a child's nose must be removed at the Accident and Emergency Department of a hospital with special instruments designed for this purpose It is all too easy to push the foreign body further up the nose and, more dangerously, into the lungs by unskilled attempts to remove it.

Heat stroke

In unexpected hot weather, or on visits to hot climates, children can suffer from heat stroke, or heat exhaustion, if sufficient care is not taken to keep them cool. Obviously prevention of overheating should be the aim, but if the child feels sick, giddy, listless or headachy, the following action should be taken:

1. Remove the child to the shade, or a cool room; use an electric fan if available.
2. Sponge down with cool water.
3. Give cold drinks.
4. If the child becomes unconscious, take to hospital immediately.

Hiccups

Most babies and young children suffer from hiccups at some time or other. Hiccups are caused by an irritation of the diaphragm causing a sharp intake of breath with the well-known (and comical!) hiccuping sound. Usually this spasm passes spontaneously and quickly. A drink of cold water or holding the breath for as long as possible will often help.

Stings

Nettle stings frequently occur on country walks. Painful blistery lesions result from this. If cold water is available this will relieve the initial pain as will antihistamine cream if available in the rucksack. Children should be dissuaded from scratching the lesion as this can introduce infection.

Bee and wasp stings often happen in the summertime. These can be very painful initially. Antihistamine cream is the mainstay of treatment. Avoid rubbing the area. If a child, or adult, is allergic to bee or wasp stings this will be an emergency as anaphylactic shock can result. Under these circumstances the child will become shocked, with all the attendant signs, and will lapse into unconsciousness unless rapid action is taken. Medical help is urgent under these conditions and a 999 call life-saving. If the child stops breathing the routine resuscitation measures should be instituted. Fortunately this condition is rare, but is extremely frightening when it does occur.

Further details on these and other conditions causing ill-health can be found in Chapter 9.

Children can be taught about road safety from RoSPA (see Appendix), who have recently introduced further characters into their 'Tufty Club'. Willy, Watchit and friends all appeal to young school-age children, and are very up-to-date, Watchit being a friendly cybersaur from cyberspace.

HEALTH AND SAFETY AT WORK ACT, 1981

A few changes were made to this document in 1990 and further changes in 1996. For further detailed information consult *First Aid at Work: Health and Safety (First Aid) Regulations 1981 and Guidance* (see Further reading).

Every employer, under the Health and Safety at Work Act, is under obligation to make provision for first aid to be given in the workplace.

'An employer shall provide, or ensure that these are provided, such equipment and facilities as are adequate and appropriate to the circumstances for enabling first aid to be rendered to employees if they are injured or become ill at work.'

In other words adequate facilities must be available at workplaces as well as adequately trained staff able to make use of these.

'. . . an employer shall provide, or ensure that there is provided, such a number of suitable persons as is adequate and appropriate to the circumstances for rendering first aid.'

A 'suitable person' to render first aid is:

'a first-aider holding a current first aid certificate issued by an organization whose training and qualifications are approved by the Health and Safety Executive.'

Organizations offering acceptable qualifications include The Red Cross and St John Ambulance as well as approved first-aid courses held in colleges, schools and workplaces. The 'First Aid at Work' course run by St John Ambulance, for example, covers all aspects of first aid over four days with a theoretical and practical examination at the end of the course. The certificate gained will need to be renewed by a two-day 'refresher' course after three years. St John also run shorter courses for 'appointed persons' and a half-day 'emergency aid' course. These courses are constantly under review and up-dated with a view to modern needs.

Regulation 4 of the HSE *Code of Practice* states:

'An employer shall inform his employees of the arrangements that have been made in connection with the provision of first aid, including the location of equipment, facilities and personnel.'

To conform to this all new employees must be told of the first-aid facilities available in their work places. There should be at least one notice posted in a conspicuous position in all places of work. This notice should be in English, together with a version in any language which is commonly used in the specific workplace.

First-aiders, as well as being available and trained to give first aid must be responsible for overseeing the stocking and easy access of first-aid boxes and kits. These kits must contain 'a sufficient quantity of suitable first aid materials and nothing else.'

- Supplies must be replaced as soon as possible after use.
- First-aid boxes must be of suitable material to protect the contents from dust and damp.
- The boxes must be clearly labelled with a white cross on a green background. The contents should include, as a minimum:

- 20 individually wrapped sterile adhesive dressings in assorted sizes;
- 2 sterile eye pads;
- 6 individually wrapped triangular bandages;
- 6 safety pins;
- 6 medium sized individually wrapped sterile wound dressings;
- 2 large individually wrapped sterile wound dressings;
- 3 extra large individually wrapped sterile wound dressings;
- pair of plastic gloves;
- pair blunt-ended scissors.

These are the basic requirements laid down by the HSE, but each work place will obviously adapt this to their own individual needs. For example, nurseries could easily need extra numbers of small dressings of both adhesive and wound type. Blankets for covering casualties and plastic disposal bags for used dressings should also be available as part of the first-aid equipment.

In addition, the appointed first-aider has a duty to record any first aid given. This record should be kept alongside the first-aid box and always be available for inspection.

(It is strongly advised that students should have the opportunity to see a copy of the Health and Safety Commission's *Approved Code of Practice*.)

Student Exercise

Find out, and record:
- the first-aid facilities in your place of work;
- who is responsible for the first-aid box and its contents;
- the location of the first-aid box and its accessibility;
- who are the first-aiders;
- the training arrangements and their frequency;
- comments on any other factors you think important.

FURTHER READING

First Aid Manual (6th edn), London: Dorling Kindersley.
First-aid texts, and leaflets from St John Ambulance or Red Cross.
Levine, S. (1992), *Play it Safe*, London: BBC Books.

Glossary

Achondroplasia	very short stature – genetically acquired
Adenoids	mass of lymphoid tissue at back of throat and nose
Alveoli	part of lungs where gaseous exchange takes place
Amniocentesis	withdrawal of fluid from uterus
Anatomy	study of body structure
Apgar score	scoring scheme to determine condition of newborn baby
Areola	coloured part around nipple
Astigmatism	condition where lens of the eye is not smooth
Bile	digestive fluid secreted by liver and stored in gall-bladder
Breech birth	baby's bottom born first
Bronchi	part of lung structure
Bronchiolitis	inflammation of tiny bronchi in a young baby
Cataracts	clouding of the lens of the eye
Cells	smallest unit of body tissues
Centile charts	charts used for serial measurements of aspects of growth
Cervix	lower part of uterus
Chorionic gonadotrophins	hormones concerned with reproduction
Chorionic villus sampling	specialised test, during pregnancy, for genetic disorders
Coccyx	base of spine
Cochlea	inner ear concerned with hearing
Colostrum	fluid secreted from breasts for 2–3 days after birth
Cot death	unexpected, unexplained death of young baby
Cystic fibrosis	inherited lung disease
Dermis	inner layer of skin
Duodenum	part of small intestine
Dura mater	a covering of the brain
Ectopic pregnancy	pregnancy occurring mainly in Fallopian tube
Eczema	skin condition
Elective surgery	planned surgery
Endocrine glands	ductless glands pouring secretions directly into blood
Epidermis	outer layer of skin
Epidural anaesthesia	anaesthetic administered into spine
Epiglottis	flap of tissue at back of throat
Epiphyseal plates	growing parts of children's bones
Episiotomy	cut to enlarge vaginal opening

Fallopian tubes	outer ends of uterus
Febrile convulsions	convulsions due to a rapid rise in body temperature
Fontanelles	'soft' parts of baby's head
Gastroenteritis	infection of gastrointestinal tract
Genes	units of inheritance
Glycogen	a form of starch
Gonads	sex organs
Haemoglobin	oxygen-carrying substance in red blood cells
Hormones	secretions from ductless glands
Hydrocephalus	excess fluid in brain
Hypoglycaemia	low blood sugar
Ileum	part of small intestine
Impetigo	bacterial skin infection
Incubation period	time between infection and onset of symptoms
Insulin	substance, secreted by pancreas, controlling blood sugar
Jaundice	yellow coloration of the skin
Masturbation	handling of genitals for pleasure
Menstruation	monthly periods
Miscarriage	loss of developing baby
Montgomery's tubercles	small swellings in breast areola
Oestrogen	female sex hormone
Ossicles	small bones in middle ear
Oxytocin	hormone concerned with onset of labour
Periosteum	membrane surrounding bones
Physiology	study of body function
Pia mater	inner covering of brain
Pituitary gland	ductless gland
PKU test	test for phenylketonuria done at 10 days following birth
Pneumonia	infection in the lungs
Portage	system of helping disabled children
Post-natal depression	severe 'baby blues'
Pre-eclamptic toxaemia	abnormal condition occurring in pregnancy
Progesterone	female sex hormone
Prolactin	hormone concerned with breast feeding
Psychiatrist	doctor specialising in mental illness
Puberty	onset of sexual maturity
Retina	visual structure at back of eye
Rhesus	type of blood group of importance during pregnancy
Ringworm	fungal infection
Sacrum	lower part of vertebral column
Salmonella	type of food poisoning
Scabies	skin infection by a mite
Sclera	outer covering of eye-ball

Semicircular canals	structures in ear concerned with balance
Surma	cosmetic containing lead
Sutures	places where skull bones join
Synapses	concerned with nerve impulses
Testes	male sex organs
Tonsillitis	infection of tonsils
Tonsils	lymphoid tissue at back of throat
Trachea	windpipe
Tympanic membrane	eardrum
Ultrasonic scan	special test used during pregnancy
Umbilical cord	structure joining baby to placenta
Vas deferens	structures associated with male reproductive organs
Vertex position	when baby is born head first
Viruses	organisms causing infection
White cells	specialised blood cells which fight infection

Appendix: Addresses

Action for Sick Children
Argyle House
29–31 Euston Road
London NW1 2SD

British Agencies for Fostering and
    Adoption
11 Southwark Street
London SE1 1RQ

Brittle Bone Society
112 City Road
Dundee DD2 2PW

British Epilepsy Association
Anstey House
40 Hanover Square
Leeds LS3 1BE

Child Growth Foundation
2 Mayfield Road
London W4 1PW

Children's Accident Prevention
    Trust
Clerk's Court
18–20 Farringdon Lane
London EC1R 3AU

Coeliac Society
PO Box 220
High Wycombe
Bucks HP11 2HY

'Contact-a-Family' (CaF)
    (Organisation giving advice and
    support to parents with a disabled
    child. They have a comprehensive
    list of self-help groups from
    which information on the specific
    condition can be obtained.)
170 Tottenham Court Road
London W1P 0HA

Cry-sis, BM Cry-sis
London WC1N 3XX

Cystic Fibrosis Trust
Alexandra House
5 Blythe Road
Bromley
Kent BR1 3RS

Diabetic Association
10 Queen Anne Street
London W1M 0BD

Down's Syndrome Association
155 Mitcham Road
London SW17 9PG

Duchenne Family Support Group
37a Highbury New Park
Islington
London N5 2EN

Foundation for the Study of Infant
    Deaths
35 Belgrave Square
London SW1X 8QB

Haemophilia Society
123 Westminster Bridge Road
London
SE1 7HR

Health and Safety Executive
PO Box 1999
Sudbury
Suffolk CO10 6FS

International Centre for Inquiring
    Children
Chace Community School
Churchbury Lane
Enfield EN1 3HQ

The Left Centre
Three Tuns House
31 High Street
Ironbridge
Telford
Shropshire TF8 7AE

National Association for Gifted
  Children
Park Campus
Broughton Green Road
Northampton NN2 7AL

National Asthma Campaign
Providence House
Providence Place
London N1 0NT

National Autistic Society
276 Willesden Lane
London NW2 5RB

National Child Minders
  Association
8 Masons Hill
Bromley
Kent BR2 9EY

National Deaf Children's Society
24 Wakefield Road
Leeds LS26 0SF

National Meningitis Trust
Fern House
Bath Road
Stroud
Glos GL5 3TJ

National Society for Prevention of
  Cruelty to Children
67 Saffron Hill
London EC1N 8RS

National Stepfamily Association
Chapel House
18 Hatton Place
London EC1N 8JH

Professional Association of Nursery
  Nurses
2 St James' Court
Friar Gate
Derby DE1 1BT

Royal National Institute for the Blind
224 Great Portland Street
London W1N 6AA

Royal Society for the Prevention of
  Accidents
Cannon Hill
The Priory Queensway
Birmingham B4 6BS

SCOPE (Cerebral Palsy)
12 Park Crescent
London W1N 4EQ

St John Ambulance
1 Grosvenor Crescent
London SW1X 7EF

INDEX

Numbers in square brackets [ ] indicate side panels which summarise key points and are a useful indicator as to where particular information might be found.

Numbers in round brackets ( ) indicate drawings or tables and are also useful indicators to major entries.